Color Atlas of O

The Quick-Reference
for Diagnosis and Treatment

Second Edition

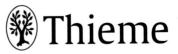

Color Atlas of Ophthalmology

The Quick-Reference Manual for Diagnosis and Treatment

Second Edition

Amar Agarwal, MS, FRCS, FRCOphth
Professor of Ophthalmology
Ramachandra Medical College
Private Practice
Chennai, India

Soosan Jacob, MS, FRCS, DNB, MNAMS
Private Practice
Chennai, India

Thieme
New York • Stuttgart

Thieme Medical Publishers, Inc.
333 Seventh Ave.
New York, NY 10001

Editorial Director: Michael Wachinger
Managing Editor: J. Owen Zurhellen IV
Editorial Assistant: Dominik Pucek
Vice President, Production and Electronic Publishing: Anne T. Vinnicombe
Production Editor: Kenneth L. Chumbley, Publication Services
Vice President, International Marketing and Sales: Cornelia Schulze
Chief Financial Officer: Peter van Woerden
President: Brian D. Scanlan
Cover illustration drawn by Karl Wesker
Compositor: MPS Content Services
Printer: Gopsons Papers Ltd.

Library of Congress Cataloging-in-Publication Data

Color atlas of ophthalmology : the quick-reference manual for diagnosis and treatment / [edited by] Amar Agarwal, Soosan Jacob.—2nd ed.
        p. ; cm.
    Includes index.
    Prev. ed. has subtitle: Manhattan Eye, Ear & Throat Hospital pocket guide.
    ISBN 978-1-60406-211-3 (alk. paper)
  1. Eye—Diseases—Atlases.   2. Eye—Diseases—Handbooks, manuals, etc.
3. Ophthalmology—Atlases.   4. Ophthalmology—Handbooks, manuals, etc.
I. Agarwal, Amar.   II. Jacob, Soosan.
    [DNLM: 1. Eye Diseases—diagnosis—Atlases.   2. Eye Diseases—diagnosis—Handbooks.
3. Eye Diseases—pathology—Atlases.   4. Eye Diseases—pathology—Handbooks.   5. Eye—
pathology—Atlases.   6. Eye—pathology—Handbooks.   7. Opthalmologic Surgical Procedures—
Atlases.   8. Ophthalmologic Surgical Procedures—Handbooks.   WW 17 C7195 2009]
    RE71.C65 2009
    617.70022'3—dc22

                                                                                        2009020093

Important note: Medical knowledge is ever-changing. As new research and clinical experience broaden our knowledge, changes in treatment and drug therapy may be required. The authors and editors of the material herein have consulted sources believed to be reliable in their efforts to provide information that is complete and in accord with the standards accepted at the time of publication. However, in view of the possibility of human error by the authors, editors, or publisher of the work herein or changes in medical knowledge, neither the authors, editors, nor publisher, nor any other party who has been involved in the preparation of this work, warrants that the information contained herein is in every respect accurate or complete, and they are not responsible for any errors or omissions or for the results obtained from use of such information. Readers are encouraged to confirm the information contained herein with other sources. For example, readers are advised to check the product information sheet included in the package of each drug they plan to administer to be certain that the information contained in this publication is accurate and that changes have not been made in the recommended dose or in the contraindications for administration. This recommendation is of particular importance in connection with new or infrequently used drugs.

    Some of the product names, patents, and registered designs referred to in this book are in fact registered trademarks or proprietary names even though specific reference to this fact is not always made in the text. Therefore, the appearance of a name without designation as proprietary is not to be construed as a representation by the publisher that it is in the public domain.

Printed in India

5 4 3 2 1

ISBN 978-1-60406-211-3

Nothing in this world moves without Him,
and so also this book was only written by Him.

This book is dedicated to

a great friend,

Brian S. Boxer Wachler, MD

Contents

Foreword

For some authors of ophthalmology, writing or editing 50 book chapters is a sizeable accomplishment over a lifetime, let alone a decade. This is not true for Professor Agarwal. Since 1998, Amar Agarwal has edited on average more than four books a year, which is an unprecedented and virtually unimaginable yearly number for any one person. His books span topics from diagnostics and imaging (such as aberrometry, angiography, topography, dry eyes, and neuro-ophthalmology) to therapeutics and surgery (including contact lenses, lasers, LASIK, strabismus, oculoplastics, cataracts, phako, and more), and many have been bestsellers. He has authored several comprehensive handbooks and textbooks of ophthalmology, and *Color Atlas of Ophthalmology* stands out as one of his best. In its 19 subspecialty chapters, this second edition illustrates over 500 diagnostics and therapeutic conditions. The comprehensive and systematic format helps the reader find and view the facts about any condition in ophthalmology instantly, making it an essential resource for both the student and the practitioner in the field.

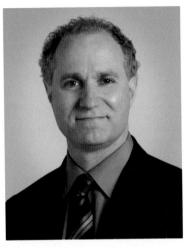

Anyone who knows Professor Agarwal can tell you that he is a consummate innovator and teacher. As a professor of ophthalmology and internationally renowned lecturer, his experience and dedication to teaching speak for themselves. Over the years, I have participated in several American Academy of Ophthalmology and American Society of Cataract and Refractive Surgery courses with Professor Agarwal and have learned a great deal about microincision cataract surgery and the management of challenging LASIK cases from them. Personally, I look forward to reviewing and referring to the content of this book on a regular basis. I recommend that you do so as well!

Ronald R. Krueger, MD, MSE
Medical Director,
Department of Refractive Surgery
Cole Eye Institute
Cleveland Clinic
Cleveland, Ohio

Preface

Every day you may make progress. Every step may be fruitful. Yet there will stretch out before you an ever-lengthening, ever-ascending, ever-improving path. You know you will never get to the end of the journey. But this, so far from discouraging, only adds to the joy and glory of the climb.

Winston Churchill (1874–1965)

What is an ophthalmologist? One who has graduated from medical school and is interested in the eye. One who has completed three years of specialized ophthalmic training. One who has spent a further two years in sub-specialization. One who has mentored the next generation of ophthalmologists. One who has innovated and changed preferred practice patterns in ophthalmology. All these classes of ophthalmologists need solid knowledge combined with patient empathy to best serve patients.

The purpose of this fully revised second edition of the successful *Color Atlas of Ophthalmology: The Quick-Reference Manual for Diagnosis and Treatment* is to give you the knowledge needed to face with confidence the full range of patients' ophthalmic disorders. In our field, where we necessarily learn, diagnose, and teach visually, top-flight clinical photographs, like the hundreds in this book (all new to this edition), are essential. The nineteen chapters, written by expert contributors from North America, Europe, and India, are well-organized and concise, and the format of "Presentation-Differential Diagnosis-Management" is designed for easy and speedy reference, so you don't have to wade through extraneous material to find what you need. This pocket atlas is intended for the resident on rounds or studying for an exam, the practicing ophthalmologist who needs confirmation of an unusual finding, or the primary physician who requires a reliable guide to eye disorders.

We are grateful to the people at Thieme Publishers, especially to J. Owen Zurhellen and Dominik Pucek. We and Thieme hope and expect that our pocket atlas aids you in providing patients with the best care possible.

Amar Agarwal, MS, FRCS, FRCOphth
Soosan Jacob, MS, FRCS, DNB, MNAMS
Chennai, India

About the Editors

Amar Agarwal, MS, FRCS, FRCOphth

Dr. Agarwal's Group of Eye Hospitals and Eye Research Centre
Chennai, India

Prof. Amar Agarwal is the pioneer of phakonit, which is phako with needle incision technology. This technique became popularized as bimanual phaco, microincision cataract surgery (MICS), or microphaco. He is the first to remove cataracts through a 0.7 mm tip with the technique called microphakonit. He is also the first to have discovered and developed cataract surgery without anesthesia. Another of his innovations is FAVIT (fallen vitreous), a new technique for removing dropped nuclei. The air pump, based on the simple idea of using an aquarium pump to increase the fluid infusion into the eye in bimanual phaco and coaxial phaco, has helped prevent unstable anterior chamber and surge during cata-

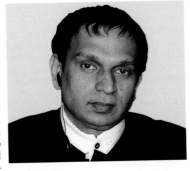

ract surgery. This provided the basis for various techniques of forced infusion for small incision cataract surgery. Dr. Agarwal was also the first to use trypan blue for staining epiretinal membranes and published the details in his four-volume textbook of ophthalmology. He has also discovered a new refractive error called aberropia. He has been the first to do a combined surgery of microphakonit (700 μm cataract surgery) with a 25-gauge vitrectomy in the same patient, thus using the smallest incisions possible for cataract and vitrectomy. And he is the first surgeon to implant a new mirror telescopic intraocular lens (IOL) Lipshitz Macular Implant (LMI) for patients suffering from age-related macular degeneration. The Malyugin ring for small pupil cataract surgery was also modified by him and is known as the Agarwal modification of the Malyugin ring for miotic pupil cataract surgeries with posterior capsular defects. He has been the world's first to implant a glued IOL. In this procedure a posterior chamber (PC) IOL is fixed in the eye without any capsules, using fibrin glue.

Anterior segment optical coherence tomography was used for the first time in Dr. Agarwal's eye hospital to quantify changes in anterior chamber (AC) morphology in inflammation, assessing all the parameters. The hyperreflective spots detected in the AC were counted manually and with an automated computer algorithm. Also for the first time, pseudophakic bullous keratopathy was managed by a combination of IntraLase (Abbott Medical Optics, Santa Ana, CA) keratoplasty, explantation of the AC IOL, vitrectomy, and implantation of a glued PC IOL. A new surgical technique, Jacob-Agarwal sling surgery, was devised for acquired and congenital ptosis with poor levator function in which the Seiff silicone suspension set is used in a frontalis sling procedure. The entire length of the silicone set is guided in the muscle plane through a single stab incision.

Prof. Agarwal has received many awards for his work in ophthalmology, the most significant being the Barraquer Award and the Kelman Award. His videos have won many awards at film festivals of the American Society of Cataract and Refractive Surgery, American Academy of Ophthalmology, and European Society of Cataract and Refractive Surgery. He has also written more than 40 books, which have been published in various languages, including English, Spanish, and Polish. He trains doctors from all over the world in his center on phaco, bimanual phaco, LASIK, and vitreo-retinal surgery. He is a professor of ophthalmology at Ramachandra Medical College in Chennai, India, and can be contacted through the hospital's Web site at http://www.dragarwal.com.

Soosan Jacob, MS, FRCS, DNB, MNAMS

Dr. Soosan Jacob is a senior consultant ophthalmologist in Dr. Agarwal's Group of Eye Hospitals and Eye Research Centre, Chennai, India. She is a gold medalist in ophthalmology. She has won many inter-national awards at prestigious international conferences in the United States. She is a noted speaker and has conducted courses and delivered lectures in numerous national and international conferences. She has a special interest in cutting-edge surgical techniques for cataract, cornea, glaucoma, and refractive surgery, including deep lamellar endothelial keratoplasty, ocular surface reconstruction, new refractive solutions, and so on.

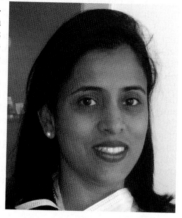

Dr. Jacob was the first to bring out the concept of anterior segment transplantation. In this, the cornea, sclera, and an artificial iris, pupil, and IOL are transplanted enbloc in patients with anterior staphyloma. She also devised a new technique for ptosis, wherein the sling surgery can be done primarily with a one stab incision rather than three, thus improving the postoperative cosmetic appearance of the patient, while still retaining excellent functional outcome.

She has authored many articles and numerous chapters in 27 textbooks by international and national publishers and is also the editor for three textbooks in ophthalmology. She is among the senior faculty for the Diplomate of National Board (DNB) postgraduate training program and phacoemulsification and the LASIK training program for overseas doctors.

Contributors

Marie D. Acierno, MD
Associate Professor
Department of Ophthalmology
Director, Ophthalmology Residency Program
Chief of Ophthalmology
Earl K. Long Medical Center
LSU Health Sciences Center
New Orleans, LA

Amar Agarwal, MS, FRCS, FRCOphth
Professor of Ophthalmology
Ramachandra Medical College
Dr. Agarwal's Group of Eye Hospitals & Eye Research Centre
Chennai, India

Athiya Agarwal, MD, FRSH, DO
Director
Dr. Agarwal's Group of Eye Hospitals & Eye Research Centre
Chennai, India

Donald R. Bergsma, MD
Herbert E. Kaufman Professor and Chairman
Department of Ophthalmology
LSU Health Sciences Center
Director
LSU Eye Center of Excellence
New Orleans, LA

Blake A. Booth, MD
Resident
Department of Ophthalmology
University of Alabama at Birmingham
Birmingham, AL

Francesco Boscia, MD
Dirigente Medico I Livello
Department of Ophthalmology and Otolaryngology
University Bari
Bari, Italy

Samuel Boyd, MD
Chief
Vitreoretinal Department
Boyd Eye Center
Panama City, Republic of Panama

Clement K. Chan, MD
President and Medical Director
Southern California Desert Retina Consultants
Associate Clinical Professor
Department of Ophthalmology
Loma Linda University
Loma Linda, CA

Kimberly P. Cockerham, MD, FACS
Adjunct Clinical Professor
Department of Ophthalmology
Stanford University School of Medicine
Private Practice
Cockerham Eye Consultants
Los Altos, CA

Kenneth M. Daniels, OD, FAAO
Adjunct Assistant Clinical Professor
Center for International Studies
Pennsylvania College of Optometry at Salus University
Philadelphia, PA
Private Practice
Hopewell-Lambertville Eye Associates
Hopewell, NJ

Lori Vidal Denham, MS
Research Assistant
Department of Biochemical Engineering
Tulane University
New Orleans, LA

Noa Ela-Dalman, MD
Clinical Instructor
Department of Ophthalmology
Jules Stein Eye Institute
UCLA School of Medicine
Los Angeles, CA

Duncan A. Friedman, MD, MPH
Resident Physician
Department of Ophthalmology
University of Alabama at Birmingham
Birmingham, AL

Pablo Gili-Manzanaro
Department of Ophthalmology
Fundación Hospital de Alcorcón
Barcelona, Spain

Santosh Hanovar, MD
LV Prasad Eye Institute,
Hyderabad, India

David R. Hardten, MD, FACS
Adjunct Associate Professor
Department of Ophthalmology
University of Minnesota
Minnesota Eye Consultants
Minneapolis, MN

James M. Hill, PhD
Assistant Professor
Department of Microbiology, Immunology, and Parasitology
LSU Health Sciences Center
New Orleans, LA

Jeffery A. Hobden, PhD
Assistant Professor
Department of Microbiology, Immunology, and Parasitology
LSU Health Sciences Center
New Orleans, LA

Jean T. Jacob, PhD
Professor of Ophthalmology and Neuroscience
Department of Ophthalmology
LSH Health Sciences Center
Director of Research
LSU Eye Center
New Orleans, LA

Soosan Jacob, MS, FRCS, DNB, MNAMS
Dr. Agarwal's Group of Eye Hospitals & Eye Research Centre
Chennai, India

Herbert E. Kaufman, MD
Emeritus Boyd Professor of Ophthalmology, Pharmacology, and Microbiology
LSU Health Sciences Center
New Orleans, LA

Natalia Kramarevsky, MD
Virginia Beach Eye Center, P.C.
Sentara Virginia Beach General Hospital
Virginia Beach, VA

Dhivya Ashok Kumar, MD
Consultant
Department of Ophthalmology
Dr. Agarwal's Group of Eye Hospitals & Eye Research Centre
Chennai, India

Mandeep Lamba, MBBS, DNB, FERC
Consultant, Retina Foundation
Dr. Agarwal's Group of Eye Hospitals & Eye Research Centre
Chennai, India

Paolo Lanzetta, MD
Associate Professor
Department of Ophthalmology
University of Udine
Udine, Italy

W. Barry Lee, MD
Private Practice
Cornea, External Disease, and Refractive Surgery
Eye Consultants of Atlanta, Piedmont Hospital
Atlanta, GA

Richard L. Lindstrom, MD
Adjunct Professor Emeritus
Department of Ophthalmology
University of Minnesota
Founder and Attending Surgeon
Minnesota Eye Consultants
Minneapolis, MN

Andrea T. Murina, MD
Resident
Department of Internal Medicine
LSU Health Sciences Center
New Orleans, LA

Andrea Olmos, BS
Department of Ophthalmology
University of California, San Francisco
San Francisco, CA

Louis E. Probst, MD
National Medical Director
TLC The Laser Eye Centers
Chicago, IL

Swati Ravani, MS
Associate Professor
BMJ Regional Institute of Ophthalmology
Ahmedabad, India

Arthur L. Rosenbaum, MD
Brindell and Milton Gottlieb Professor of Ophthalmology
Chief, Division of Pediatric Ophthalmology and Strabismus
Vice Chairman
Department of Ophthalmology
Jules Stein Eye Institute
UCLA School of Medicine
Los Angeles, CA

Praveen Saluja, MS
Dr. Agarwal's Group of Eye Hospitals & Eye Research Centre
Chennai, India

Carlo Sborgia, MD
Chair, Institute of Ophthalmology
Department of Ophthalmology and Otolaryngology
University of Bari
Bari, Italy

Ivan R. Schwab, MD, FACS
Professor
Department of Ophthalmology
University of California, Davis Health System Eye Center
Sacramento, CA

Cristina Simón-Castellví
Simon Eye Clinic
Barcelona, Spain

Guillermo Simón-Castellví
Chief, Anterior Segment Surgeon
Simon Eye Clinic
Department of Ophthalmology
University of Barcelona
Barcelona, Spain

José María Simón-Castellví
Anterior Segment Consultant
Emergency Room
Simon Eye Clinic
President
World Federation of Catholic Medical Associations
Barcelona, Spain

Sarabel Simón-Castellví
Chief, Posterior Segment Surgeon
Simon Eye Clinic
Barcelona, Spain

José María Simón-Tor
Chairman
Glaucoma Senior Consultant
Simon Eye Clinic
Barcelona, Spain

Giuseppe Smaldone, MD
Resident
Department of Ophthalmology and Otolaryngology
University of Bari
Bari, Italy

Dariusz G. Tarasewicz, MD, PhD
Retina Section Chief
Department of Ophthalmology
Kaiser Permanente
Sacramento, CA

Federico G. Velez, MD
Assistant Clinical Professor
Department of Ophthalmology
Jules Stein Eye Institute
UCLA School of Medicine
Los Angeles, CA
Director
Division of Pediatric Ophthalmology and Strabismus
Olive View–UCLA Medical Center
Sylmar, CA

Daniele Veritti, MD
Registrar
Department of Ophthalmology
University of Udine
Udine, Italy

Christopher I. Zoumalan, MD
Clinical Instructor
Department of Ophthalmology
Division of Ophthalmic Plastic and Reconstructive Surgery
New York University
Langone Medical Center
Manhattan Eye, Ear, and Throat Hospital
New York, NY

1 Ocular Trauma

Daniele Veritti, Carlo Sborgia, Francesco Boscia, Giuseppe Smaldone, and Paolo Lanzetta

◆ Anterior Segment Trauma

Eyelid Laceration

Blunt and penetrating facial trauma may result in eyelid laceration. The laceration may be extramarginal, may involve the eyelid margin, or may cause tissue loss. Eyelid trauma is often associated with vehicle accidents, falls, sport-related traumas, and assaults. Eyelid laceration is more common in young males due to occupational and recreational preferences. Proper management is necessary to preserve correct lid dynamics and cosmetic appearance.

◆ Presentation

Patients usually complain of mild pain and epiphora. Displacement or abnormalities of the canthal angles may indicate canthal ligament injury. Lacerations of the deep head of the medial canthal ligament may cause telecanthus. Hyphema, other ocular adnexa traumas, and orbital fractures may be present (**Fig. 1.1**).

◆ Management

The mechanism of injury should be investigated first, followed by a complete ocular examination to rule out injuries to the globe. If no globe rupture is present, lids should be everted, palpated, and examined for foreign bodies. The laceration should be carefully examined to determine depth, extension, and margin involvement. Photography of the lesions is recommended. Canalicular involvement and injury to the levator and the supraorbital nerve should be excluded. A computed tomographic scan should be obtained when globe rupture and foreign bodies are

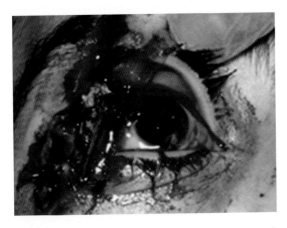

Fig. 1.1 Eyelid laceration involving the eyelid margin with loss of tissue.

suspected. Tetanus prophylaxis and baseline serology for human immunodeficiency virus (HIV) and hepatotropic viruses should be considered. Surgical repair
should be performed under local anesthesia, with good lighting and magnification.
After adequate anesthesia, wound cleaning, and decontamination, the laceration
should be repaired using Vicryl (Ethicon, Inc., Somerville, NJ) or silk 6–0 suture.
Posterior tendon repair and canalicular repair should precede lid suturing. Eyelid
margin laceration should be sutured with a vertical mattress technique. Finally,
antibiotic ointment should be applied to the wound, and systemic antibiotic therapy should be considered if contamination is suspected. Possible complications
include posttraumatic upper lid ptosis and corneal ulceration due to corneal exposure or an exposed suture.

Lacrimal System Trauma

The lacrimal drainage apparatus consists of the lacrimal puncta on the upper lid
and the lower lid, the canaliculi, the common canaliculus, the lacrimal sac, and
the nasolacrimal duct. From their origin at the puncta, the canaliculi run medially toward the internal angulus of the eye, where they join to form the common
lacrimal canaliculus that opens in the lacrimal sac. Canalicular lacerations are the
most frequent cause of injury to the lacrimal system and occur in up to 16% of all
eyelid injuries. Common causes of canalicular laceration include vehicle accidents,
falls, assaults, sharp trauma, and animal bites. Successful management of these
injuries depends on prompt intervention and good surgical technique to minimize
the incidence of posttraumatic epiphora due to scarring and stenosis in any tract
of the lacrimal drainage system.

◆ Presentation

Patients usually present with a history of trauma and mild pain. The lacrimal
drainage system lesion may be obvious or occult. The use of methylene blue or flu-
orescein-tinged water irrigation through the puncta and subsequent visualization
of the dye in the wound may be helpful in identifying the cut end (**Fig. 1.2A,B**).

◆ Differential Diagnosis

Lid laceration not involving the lacrimal drainage system, preexisting epiphora

◆ Management

The mechanism of injury should be investigated, and a complete ophthalmic examination should be performed. The injury to the lacrimal drainage system can
be proven with Bowman probe insertion in the puncta or by irrigation with fluo-
rescein-stained saline solution. Tetanus prophylaxis should be considered. Surgical repair should provide accurate approximation of the severed ends to promote
mucosal healing. Most surgeons use silicone intubations of the system, followed
by apposition of the pericanalicular tissues with microscopically assisted 7–0 suture. The medial canthal ligament is often injured from the trauma and must be
repaired to restore lid function and anatomy. The success rate with silicone intubation and microscopic reanastomosis ranges from 86 to 95%.

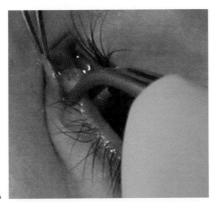

 A

Fig. 1.2 **(A)** Lacrimal system trauma with laceration of the inferior canaliculus. **(B)** Canalicular injury with eyelid laceration.

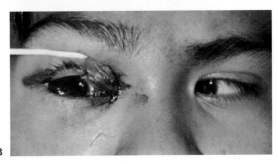

B

Subconjuctival Hemorrhage

Subconjunctival hemorrhage follows the bleeding of conjunctival and episcleral blood vessels into the subconjunctival space. It is usually associated with minor trauma or arises spontaneously with increased venous pressure due to violent Valsalva maneuvers. Less frequently subconjunctival hemorrhage can be associated with severe hypertension and coagulopathies. Various drugs, such as warfarin, nonsteroidal antiinflammatory drugs (NSAIDs), and steroids can make conjunctival vessels more susceptible. It is also a normal sequela of ocular surgery.

◆ Presentation

A bright red and flat collection of blood is seen underneath the conjunctiva; it is usually sharply demarcated at the limbus and surrounded by normal conjunctiva. This condition is usually asymptomatic. If pain, photophobia, or diminished visual acuity occurs, a more serious pathological condition should be considered (**Fig. 1.3**).

◆ Differential Diagnosis

The differential diagnosis of subconjunctival hemorrhage includes other causes of red eye, such as conjunctivitis, episcleritis, iritis, acute glaucoma, and dendritic ulcer. Kaposi sarcoma, or other conjunctival neoplasms with secondary hemorrhage should be taken into consideration.

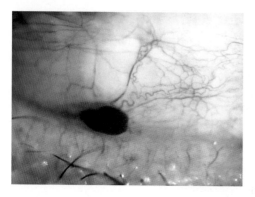

Fig. 1.3 Subconjunctival hemorrhage. A bright red and flat collection of blood is seen underneath the conjunctiva; it is sharply demarcated and surrounded by normal conjunctiva.

◆ Management

Blood pressure should be checked in all patients, and if there is a history of recurrent, unprovoked subconjunctival hemorrhages, a bleeding diathesis should be investigated. The uncomplicated hemorrhage, not associated with any significant trauma or bleeding diathesis, is typically a self-limiting condition that requires only reassurance. Cold compresses for 24 hours and artificial tears can be used for mild irritation. Hemorrhage clears spontaneously in 1 to 2 weeks. Elective use of NSAIDs is typically discouraged.

Conjunctival Laceration

The conjunctiva is a strong and resilient tissue, but it may be lacerated in cases of ocular trauma with pointed and sharp objects, such as broken glass. It may be isolated or part of more severe intraocular injuries.

◆ Presentation

Patients usually present with a history of ocular trauma and complain of red eye, mild pain, and foreign body sensation. Slit-lamp examination reveals a conjunctival surface defect. The edges are usually retracted and rolled up, disclosing the underlying white sclera. Subconjunctival hemorrhages and chemosis are often present. Fluorescein staining under the cobalt filter will enhance the visualization of the defect (**Fig. 1.4**).

◆ Management

An accurate history of ocular trauma and a complete ophthalmic examination are necessary: topical anesthesia may be used to accurately investigate the underlying sclera in search of injuries and subconjunctival foreign bodies. However, patients under topical anesthesia may lose symptoms associated with the presence of a foreign body. A Seidel test should be performed to rule out a ruptured globe.

B-scan ultrasonography and a computed tomographic scan of the orbit may be useful to exclude intraocular or intraorbital foreign bodies.

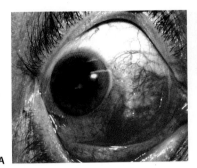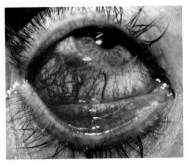

A   B

Fig. 1.4 Conjunctival laceration and foreign body. (Courtesy Pablo Gili M.D.)

In the absence of a ruptured globe or perforating injuries, small conjunctival lacerations heal without surgical repair. Large lacerations (e.g., greater than 1.0 to 1.5 cm) may be sutured (e.g., Vicryl 8–0). Pressure patching for 24 hours and prophylactic antibiotic ointment (e.g., gentamicin) three times a day for 4 to 7 days should suffice.

Chemical Exposure

Chemical burns constitute a true ocular emergency and should be treated promptly. Chemical burns may be caused by either acidic or alkaline agents. Acid burns cause coagulative necrosis of the corneal epithelium. The formation of a coagulum limits penetration and corneal damage. Hydrofluoric acid is an exception because it causes liquefactive necrosis. Common acids causing ocular burns include sulfurous acid (present in some bleaches), sulfuric acid (present in car batteries), hydrochloric acid (used in swimming pools), nitric acid, chromic acid, and acetic acid. Alkali burns are typically more severe because alkaline agents are lipophilic and penetrate more rapidly than acids. They combine with cell membrane lipids and cause saponification of cell membranes, cell death, and disruption of the extracellular matrix. The release of collagenases and proteases after the injury leads to corneoscleral melting. Alkali substances that commonly cause ocular burns contain sodium hydroxide (caustic soda), ammonium hydroxide (fertilizer production), potassium hydroxide, and calcium hydroxide. Chemical burns are often bilateral and are frequently due to industrial and occupational exposures.

◆ Presentation

The diagnosis of ocular chemical burn is typically based on history of contact with alkaline or acid agents. The symptoms usually include pain, photophobia, blepharospasm, reduced vision, and excessive tearing. If the burn is mild or moderate, the conjunctiva is hyperemic. Focal conjunctival chemosis, hyperemia, or hemorrhages can be present. Eyelid edema and first- to second-degree periocular skin burns can be seen. Corneal findings may range from superficial punctate keratitis (SPK) to focal epithelial defects. In severe conditions white areas of conjunctival and limbal ischemia can be seen. Corneal findings usually consist of total epithelial loss, stromal hazing, and, in same cases, complete opacification. Other signs include anterior chamber reaction and second- or third-degree periocular burns. (**Fig. 1.5A,B**).

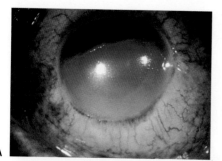

A

Fig. 1.5 (A) A moderate chemical injury with 6 hours of limbal blanching, a large epithelial defect, and stromal haze. **(B)** The sequelae of a severe chemical injury demonstrating a scarred and vascularized cornea. This eye underwent a permanent keratoprosthesis. (Courtesy of Christopher Rapuano)

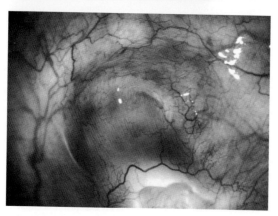

B

◆ Differential Diagnosis

Thermal burns, ultraviolet (UV) keratitis, ulcerative keratitis

◆ Management

Chemical burns are considered a true ophthalmologic emergency and require immediate care. The first priority is immediate and copious irrigation with sterile irrigating solution or saline solution. If these solutions are not available, tap water can be used. Irrigation should be continued until neutral pH is reached. Insertion of a lid speculum and topical anesthetic prior to irrigation facilitates the procedure. After irrigation a good history with an exact identification of the chemical agent should be obtained. Slit-lamp examination with fluorescein staining should be performed. Eyelids should be everted to search for residual chemicals and foreign bodies. The goal of therapy is to reduce pain, inflammation, and risk of infection. Thus cycloplegic agents (avoid phenylephrine because it is a vasoconstrictor), oral analgesics (avoid repeated applications of topical anesthetics because they can delay epithelial healing), and ophthalmic antibiotics (avoid aminoglycoside antibiotics because they impair epithelial healing) should be administered. The use of topical steroids remains controversial. They can limit inflammation-mediated ocular damage, but they retard wound healing and predispose to infection. Severe burns can be managed with adjunctive therapy: ocular hypotensive medications if the intraocular pressure is elevated, collagenase inhibitors if any melting of the cornea occurs, lysis of conjunctival adhesions if present, and active surgical removal of necrotic tissue. Long-term complications of chemical burns include perforation, scarring, corneal neovascularization, symblepharon, glaucoma, cataracts, and retinal damage. Ultimate prognosis is related to the degree of limbus ischemia, the depth of the corneal injury, and the presence of symblepharon.

Corneal Abrasion

Corneal abrasions represent one of the most common ophthalmic problems seen in emergency departments. A corneal abrasion is the disruption of the protective epithelium covering the cornea; it may be caused by direct or tangential impact. Common causes are scratches from fingernails, animal paws, tree branches, or a paper cut. Another common cause is contact lens overwear. A large number of corneal abrasions are preventable. High-risk workers (e.g., woodworkers, metal workers) and players of certain sports (e.g., hockey, racquetball, cross-country skiing, mountain biking) should wear appropriate eye protection.

◆ Presentation

The patient's history typically includes eye trauma and subsequent acute pain. Presenting symptoms usually include severe pain, excessive tearing, photophobia, foreign body sensation, blepharospasm, and blurred vision. At slit-lamp examination diffuse corneal edema, epithelial disruption, and circumcorneal injection can be seen (**Fig. 1.6**).

◆ Differential Diagnosis

Acute angle glaucoma, herpes ulcers and other corneal ulcers, corneal foreign body, and corneal perforation

◆ Management

Visual acuity should be assessed because it may be significantly reduced if the abrasion is on the optic axis. Upper and lower tarsal conjunctiva should be inspected carefully for foreign bodies. If examination is limited by excessive pain, one drop of topical anesthetic could be administered for diagnostic purposes. At slit-lamp ex-

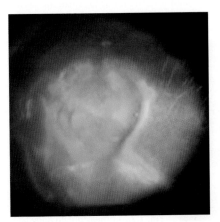

Fig. 1.6 Corneal defect stained with fluorescein. (Courtesy of Nibaran Gangopadhyay)

amination the visualization of the corneal abrasion can be improved using fluorescein staining under blue-cobalt filtered light. The abrasion should be documented in size, shape, depth, and localization. A Seidel test should be performed to rule out possible full-thickness injury. Intraocular pressure should be measured in both eyes, and the anterior chamber should be carefully investigated for evidence of iritis. Prevention of infection is a key point in corneal abrasion treatment. An antibiotic ointment should be used; consider antipseudomonas coverage for abrasions due to contact lens overwear. Patients with contact lens–associated corneal abrasion or a wound that is caused by vegetable matter should have antipseudomonas coverage (e.g., tobramycin, ciprofloxacin, gentamicin, ofloxacin). Oral analgesics are often necessary owing to the severity of pain. Topical NSAIDs (e.g., diclofenac, ketorolac) may be useful in reducing pain. Patients using topical NSAIDs may take fewer oral analgesics. Never provide topical anesthetics to take home because they can delay wound healing. One drop of topical cycloplegic can be used if the patient is really photophobic. This relieves ciliary spasm, reduces pain, and improves comfort. Pressure patching is no longer recommended. It should be used for 6 hours only if pain is severe. Given the risk of infection, do not patch if the lesion is caused by vegetable matter or contact lenses. Healing of small abrasions is expected within 24 to 48 hours. Deep and large abrasions may require 5 to 7 days to heal. Most corneal abrasions (small and peripheral) do not need any follow-up. However, contact lens wearers or patients with a central or large abrasion should be reevaluated in 24 hours and every 2 to 3 days until abrasion clears. Patients should return sooner if symptoms worsen.

Corneal Foreign Body

A corneal foreign body is a common cause of visits for ophthalmic emergencies. It frequently occurs when one is grinding and drilling steel without wearing protective goggles.

◆ Presentation

The patient's history usually includes an ocular trauma. The more frequent symptoms are mild or moderate pain, foreign body sensation, excessive tearing, photophobia, and blurred vision. At slit-lamp examination one or more objects can be seen lodged superficially or embedded within the cornea. Metallic foreign bodies may leave rust rings in the surrounding cornea. Other signs include a circumlimbal conjunctival injection, eyelid edema, and a sterile infiltrate surrounding the foreign body (**Fig. 1.7**).

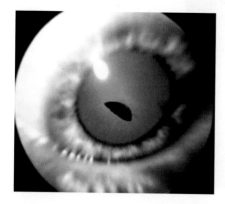

Fig. 1.7 Corneal foreign body.

◆ Differential Diagnosis

Corneal abrasion, intraocular foreign body, bacterial or fungal keratitis

◆ Management

After having assessed visual acuity, it is important to rule out a possible perforating injury. This can be done using a Seidel test (instill fluorescein to inspect for aqueous leakage), measuring intraocular pressure, and paying attention to anterior chamber reaction. Consider a b-scan ultrasound and an orbital computed tomographic scan to exclude intraocular and intraorbital foreign bodies. If there is no perforation, the object can be removed under topical anesthesia (e.g., proparacaine 0.5%) using a foreign body spud or a 25-gauge needle. This operation can be facilitated by sterile irrigation. The rust ring can be removed using an ophthalmic drill. These procedures should be performed at slit lamp by well-trained and experienced physicians. Before and after the removal, antibiotic drops should be applied until healing. A topical cycloplegic can be used to reduce photophobia and pain. Patients should be reevaluated every 2 to 3 days until the wound is healed and the infiltrate resolved.

Corneal Laceration

The laceration can be partial thickness or full thickness.

◆ Presentation

In partial-thickness laceration, the anterior chamber is not entered, and, therefore, the cornea is not perforated. If the Seidel test is positive, a full-thickness laceration is present. In full-thickness laceration the patient presents with tearing, pain, and loss of vision. Associated findings include: shallow anterior chamber, anterior synechiae, corneal opacity with endothelial dysfunction, or cataract. Intraocular pressure may be very low (**Fig. 1.8**).

◆ Management

A history and complete ophthalmic examination are required to ascertain the diagnosis. While managing a partial-thickness laceration, a cycloplegic (e.g., scopol-

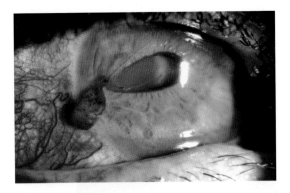

Fig. 1.8 Penetrating corneal laceration with iris prolapse.
(Courtesy Pablo Gili M.D.)

amine 0.25%) and an antibiotic (e.g., frequent polymyxin B/bacitracin ointment such as polysporin) or fluoroquinolone drops, depending on the nature of the wound, are started immediately.

When a moderate to deep corneal laceration is accompanied by wound gape, it is often best to suture the wound closed in the operating room to avoid excessive scarring and corneal irregularity, especially in the visual axis. Tetanus toxoid for dirty wounds is a must.

Note that small, self-sealing, or slow-leaking lacerations may be treated with aqueous suppressants, bandage soft contact lenses, fluoroquinolone drops four times a day. Alternatively, a pressure patch and twice-daily antibiotics may be used. Avoid topical steroids.

Traumatic Iritis

A blunt trauma to the eye can cause traumatic inflammation of the iris or, more accurately, of the anterior uveal tract. This leads to the presence of inflammatory cells in the anterior chamber of the eye. Traumatic iritis generally develops quickly after the trauma and usually affects only the injured eye.

◆ Presentation

Patients usually present with a history of ocular trauma. Symptoms include pain, photophobia, and possibly headache. Pain typically worsens when either the injured eye or the uninvolved eye is exposed to bright light (due to consensual pupillary constriction). Signs include cells and flare in the anterior chamber and perilimbal injection (**Fig. 1.9**). The iris pupillary margin of the involved eye may be different in shape compared with the contralateral.

◆ Differential Diagnosis

Traumatic corneal abrasion, traumatic microhyphema, other causes of anterior uveitis

◆ Management

Posttraumatic pain without corneal abrasion or ulcer should suggest the diagnosis of traumatic iritis. This diagnosis can be confirmed by the presence of cells and

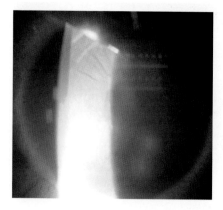

Fig. 1.9 Posttraumatic hyphema and iritis. (Courtesy of Amar Agarwal, Dr. Agarwal's Eye Hospital, Chennai, India)

flare in the anterior chamber at slit-lamp examination. A complete ophthalmic evaluation should be performed, including tonometry and fundus examination. Treatment typically consists of cycloplegic agents. In refractory cases and if no corneal epithelial defect is detected, a steroid drop could be given. Patients should be re-evaluated within a week; if iritis is resolved, medication can be discontinued.

Iris Sphincter Tear

Blunt injury often causes tears in the sphincter pupillae of the iris.

◆ Presentation

The patient may be asymptomatic or may have glare and photophobia. The tears in the pupillary margin can be visualized on slit lamp examination (**Fig. 1.10**)

◆ Differential Diagnosis

Other causes of a dilated pupil (e.g., pharmacological mydriasis)

◆ Management

A thorough ocular examination is done to rule out any other coexisting damage. It may be left alone untreated. If causing symptoms, and if cataract extraction is also being planned, one may perform a pupilloplasty or use aniridia segments.

Traumatic Cataract

Traumatic cataract can develop after various types of insult: blunt or perforating trauma, electric shock, infrared, UV, and ionizing radiation. Blunt trauma is the most common cause, and coup and contrecoup injuries, along with equatorial expansion, are the pathophysiological mechanism responsible for ocular damage. As regards lens injury, "coup" is the cause for Vossius ring (iris pigment remains imprinted on the anterior capsule), and "contrecoup" is responsible for the shock waves that may lead to anterior or posterior capsular rupture and subsequent lens opacification. The equatorial stretching can disrupt the zonules and capsule. The

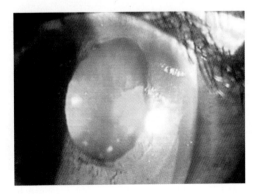

Fig. 1.10 Sphincter tear. (Courtesy of Amar Agarwal, Dr. Agarwal's Eye Hospital, Chennai, India)

release of lens proteins due to capsule rupture can lead to phacoanaphylactic uveitis, characterized by the presence of polymorphonuclear leukocyte (eosinophils) and giant cell infiltration surrounding lens materials. The occlusion of the trabecular meshwork due to lens proteins and macrophages can lead to an acute rise in intraocular pressure. Glaucoma can also be secondary to relative pupillary block due to posterior synechiae or lens swelling (phacomorphic glaucoma).

◆ Presentation

If no perforating trauma or trauma-related symptomatic iritis occurs, the patient could wait for days, weeks, or months before searching for medical care. The patient usually presents with a history of trauma and may complain of decreased vision and monocular diplopia. At slit lamp examination, cataract associated with blunt trauma usually appears as stellate or rosette-shaped "visual axis" opacification located in-axis and involving the posterior capsule. Perforating trauma leads to cortical opacification at the site of injury. This opacification usually remains localized, but if the capsular tear is large enough, the entire lens may opacify. Hyphema, signs of iritis, and lens dislocation or subluxation may be present (**Fig. 1.11A,B**).

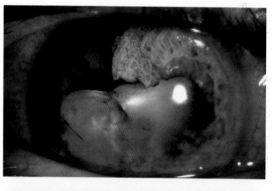

A

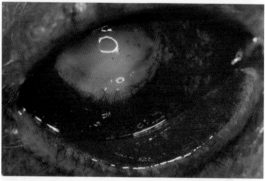

B

Fig. 1.11 **(A)** Cataract and iridodialysis secondary to severe penetrating trauma. **(B)** Posttraumatic endophthalmitis.

◆ **Differential Diagnosis**

Senile cataract, ectopia lentis, angle recession glaucoma, and hyphema

◆ **Management**

Mechanism of injury and past ocular history should be investigated first. Then a ruptured globe and intraocular foreign body should be ruled out and a complete ophthalmic examination should be performed. Type and extent of lens opacification and the presence of ocular inflammation, hyphema, phacodonesis, iridodonesis, angle recession, lens swelling, lens dislocation, or subluxation should be documented. Zonular disruption may be detected gonioscopically through a dilated pupil. Posterior segment trauma-related pathology should be investigated by funduscopy. If opacification obstructs the view of the posterior segment, ultrasonography may be helpful. Medical treatment should be directed to focal and off-axis opacities, inflammation, and intraocular pressure rise. Miotics can help to obtain a clear visual axis, inflammation can be controlled with corticosteroids, increased intraocular pressure can be treated with standard ocular hypotensive medications. However, surgical removal of the lens usually resolves these complications. Decreased visual acuity, lens-induced inflammation or glaucoma, capsular rupture with lens swelling, and poor visualization of posterior segment pathology are indications for surgery. Standard phacoemulsification is preferred if the lens capsule is intact and there is sufficient zonular support; intracapsular extraction is indicated for zonular instability or anterior dislocation. In cases of posterior dislocation or posterior capsular rupture, pars plana lensectomy and vitrectomy may be preferred. As regards lens implantation, capsular fixation is indicated if zonular support and the lens capsule are intact; capsular tension rings may help in cases of limited zonular dialysis. If the posterior capsule is compromised but sufficient zonular support remains, sulcus fixation should be chosen. A suture fixation approach would be the best if both zonular and capsular support are inadequate. If no posterior support is maintained, anterior chamber positioning should be considered. Complications associated with traumatic cataract include glaucoma (pupillary block glaucoma, phacolytic glaucoma, phacomorphic glaucoma, angle recession glaucoma), phacoanaphylactic uveitis, hyphema, retinal detachment, choroidal rupture, traumatic optic neuropathy, and globe rupture.

Lens Dislocation/Subluxation

Subluxation is partial disruption of the zonular fibers; the lens is decentered but remains partially in the pupillary aperture. Dislocation is complete disruption of the zonular fibers; the lens is displaced out of the pupillary aperture. Trauma (most common cause), Marfan syndrome, homocystinuria, Weill–Marchesani syndrome, acquired syphilis, congenital ectopia lentis, aniridia, Ehlers–Danlos syndrome, Crouzon disease, hyperlysinemia, sulfite oxidase deficiency, high myopia, chronic inflammations, and hypermature cataract are some of the causes of lens subluxation.

◆ **Presentation**

Decreased vision and double vision that persist when covering one eye (monocular diplopia) are the main symptoms. Critical signs are decentered or displaced lens, iridodonesis (quivering of the iris), and phacodonesis (quivering of the lens). Other signs include marked astigmatism, cataract, angle closure glaucoma as a result of pupillary block, acquired high myopia, vitreous in the anterior chamber, and asymmetry of the anterior chamber depth (**Fig. 1.12**)

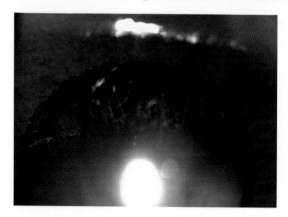

Fig. 1.12 Lens subluxation and zonular disruption.

◆ **Management**

Family, personal, medical, and trauma history is very important. Systemic examination should evaluate stature, extremities, hands, and fingers as necessary. Rapid plasma reagin test and fluorescent treponemal antibody absorption test, sodium nitroprusside test, echocardiography, and urine chromatography to rule out homocystinuria are needed.

◆ *Lens dislocated into the vitreous*: Surgically remove the lens.
◆ *Lens capsule intact, patient asymptomatic no signs of inflammation*: Observe.
◆ *Lens capsule broken eye inflamed*: Lensectomy is done either through the pars plana or by using a limbal approach
◆ *Subluxation*
  ◆ *Asymptomatic*: Observe.
  ◆ *High uncorrectable astigmatism or monocular diplopia*: Surgical removal of the lens.
  ◆ *Symptomatic cataract*: Options include surgical removal of the lens.
  ◆ *Pupillary block*: Treatment is identical to that for aphakic pupillary block.
  ◆ *Marfan syndrome is present*: Refer the patient to a cardiologist for an annual echocardiogram and management of any cardiac-related abnormalities. Prophylactic systemic antibiotics are required if the patient undergoes surgery (or a dental procedure) to prevent endocarditis.
  ◆ *Homocystinuria is present*:
    ◆ Administer pyridoxine, 50 to 1000 mg by mouth four times a day.
    ◆ Reduce dietary methionine.
    ◆ Avoid surgery if possible because of the risk of thromboembolic complications. If surgical intervention is necessary, anticoagulant therapy is indicated.

Microhyphema/Hyphema

Traumatic hyphema is defined by postinjury accumulation of blood within the anterior chamber. Microhyphema consists of suspended erythrocytes in the anterior chamber, generally visible at slit lamp. Equatorial expansion after blunt trauma induces stress to angle structures, which can lead to rupture of iris and ciliary body vessels with subsequent hemorrhage. Lacerating injury can be associated with direct damage of blood vessels and hypotony. Some conditions such as rubeosis iridis, juvenile xanthogranuloma, hemophilia, leukemia, and the use of drugs that alter platelet or thrombin function may facilitate the onset of hyphema. A significant number of sight-threatening complications may develop, which requires careful follow-up for hyphema patients.

◆ Presentation

Patients usually present with a history of blunt trauma. Pain and blurred vision are common symptoms. Hyphemas are graded on the amount of blood within the anterior chamber: grade I is less than one third filling of the anterior chamber, grade II hyphemas have more than one third but less than one half of the anterior chamber filled with blood, grade III is more than one half but less than total filling, grade IV is a total hyphema, also known as eight-ball hyphema (**Fig. 1.13**).

◆ Differential Diagnosis

Uveitic glaucoma and causes of spontaneous hyphema such as juvenile xanthogranuloma, iris cavernous hemangioma, hypertension, and bleeding disorders

◆ Management

Mechanism and time of injury should be investigated carefully. A history of sickle cell trait or disease should be sought out. Inspection for gross ocular injury and evaluation of the adnexa should be performed. A ruptured globe should be ruled out. A complete ocular examination is imperative and must include intraocular pressure measurement and dilated funduscopic evaluation. Gonioscopy should be deferred until hyphema resolves to detect potential rebleeding sites and angle recession. A drawing of the hyphema documenting shape and size should be recorded at every ophthalmic evaluation. Depending on the patient's history, hemoglobinopathies and bleeding disorders should be investigated. B-scan ultrasonography may be useful in patients with large hyphemas, when ophthalmoscopy is not feasible. Noncompliant patients or those with increased risk of rebleeding, uncontrolled

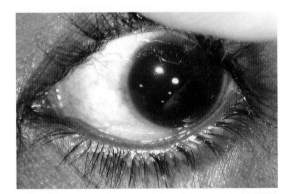

Fig. 1.13 Posttraumatic hyphema. Grade II hyphemas have more than one third but less than one half of the anterior chamber filled with blood.

glaucoma, positive sickle cell trait, or anemia should be considered for inpatient hospitalization. The elevation of the patient's head to 30 to 45 degrees while lying supine may facilitate the settling and layering of the hyphema in the inferior anterior chamber, allowing an easier classification of the hyphema, an earlier evaluation of the posterior pole, and a more rapid improvement in visual acuity. A transparent plastic shield should be used to protect the involved eye from further injury. Its transparency allows recognizing rebleeding or sudden visual loss.

Medical treatment includes topical cycloplegics (1 drop of 1% atropine three times a day for up to 5 days) to increase the patient's comfort (consider the risk of precipitating acute glaucoma in patients with a narrow chamber angle) and topical steroids (0.1% dexamethasone) to decrease inflammation, reduce anterior chamber reaction, and prevent the incidence of secondary hemorrhage (caution should be exerted if steroids are used for a prolonged period because they can increase the risk of cataract and glaucoma). Topical and systemic antifibrinolytics, such as aminocaproic acid, could be used to prevent rebleeding and retarding clot lysis. The more common side effects of aminocaproic acid include vomiting, diarrhea, and postural hypotension. Its systemic use should be avoided in patients with hepatic or renal disease. Persistent increased intraocular pressure should be treated initially with topical β-blockers. If this treatment is unsuccessful, topical α-agonist or carbonic anhydrase inhibitor may be added in patients without sickle cell trait or disease. Aspirin and other NSAIDS should be discontinued. Uncontrolled elevated intraocular pressure (at least 45 mm Hg for 5 days) could be surgically treated with paracentesis and anterior chamber washout. Other indications to surgery are early corneal staining or rebleeding hyphemas. Smaller hyphemas are usually self-limiting and clear within 5 days. Large hyphemas are associated with complications and the worst prognosis. Such complications are secondary hemorrhage, corneal blood staining, glaucoma, anterior and posterior synechiae, cataract, and optic atrophy.

Ruptured Globe

A ruptured globe is a devastating injury with significant long-term consequences for the patient. It represents a discontinuity of the eye's outer membranes caused by blunt or penetrating trauma. Ruptures resulting from blunt trauma usually occur at the sites where the sclera is weakest, such as at the insertion of the extraocular muscles, around the optic nerve, and at the limbus. Sharp objects with sufficient momentum may directly perforate the globe. Globe rupture is more common in young males owing to their occupational and recreational preferences. High myopia and previous eye surgery can make tissues more vulnerable to rupture. A ruptured globe is an ophthalmic emergency and requires surgical repair as soon as possible. The visual outcome depends largely on early recognition and prompt intervention.

◆ Presentation

The patient usually presents with a history of ocular trauma. Symptoms include pain, which can be not extremely severe in the case of sharp injury, and decreased vision. Diplopia may be present due to extraocular muscle entrapment or dysfunction and trauma-associated cranial nerve palsy. At physical examination the globe rupture may be obvious or occult. A full-thickness corneal or scleral laceration is a sign of globe perforation. Prolapse of the iris or extrusion of ocular contents may be present. Severe conjunctival hemorrhage, usually involving 360 degrees of bulbar conjunctiva, typically indicates globe rupture. Other accompanying signs include irregular pupil, hyphema, lens injury, commotio retinae, vitreous hemorrhage, choroidal rupture, retinal tears and detachments, and traumatic optic neuropathy. A ruptured globe may present with both enophthalmos and exophthalmos, depending on the presence of an associated retrobulbar hemorrhage (**Fig. 1.14**).

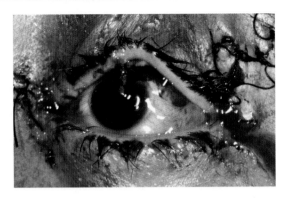

Fig. 1.14   Perforating ocular trauma.

◆ Management

The mechanism and the circumstances of injury and the nature of the traumatizing object should be investigated. Visual acuity should be documented and extraocular muscle function should be evaluated. Pupils should be examined for size, shape, and light reflex. The diagnosis of a ruptured globe should be made by slit lamp or penlight. The orbit and adnexa should be examined for injuries, foreign bodies, bone deformity, and eyeball displacement. Intraocular pressure measurement is contraindicated to avoid pressure on the globe. The eye should be protected with a shield. Systemic prophylactic antibiotics and analgesics, if advisable, should be administered. The patient should receive tetanus immunization if indicated and be kept nothing per os. The imaging study of choice is computed tomography; if it is not available a plain x-ray film should be obtained. Magnetic resonance imaging may be useful to identify soft tissue and globe injuries, but it is contraindicated if a metallic foreign body is suspected. Careful B-scan ultrasonography may be useful to identify the site of rupture and intraocular foreign bodies. Surgical repair should be prompt. If there is no expectation to restore vision, enucleation should be considered. Endophthalmitis and sympathetic ophthalmia are possible sight-treating complications that should be borne in mind.

◆ Posterior Segment Trauma

Posttraumatic Vitreous Hemorrhage

Vitreous hemorrhage results from bleeding into one of the several potential spaces formed around and within the vitreous body. This condition can follow injuries to the retina and uveal tract and their associated vascular structures. Neovascularization occurring in diseases like proliferative diabetic retinopathy may predispose to bleeding, even if the trauma is mild. Other disorders that promote the release of angiogenic vasoactive factors and subsequent formation of neovascular and fragile vessels that can easily bleed are ischemic retinopathy secondary to retinal vein occlusion, retinopathy of prematurity, and proliferative sickle cell retinopathy. Traumatic vitreous hemorrhage in children may be a sign of child abuse (shaken baby syndrome).

◆ Presentation

Patients with traumatic vitreous hemorrhage usually present with a complaint of decreased visual acuity, floaters, cloudy vision, perception of shadows, visual haze, and photophobia. Patients may not remember the traumatic insult. Direct ophthalmoscopy reveals a diminished red reflex that can be black in severe cases. Indirect ophthalmoscopic examination discloses the presence of blood in the anterohyaloid or retrohyaloid spaces or within the vitreous gel. Usually a subhyaloid hemorrhage suggests a source of bleeding anterior to the retina, whereas a hemorrhage posterior to the internal limiting membrane implies a source of bleeding within the retina. Long-standing hemorrhages can evolve in white masses (**Fig. 1.15**).

◆ Differential Diagnosis

Differential diagnosis of traumatic vitreous hemorrhage includes other vitreous hemorrhages not related to trauma. Spontaneous vitreous hemorrhage may occur in conditions like proliferative retinopathies, choroidal or ciliary body melanoma, retinoblastoma, uveitis, sarcoidosis, ocular manifestation of syphilis, or histoplasmosis.

◆ Management

A detailed history is very important. Underlying pathologies and mechanism of trauma should be documented. A complete eye examination should be performed, including slit lamp examination, intraocular pressure measurement, and dilated fundus evaluation. Globe perforation and intraocular foreign body should be ruled out. B-scan ultrasonography can be used when the fundus is difficult to visualize, disclosing the presence of retinal detachment, retinal tears, intraocular foreign body, or intraocular tumor. Initial therapy consists of bed rest with 30- to 45-degree head elevation (allows the blood to settle inferiorly) and avoidance of anticoagulative drugs and intense Valsalva maneuvers. Conclusive therapy is fired at the underlying cause: retinal breaks can be closed with laser photocoagulation, and surgery can resolve retinal detachments. Vitrectomy is also indicated in long-standing vitreous hemorrhage (> 2 to 3 months) and when vitreous hemorrhage is associated with rubeosis and ghost-cell glaucoma. Complications of vitreous hem-

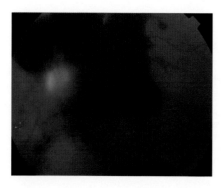

Fig. 1.15 Posttraumatic vitreous hemorrhage.

orrhage usually develop when large amounts of blood remain for long periods in the vitreous cavity and include enhanced proliferative retinopathy, hemosiderosis bulbi and consequent iron toxicity, ghost-cell glaucoma, amblyopia (resulting from visual deprivation), and myopic shift in infants.

Commotio Retinae

Commotio retinae is a clinical entity first described in 1873 by Berlin and is characterized by a transient whitening at the deep sensory retina. This condition is common; it has been shown to be responsible for 9.4% of all posttraumatic fundus changes. The mechanism of injury is the contrecoup force following blunt ocular trauma that causes degeneration of the photoreceptors' outer segments and subsequent phagocytosis by retinal pigment epithelium cells. The presence of edema in the outer plexiform layers, nuclear layers, and subretinal space has been demonstrated. Angiographic evidence has supported the belief that retinal and choroidal vessels do not play a significant role in the pathogenesis of this condition.

◆ Presentation

Patients may be asymptomatic if commotio retinae is limited to the peripheral retina, or they may complain of decreased vision if the whitening occurs in the foveal region. Visual acuity may be variably affected and does not always relate to the degree of opacification. Ophthalmoscopic examination reveals a cloudy opacification of the retina, usually with poorly defined margins. It can be located anywhere within the posterior segment. In some cases the entire posterior pole can be involved, and it may appear as a pseudocherry red spot. Retinal vessels are clearly visible and appear undisturbed. Other associated traumatic pathology may be present, such as subretinal, intraretinal, and preretinal hemorrhages; macular holes; macular detachments, and choroidal ruptures (**Fig. 1.16**).

◆ Differential Diagnosis

Differential diagnosis of commotio retinae includes retinal detachment, central artery occlusion, branch retinal artery occlusion, and retinal white without pressure.

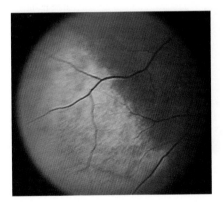

Fig. 1.16 Peripheral commotio retinae with undefined posterior borders.

◆ **Management**

The mechanism of trauma should be documented. A complete ophthalmic examination should be performed, including dilated fundus evaluation and scleral depression if there is no evidence of hyphema, microhyphema, or iritis. The retinal whitening usually fades within some weeks, and no treatment is available, only observation. About 60% of patients fully recover vision, and 40% sustain permanent visual loss. Complications of commotio retinae include cystoid areas that may degenerate into macular holes, photoreceptor loss, retinal pigment epithelium (RPE) migration, degeneration, atrophy, or hyperplasia.

Choroidal Rupture

Traumatic choroidal rupture is a common occurrence after a blunt ocular trauma (5 to 10%). It is a defect in the Bruch membrane, the choroid, and the retinal pigment epithelium. When sudden anteroposterior compression and equatorial expansion subsequent to ocular blunt trauma take place, the sclera has enough tensile strength and the retina has enough elasticity to be relatively protected. Because the Bruch membrane does not have these properties, it is prone to break. The damage at the choriocapillaris vessels may lead to subretinal, sub-retinal pigment epithelium, or intrachoroidal hemorrhage. In the acute phase the overlying hemorrhage and the retinal edema may obscure the choroidal rupture itself. Typically, during the healing phase, choroidal neovascularization occurs and in most cases resolves spontaneously. Conditions associated with an increased fragility of the Bruch membrane, such as angioid streaks, are risk factors for traumatic choroidal rupture.

◆ **Presentation**

Patients usually present with a history of ocular blunt trauma, decreased vision, and a variety of visual field defects (paracentral, central, sector scotomas). At ophthalmoscopic examination the choroidal lesion appears as a yellow-white, crescent-shaped, subretinal streak, concentric to the optic disc. The border of the rupture may be hyperpigmented or hypopigmented. Often the overlying hemorrhage may obscure the choroidal rupture (**Fig. 1.17A,B**).

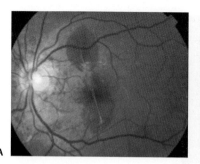
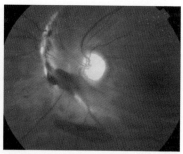

A

B

Fig. 1.17   **(A)** Traumatic choroidal rupture. **(B)** Traumatic choroidal rupture.

◆ **Differential Diagnosis**

Angioid streaks, high myopia, subretinal neovascular membranes, ocular histo-plasmosis syndrome, choroidal neovascularization, pseudoxanthoma elasticum

◆ **Management**

A complete ocular examination is mandatory. Fluorescein angiography may be considered to confirm the presence of choroidal rupture and to detect choroidal neovascularization. Indocyanine green angiography may be useful when subretinal hemorrhage obscures choroidal neovascularization recognition. Conservative treatment is advised for most traumatic choroidal ruptures. Extrafoveal choroidal neovascularization may be treated with laser photocoagulation. Pars plana vitrectomy and membrane extraction may be considered for subfoveal and juxtafoveal choroidal neovascularization. Good visual outcomes are expected if the rupture does not involve the fovea. Possible complications are hemorrhagic or serous macular detachment.

Posttraumatic Retinal Tears and Detachment

Ocular trauma is responsible for ~10% of retinal detachments. Usually the traumatic injury causes an anterior-posterior compression of the globe and a lateral expansion of the equator. This results in a tractional force on the vitreous base, where the vitreous body is physiologically adherent to the peripheral retina. Retinal breaks are the result of vitreous traction at the ora serrata or in sites of focal vitreoretinal adhesion (such as corioretinal scars and lattice degeneration). In the presence of vitreous syneresis, fluid dissects the retina, giving rise to retinal detachment. Common abnormalities causing posttraumatic retinal detachments are retinal dialysis and giant retinal tears. Another mechanism of injury is retinal necrosis as a result of direct trauma to the sclera. It is often associated with retinal hemorrhages and edema and leads to large and irregularly shaped retinal tears. High myopia and sites of focal vitreoretinal adherence are risk factors for traumatic retinal detachment.

◆ **Presentation**

Retinal detachments and retinal tears can be diagnosed months or years after the trauma, so the causal nexus is not always easy to identify. Patients can present complaining of mild blurring of vision, floaters, photopsia, and visual-field defects. Ophthalmoscopic findings that suggest a vitreoretinal interface involvement after a trauma include vitreous base avulsion, retinal dialysis, retinal tears of various shapes and dimensions (giant, round, horseshoe), and retinal detachment. Once the retina becomes detached, it appears as an elevated, slightly opaque, corrugated surface that undulates freely with eye movements. In the cases of retinal detachment intraocular pressure is usually lower than that of the fellow eye (**Fig. 1.18**).

◆ **Differential Diagnosis**

Penetrating trauma, retinal detachments caused by other conditions (proliferative, tractional, postoperative, exudative), acute retinal necrosis, senile retinoschisis

◆ **Management**

A complete ophthalmic evaluation should be performed, including intraocular pressure measurement and accurate retinal examination. Retinal abnormalities, vitreo-

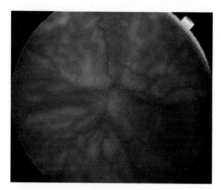

Fig. 1.18 Retinal detachment secondary to a retinal dialysis.

retinal tractions, tears, and detachments must be recorded. B-scan ultrasonography and optical coherence tomography are useful imaging studies when media opacities impair a complete ophthalmoscopic retinal examination. Retinal tears may be treated successfully by laser photocoagulation and cryopexy. However, some giant retinal tears may progress to retinal detachment regardless of therapy. For this reason a prophylactic scleral buckle may be considered in the cases of an elevated tear flap or focal vitreoretinal traction. Retinal detachments are essentially managed with surgery. Common procedures are vitrectomy, pneumatic retinopexy, and scleral buckling to support the dialysis. Perfluorocarbonate liquids or gas bubbles can be used intraocularly to facilitate the retina's adherence. The final postsurgery visual acuity depends primarily on whether the macula was involved in the retinal detachment: once the macula is detached, photoreceptors start to degenerate, impairing visual recovery. Other concurrent damages to the macula, such as macular holes, commotio retinae, or choroidal rupture, may limit final visual acuity.

Traumatic Macular Hole

A macular hole is a full-thickness defect of the retina involving the foveal region. Traumatic macular hole was first described in 1869 by Knapp. Since then a large number of cases have been reported and, despite several publications, the exact mechanism of traumatic macular hole formation remains controversial. Some theories have been proposed to explain development of traumatic macular holes: historical hypotheses claimed traumatic, cystic degeneration, and vitreous and vascular etiologies. In more recent times, Johnson et al advanced that equatorial expansion causes retinal flattening and tangential traction. Yamada et al observed that vitreous traction may play a role in the formation of some traumatic macular holes. Tornambe proposed the experimental hydration theory, stating that the altered homeostasis due to a break in the internal retinal layer leads to intraretinal swelling and hole formation. The incidence of traumatic macular holes varies from 1 to 9%. Patients are usually young and male. Most traumatic macular holes derive from closed-globe contusion injuries from various insults, the most common being blunt ocular trauma caused by a variety of types of balls. Traumatic macular holes can also be caused by accidental yttrium-aluminum-garnet (i.e., YAG) laser burns.

◆ Presentation

Patients usually present with a history of ocular trauma and subsequent reduction of central visual acuity, which is usually 20/80 to 20/400. Ophthalmoscopic examination normally discloses a full-thickness and well-defined hole in the center of the macula. It is usually round or elliptical and measures 300 to 500 μm. Other common findings are the presence of small yellow deposits at the level of the retinal pigment epithelium (RPE) and a ring of subretinal fluid surrounding the hole. Associated epiretinal membrane and operculum are typically missing. Erythrocytes and inflammatory cells may be present in the vitreous, and associated ocular injuries are common (**Fig. 1.19**).

◆ Differential Diagnosis

Idiopathic macular hole, epiretinal membrane

◆ Management

A complete ophthalmic examination should be performed, including intraocular pressure measurement and careful posterior segment evaluation. Useful imaging studies include fluorescein angiography, optical coherence tomography, and B-scan ultrasonography. Microperimetry may document the pattern of visual acuity loss. Vitrectomy has been shown to close traumatic macular holes effectively and improve vision. Current technique includes removal of the posterior hyaloid and all epiretinal membranes from the macular area and prolonged postoperative macular gas tamponade. Spontaneous closure of traumatic macular holes is relatively frequent. Therefore, a period of observation before deciding on surgical intervention is recommended. Associated macular RPE atrophy and choroidal injury may limit visual outcomes.

Intraocular Foreign Body

The ophthalmic pathologies caused by an intraocular foreign body arise from two mechanisms: the direct damage caused by the penetrating injury and its associated complications, depending on the size, shape, and momentum of the object; and the damage caused by the existence of an intraocular foreign body, such as metal toxicity and microbial endophthalmitis. Metallosis bulbi is an extensive ocular damage caused by the chronic presence of a reactive metallic foreign body, most commonly made of iron or copper. Siderosis is characterized by a rusty brown deposit and discoloration involving the lens and the iris, and retinal degenerative

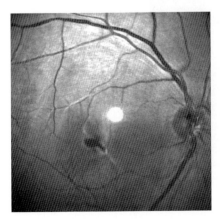

Fig. 1.19 Traumatic macular hole.

pigmentary changes. Chalcosis is made distinctive by the presence of a greenish blue ring in the peripheral cornea (Kayser-Fleischer ring), greenish coloration of the iris, anterior subcapsular cataract, and refractive deposits on the surface of the retina. Commonly, intraocular foreign bodies arise from hammering and using power tools. Protective eyewear can prevent most injuries.

◆ **Presentation**

Patients usually present with a suggestive history, but ophthalmologists should take into account that a patient may be unaware of any object penetrating the eye. Patients may be asymptomatic or complain of decreased vision and eye pain. The foreign body may be visible at slit-lamp examination of the anterior segment; other signs include corneal entry wound, iris transillumination defect, irregular pupil, lens damage, and anterior chamber reaction. Dilated indirect ophthalmoscopy may reveal a posterior segment foreign body and associated injuries, such as vitreous hemorrhage, retinal tears, and detachment (**Fig. 1.20**).

◆ **Differential Diagnosis**

Other causes of sudden visual loss

◆ **Management**

History should be carefully investigated, including mechanism of injury and foreign body composition. Ocular examination should be performed, with attention to possible sites of ocular perforation. The anterior chamber and posterior segment should be evaluated carefully. The direct visualization of the foreign body is usually very informative for the surgeon. Computed tomography is the imaging study of choice; if it is unavailable a plain x-ray may be considered in the case of a metallic foreign body. A careful use of B-scan ultrasonography may be convenient to localize the foreign body even if the globe is open. If a chronic intraocular foreign body is found, electroretinography is a useful for evaluating retinal function in the metallosis bulbi. Topical and systemic antibiotic therapy, topical steroids, and tetanus prophylaxis (if needed) are required prior to the surgical intervention. The timing of surgery depends on the nature and location of the foreign body

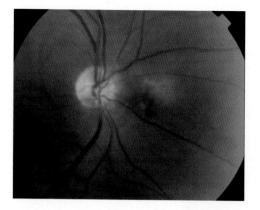

Fig. 1.20   Intraocular foreign body.

and on the risk of endophthalmitis. Foreign bodies in the anterior chamber should be extracted through a paracentesis and with the auxiliary use of viscoelastics to reduce possible damage to the lens and the corneal endothelium. Foreign bodies embedded in the lens do not automatically result in cataract. If no opacification is evident and there is no risk of siderosis, then they can be left in situ. Vitrectomy is the surgical procedure of choice for posterior segment foreign bodies. In the case of magnetic foreign bodies, they can be removed with the use of a strong intraocular magnet. Proper forceps should be used for nonmagnetic foreign bodies. Associated injuries should be treated accordingly. If possible a culture of the foreign body or of a sample of vitreous may be useful if an infection is suspected. Possible complications of intraocular foreign bodies include endophthalmitis, metallosis, corneal scarring, cataract, retinal detachment, and elevated intraocular pressure.

Traumatic Optic Neuropathy

Trauma-associated lesion of the optic nerve can occur anywhere in the course of the nerve. The injury can be due to laceration of the nerve by a foreign body or a bone fragment, compression of the nerve, and hemorrhage or perineural edema. It is usually associated with head trauma or midfacial fracture. Optic nerve trauma is often due to vehicle accidents, falls, recreational sports, assaults, or penetrating orbital trauma. The frequency of optic nerve injury in the United States occurring in closed head trauma varies from 0.5 to 5.0% (**Fig. 1.21**)

◆ Presentation

Typically, patients present with a history of head injury and report a classic sequence of events: the patient recovers consciousness after head injury and experiences a posttraumatic loss of visual function in one eye. Visual acuity and color vision may be altered, and visual field defects may be present. The critical sign is a new ipsilateral afferent pupillary defect. Optic atrophy usually occurs weeks after retrobulbar trauma. Injuries to the optic nerve may be either direct or indirect. Direct injuries include the following:

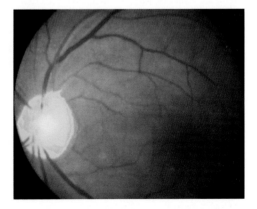

Fig. 1.21 Traumatic optic neuropathy. (Courtesy of Athiya Agarwal, Dr. Agarwal's Eye Hospital, Chennai, India)

◆ *Optic nerve avulsion*: It usually follows severe orbital trauma with an acute and serious visual loss. Ophthalmoscopy shows the absence of the optic disc and peripapillary hemorrhage.

◆ *Optic nerve transection*: The vision loss is immediate and complete, and computed tomographic scanning reveals the bone fragment or the foreign body transecting the optic nerve.

◆ *Optic nerve sheath hemorrhage*: Visual function abnormalities may vary and proptosis may not be present. Magnetic resonance imaging may be helpful in confirming the diagnosis. The visual loss associated with this condition may be reversible via sheath fenestration.

◆ *Orbital hemorrhage*: It is associated with proptosis and ophthalmoplegia. Raised intraocular pressure may be initially controlled with topical ocular hypotensive agents. If conservative measures fail, lateral canthotomy and hemorrhage drainage should be considered.

◆ *Orbital emphysema*: Injuries to the thin bones limiting the paranasal sinus may produce a one-way valve that results in an air accumulation in the orbit with subsequent compression of the optic nerve, proptosis, and elevation in the intraocular pressure. Drainage of the intraorbital air usually resolves this condition.

Indirect optic nerve injury usually results from a blunt trauma to the superior orbital rim or the frontal area. The compression forces are then transmitted via orbital bones to the orbital apex and optic canal. Compression and contusion of the nerve produce a compartment syndrome that results in localized optic nerve ischemia and edema.

◆ Differential Diagnosis

Posttraumatic intraocular lesions, preexisting neuropathies, factious amblyopia

◆ Management

The management of indirect optic nerve injury should include complete ocular examination, color vision testing, visual field testing, computed tomographic scanning of the head and orbit, and B-scan ultrasonography. Other tests that may be useful are visual evoked potential and electroretinography. The treatment of optic nerve indirect injury is somewhat controversial. Very high-dose corticosteroids have been proposed to limit free-radical amplification of the injury response. Surgery may be reserved, when indicated, for the cases of direct injury or to decompress the optic canal in indirect injuries. Nevertheless, the serious complications of surgery, such as iatrogenic damage of the optic nerve or of the adjacent structures, should be carefully considered.

◆ Orbital Trauma

Orbital Fractures

Blow-out fracture of the inferior wall of the orbit is the most common of the orbital fractures. The medial wall of the orbit is the thinnest of all and is commonly associated with multiple wall fractures of the orbit.

◆ Presentation

Patients present with pain (especially on attempted vertical eye movement), local tenderness, binocular double vision, eyelid swelling and crepitus after nose blowing, and recent history of trauma. Examination reveals restricted eye movement (especially in upward or lateral gaze), subcutaneous or conjunctival emphysema, hypoesthesia in the distribution of the infraorbital nerve (ipsilateral cheek and upper lip), and enophthalmos (may initially be masked by orbital edema). Associated signs include nosebleed, eyelid edema, and ecchymosis. Superior rim and orbital roof fractures may show hypoesthesia in the distribution of the supratrochlear or supraorbital nerve (ipsilateral forehead) and ptosis. Trismus, malar flattening, and a palpable step-off deformity of the inferior orbital rim are characteristic of tripod fractures (**Fig. 1.22A,B**).

◆ Differential Diagnosis

Orbital edema and hemorrhage without a blow-out, cranial nerve palsy

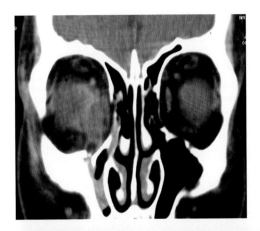

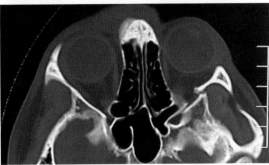

Fig. 1.22 **(A)** Blow-out fracture inferior wall. **(B)** Orbital blow-out fracture of the lateral wall. (Image (A) Courtesy of Soosan Jacob, Dr. Agarwal's Eye Hospital, Chennai, India)

◆ Management

Complete ophthalmologic examination, including measurement of extraocular movements and globe displacement. Check pupils and color vision carefully to rule out a traumatic optic neuropathy. Forced-duction testing is performed. Computed tomographic scan of the orbits is obtained in all cases of suspected orbital fractures.

Treatment includes nasal decongestants (e.g., pseudoephedrine nasal spray, twice a day); broad-spectrum oral antibiotics (e.g., cephalexin 250 to 500 mg by mouth four times a day, or erythromycin 250 to 500 mg by mouth four times a day) for 7 days may be used but are not mandatory. Apply ice packs to the orbit for the first 24 to 48 hours. Surgical repair should be considered based on the following criteria.

Immediate repair (usually within 24 hours) is required if there is evidence by computed tomographic scan of entrapped muscle or periorbital tissue in combination with diplopia and nonresolving bradycardia, heart block, nausea, vomiting, or syncope.

Repair in 1 to 2 weeks is done if there is evidence of persistent, symptomatic diplopia in primary or downgaze that has improved at 1 week, with positive forced ductions and evidence of entrapment on computed tomography or large floor fractures (more than one half of the orbital floor) that have caused or are likely to cause cosmetically unacceptable enophthalmos.

Intraorbital Foreign Body

Intraorbital foreign bodies can occur either from high-velocity injuries or from relatively minor traumas. The nature of the object is fundamental in determining the severity of ocular and orbital complications. Organic foreign bodies are poorly tolerated and often lead to inflammation. Most metals, stone, glass, and plastic are usually inert and well tolerated. Thus inorganic foreign bodies typically cause decreased vision or orbital complications due to direct trauma, whereas organic foreign bodies can easily develop orbital infections.

◆ Presentation

Patients may present with a recent history of trauma and severe pain. However, they can also be asymptomatic and do not recall the trauma at all. Pain, decreased vision, and diplopia are common presenting symptoms. Intraorbital foreign bodies can be subtle and not easily identifiable on examination. Clinical signs include palpable ocular mass, proptosis, afferent pupillary defect, edema and ecchymosis of the eyelids, laceration of the conjunctiva or the periocular tissues, and limitation of the extraocular movements. Organic foreign bodies may induce a marked inflammatory response with elevation of the serum white cell count (**Fig. 1.23**).

◆ Management

A detailed history is necessary to determine the mechanism of injury and the nature of the foreign body. A complete ophthalmologic examination should be performed, with particular attention to funduscopic examination, intraocular pressure, and pupillary reaction. Ocular and periocular inspection should be addressed to discover an entry wound. Neurological testing and attention to the patient's mental status are required to evaluate a possible neurological injury. The imaging study of choice is computed tomographic scan. It can reveal most foreign bodies, and it is safe in case of metallic foreign bodies. However, wooden or plastic foreign bodies can be missed on computed tomographic scan or can be misidentified as intraorbital air. Once a metallic foreign body has been excluded, magnetic reso-

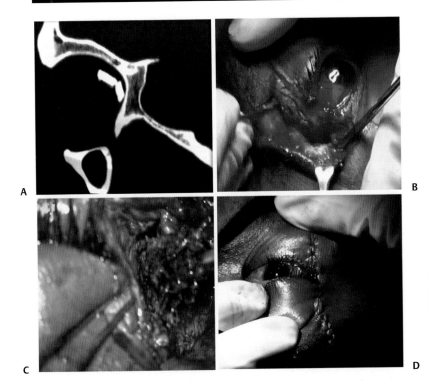

Fig. 1.23 Orbital foreign body removal. **(A)** Computed tomographic scan showing radiopaque foreign body within the orbit. **(B)** Foreign body approached through wound of entry. **(C)** Foreign body located and removed. **(D)** Final appearance after removal of both foreign bodies and closure of wound. (All images courtesy of Soosan Jacob, Dr. Agarwal's Eye Hospital, Chennai, India; courtesy, Pablo Gili)

nance imaging can be useful in diagnosing wooden and plastic foreign bodies. Ultrasonography represents a complementary test. The medical treatment consists of tetanus prophylaxis and broad-spectrum systemic antibiotic therapy. Surgical removal of the foreign body depends on the nature and the location of the object. Surgical intervention is indicated if signs of infection or optic nerve compression are evident. Moreover, all organic and poorly tolerated foreign bodies should be surgically removed. Asymptomatic patients with small, nonorganic intraorbital foreign bodies do not require any surgical intervention.

Retrobulbar Hemorrhage

Orbital hemorrhage in the potential space surrounding the globe may occur after blunt trauma and subsequent injury to the orbital vessels. The orbit is an enclosed space with limited capacity for expansion. The globe and septum can be displaced anteriorly to some extent, giving rise to proptosis. However, this forward movement is limited, and the increased volume results in increased intraorbital pressure and compression of the structures contained in the orbit. Traumatic hemorrhage in the retrobulbar space may lead to acute loss of vision due to central retinal artery occlusion, direct optic nerve compression, or compression of the optic nerve vasculature. Acute retrobulbar hemorrhage is a rare and sight-threatening complication of blunt eye trauma, but it can be reversible when diagnosed and treated promptly.

◆ Presentation

Patients usually present with a recent history of trauma or orbital surgery, pain, and decreased vision. Acute retrobulbar hemorrhage gives rise to marked clinical signs: painful exophthalmos or proptosis with resistance to retropulsion, restriction of extraocular movements, diffuse subconjunctival hemorrhage, periorbital edema, and ecchymosis. Intraocular pressure is typically raised. Congested conjunctival vessels, partial or complete ophthalmoplegia, afferent pupillary defect, and color vision disturbances may also be present. An orbital computed tomographic scan demonstrates a retrobulbar hematoma (**Fig. 1.24**).

◆ Differential Diagnosis

Orbital cellulitis, isolated orbital fracture, globe rupture, carotid cavernous fistula, and varix

◆ Management

Computed tomography is the imaging study of choice to determine retrobulbar hemorrhage and associated orbital injuries. However, it should be delayed in sight-threatening cases. Medical therapy consists of ocular hypotensive medications, but it is considered an ancillary procedure for patients presenting with increased orbital pressure and decreased vision. These patients should undergo emergent decompression of the orbital space via surgical drainage. Surgical procedure consists of lateral canthotomy and cantholysis. Early recognition and prompt surgical intervention preserve and restore vision in most cases.

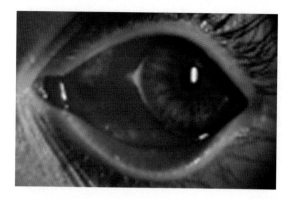

Fig. 1.24 Retrobulbar hemorrhage.

Posttraumatic Pulsating Exophthalmos

The classic clinical picture of pulsating exophthalmos, which is a rare condition, can be produced by posttraumatic carotid-cavernous fistulas. Cerebral traumas account for ~75% of carotid-cavernous fistulas, which are initiated by tears in the walls of the intracavernous internal carotid artery or its branches. Thus arterial blood may short-circuit in the venous complex of the cavernous sinuses. Other causes of pulsating exophthalmos are congenital arteriovenous malformations, arteriosclerosis-related retrobulbar aneurysms, and neurofibromatosis.

◆ Presentation

Patients typically complain, days or weeks after trauma, of a severe and sudden cephalic and orbital pain, a roaring sound in the head synchronous with the pulse, decreased vision, diplopia, and ophthalmoplegia. The pulsating exophthalmos is usually reducible. Inspection reveals engorged and chemotic conjunctiva. Palpation of the eye discloses a thrill, and auscultation reveals an ocular or cephalic bruit synchronous with the pulse. Other ocular signs include dilated retinal veins, disk edema, retinal vein occlusions, venous stasis retinopathy, and increased intraocular pressure due to altered outflow in the vortex veins (**Fig. 1.25A,B**).

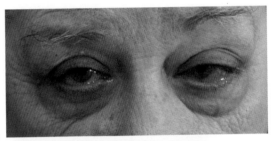

A

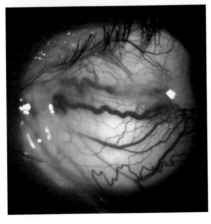

B

Fig. 1.25 (A) Posttraumatic carotid cavernous fistula. **(B)** Engorged vessels and chemotic conjunctiva in a patient with a traumatic carotid cavernous fistula.

◆ Differential Diagnosis

Pulsating exophthalmos that is not trauma related

◆ Management

A complete ophthalmological examination should be performed, including dilated funduscopic examination and intraocular pressure measurement. The function of cranial nerves III, IV, and VI should be tested. The diagnosis can be confirmed by echography, digital angiography, and computed tomography. Therapy is directed to thrombosis of the fistula and normalization of orbital hemodynamics via trans-orbital or transvenous embolization. The increase in intraocular pressure can be initially treated medically.

2 Eyelids and Lacrimal System

Christopher I. Zoumalan, Andrea Olmos, and Kimberly P. Cockerham

◆ Ectropion

Ectropion is a frequently seen condition in elderly people; it is an eyelid malposition in which the eyelid (usually lower) is everted away from the globe.

◆ Presentation

Many symptoms are a result of chronic irritation and exposure to the eye and eyelids. Patients can complain of excessive tearing, conjunctivitis, corneal epitheliopathy, and keratitis, all of which can result in decreased vision. The tarsal conjunctiva can be chronically inflamed, with secondary changes including thickening and keratinization. There are five general classifications of ectropion: involutional, cicatricial, paralytic, congenital, and mechanical:

- ◆ *Involutional:* Attributed to age-related changes that affect the lower lids. There is loss of elasticity of the lid compartments, and often there is medial and lateral canthal tendon laxity. The distraction test and the snap-back test can determine an abnormality in horizontal lid laxity. Anterior lid distraction greater than 6 to 8 mm (where the central part of the eyelid can be pulled away from the globe) suggests a positive lid distraction test. If the lower lid is pulled inferiorly, the lid should quickly return to its previous position. If not, this may be interpreted as an abnormal snap-back test result (**Fig. 2.1A**).
- ◆ *Paralytic:* Because of ipsilateral facial nerve palsy, often associated with lid retraction and subsequent lagophthalmos. Exposure keratopathy and epiphora are common complications (**Fig. 2.1B**).
- ◆ *Cicatricial:* Often, scarring from chronic inflammation such as trichiasis or sun exposure can lead to a contracture of the anterior lamellae (skin and orbicularis muscle). There is a shortage of anterior lamellae skin such that the lower lid cannot be superiorly lifted past the inferior limbus in excess of 2 mm (**Fig. 2.1C**).
- ◆ *Congenital ectropion:* May be seen in the lower lid and is generally seen in association with conditions such as blepharophimosis syndrome and ichthyosis.
- ◆ *Mechanical:* Discrete eversion of the eyelid due to a lid lesion.

◆ Differential Diagnosis

Make sure to rule out other causes of ectropion such as floppy eyelid syndrome described earlier.

◆ Management

Depends on extent of ectropion and symptoms. Conservative measures include aggressive lubrication of the ocular surface. Surgery is often needed for a definite solution.

- ◆ *Involution ectropion:* A variety of surgical options are available depending on the extent of ectropion, horizontal lid laxity, and degree of canthal tendon laxity. Generalized ectropion can be corrected by horizontal lid shortening via full-thickness excision or reattaching it to the lateral canthus through a lateral tarsal strip suspension technique.

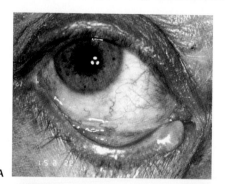

A

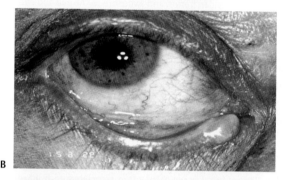

B

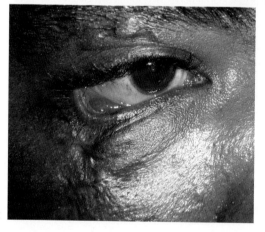

C

Fig. 2.1   **(A)** Involutional ectropion (with punctal ectropion and stenosis). **(B)** Paralytic ectropion secondary to seventh nerve palsy (brow ptosis and lagophthalmos are also present). **(C)** Cicatricial ectropion caused by a lower eyelid scar. (Courtesy of Dr. Soosan Jacob, Dr. Agarwal's Eye Hospital, Chennai, India)

◆ *Paralytic ectropion*: Temporary treatment with a tarsorrhaphy can help reduce the extent of exposure keratopathy. Permanent cases may require the use of medial canthoplasty, medial wedge resection, and/or lateral canthal suspension to reduce the horizontal and vertical dimensions of the palpebral aperture.
◆ *Cicatricial ectropion*: Use of skin grafts or transpositional flaps to restore the normal anterior lamellae
◆ *Congenital ectropion*: Reconstructing the anterior lamellae with the use of skin grafts or transpositional flaps

◆ Entropion

Inward rotation of the eyelid

◆ Presentation

The margin of the eyelid and lashes makes contact with the globe and, in certain cases, can lead to corneal epitheliopathy and subsequent ulceration or pannus formation. Irritation and epiphora are common presenting signs. They can be involutional, congenital, and cicatricial:

◆ *Involutional*: Age-related changes involving degeneration of the elastic and fibrous tissues, usually affecting the lower lid. The lateral and/or medial horizontal laxity is associated with increased orbicularis tone causing inward rotation of the eyelid (**Fig. 2.2A**).
◆ *Cicatricial*: Scarring from trauma, Stevens-Johnson syndrome and other cicatrizing conditions, chemical burns, and trachoma can lead to shortening of the posterior lamellae (**Fig. 2.2B**).
◆ *Congenital*: Often seen in lower lids, usually related to the lack of normal development of the retractor aponeurosis.

◆ Differential Diagnosis

Epiblepharon, distichiasis, trichiasis, blepharospasm, and ruling out other causes of entropion already mentioned

◆ Management

Temporary treatment can be achieved by ocular lubrication and lid taping. Botulinum toxin has been used with success in involutional or congenital cases. Surgical correction is often used in severe cases.

◆ *Involutional*: If there is little horizontal lid laxity, transverse everting sutures can provide a temporary solution. Horizontal lid splitting with insertion of everting sutures provides a lasting correction. In cases with associated horizontal lid laxity, horizontal lid shortening can provide benefit in addition to the aforementioned procedures.
◆ *Cicatricial*: Mild cases can be corrected with a transverse tarsotomy (tarsal fracture) with anterior rotation of the lid margin. More extensive cases will often employ the use of composite grafts (mucous membrane or palate) to reconstruct the damaged posterior lamellae.
◆ *Congenital*: Can be corrected with excision of a strip of skin and underlying orbicularis muscle and with possible fixation of the skin crease to the tarsal plate.

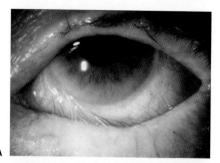

Fig. 2.2 **(A)** Involutional entropion with trichiasis. **(B)** Cicatricial entropion with associated trichiasis.

A

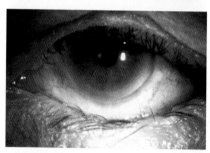

B

◆ Ptosis

An abnormally low position of the upper eyelid, which may be congenital or acquired

◆ Presentation

Patients complain of a tired appearance and deficits in their superior visual field. To overcome this, patients may elevate their chin position or subsequently contract their frontalis muscle to raise their brows. Certain measurements are key in the evaluation. Margin to lid reflex (MRD) is the distance from the margin of the upper lid to the central corneal reflex (normal is 4.0 to 4.5 mm). Levator function measures the distance of excursion of the upper eyelid margin from far downgaze to upgaze while the frontalis muscle is held still with the examiner's thumb (normal is 14 mm or more). The palpebral fissure is the distance from the upper to the lower eyelid margin when the patient is in primary gaze (normal range can vary from 7 to 12 mm and is greater in women than in men). Superior lid crease is the vertical distance of the superior lid margin from the lid crease in downgaze (normal 8 to 10 mm).

There are various causes of ptosis, including the following:

◆ *Congenital*: Failure of neuronal migration within the levator complex. Can be unilateral or bilateral with variable severity. Poor levator function and absent lid crease. Ptosis improves on downgaze. Need to be evaluated for amblyopia (**Fig. 2.3A**).

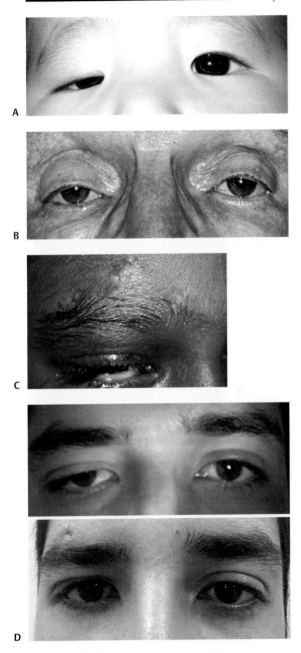

Fig. 2.3 **(A)** Congenital ptosis, right eye. **(B)** Bilateral ptosis, compensating with frontalis overaction. **(C)** Suprabrow and lid scars following conventional sling surgery **(D)** Presurgical and postsurgical pictures following Jacob Agarwal guided sling surgery. Note only a single scar over the forehead. ([A] Courtesy of Deborah Alcorn, MD; [C–D] Courtesy of Soosan Jacob, Dr. Agarwal's Eye Hospital, Chennai, India)

◆ *Aponeurotic*: Most common type of ptosis, usually seen in elderly patients. Can be bilateral or unilateral. Due to a dehiscence or disinsertion of the levator aponeurosis, usually the result of involutional changes. Normal levator function but high superior lid crease (> 12 mm) (**Fig. 2.3B**).

◆ *Neurogenic*: Innervational defect due to an oculomotor nerve palsy

◆ *Myogenic*: Seen in defects in the neuromuscular junction itself or within the levator complex; can be due to myasthenia gravis or muscular dystrophy

◆ *Mechanical*: Secondary to a gravity mass effect or contraction from a scar

◆ Differential Diagnosis

It is important to differentiate true ptosis from pseudoptosis, which can be caused by contralateral lid retraction, ipsilateral hypotropia, brow ptosis, and dermatochalasis. Other differential diagnoses include Marcus-Gunn jaw winking syndrome, aberrant third or seventh nerve regeneration, and blepharophimosis syndrome.

◆ Management

Depends on the severity of the ptosis and its etiology. Usually severe ptosis with poor levator function will need to be addressed by a frontalis-sling procedure. Levator resection is indicated in cases with fair to good levator function (at least 5 mm). Cases with reasonably good or excellent levator function can be addressed by either a posterior approach or an anterior aponeurosis repair.

◆ *Congenital ptosis*: Usually needs to be addressed early if amblyopia is a concern, especially in unilateral cases. Depending on the levator function, different procedures can effectively correct the ptosis. Poor levator function (< 4 mm) will require a frontalis-sling procedure, whereas fair levator function (> 4 mm) may be corrected with a levator resection.

◆ *Aponeurotic ptosis*: Several options are available, depending on the severity of the ptosis. For instance, a posterior approach (e.g., Fasanella-Servat procedure or Müller-conjunctival resection) can correct mild cases. Alternatively, an anterior approach with reinsertion or advancement of the aponeurosis can correct cases with excellent levator function.

Jacob-Agarwal Technique of Guided Sling Surgery with Single Stab Incision Frontalis muscle suspension procedure is the gold standard for the treatment of congenital ptosis with poor levator function. It creates a link between the frontalis muscle and the tarsus of the upper eyelid, which allows for a better eyelid position in primary gaze. The Jacob-Agarwal technique differs from the conventional procedures by the use of a single-stab incision in making the pentagon and guiding the silicone sling in the surgical plane with one external incision while suspending the frontalis muscle (**Fig. 2.3C,D**).

Surgical Technique A pentagon shape is marked over the skin with a marker. A single supraeyebrow stab incision of ~2.5 to 3.0 mm is put on the superior mark of the pentagon ~5 mm from the eyebrow, and a subperiosteal pocket is dissected upward (**Fig. 2.4**). A sterile frontalis suspension set (Seiff) dipped in antibiotic is used as the sling material. This has a long, solid silicone rod/tube with a length of 40cm (15¾ in) and a diameter if .80mm (.032 in), with a stainless steel needle on either end (20G × 2½ in). The silicone tube is provided with a silicone sleeve, which is removed from the tube before surgery begins (**Fig. 2.5**).

The needle is first passed through the epi-tarsal tissue between the marks made on the upper eyelid. The lid is everted and checked to ascertain that it has not gone through the full thickness of the tarsus. With a lid guard behind the lid, the medial end of the needle is then inserted through the medial needle exit point on

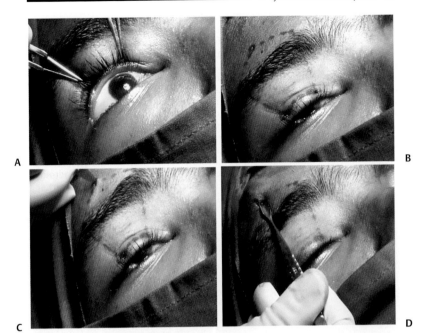

Fig. 2.4 **(A)** Upper eyelid elevation and contour checked preoperatively. **(B)** Pentagonal shape as in conventional sling surgery is marked over the skin. **(C)** Single supraeyebrow stab incision of ~2.5 to 3.0 mm is put on the superior mark of the pentagon ~5 mm from the eyebrow. **(D)** Subperiosteal pocket dissected upward. (All images courtesy of Soosan Jacob, Dr. Agarwal's Eye Hospital, Chennai, India)

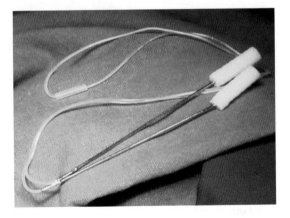

Fig. 2.5 Seiff Silicone frontalis suspension set (BD Ophthalmic Systems, Bidford on Avon, UK). (Courtesy of Soosan Jacob, Dr. Agarwal's Eye Hospital, Chennai, India)

the eyelid and advanced upward, dipping behind the septum, to the mark made on the medial eyebrow. When the upper medial corner of the pentagon is reached, the needle is then turned and guided in the same surgical plane (without exteriorizing), using a combination of visualization and palpation and is brought out through the central suprabrow incision (**Fig. 2.6**). The same procedure is repeated with the needle on the lateral side so that it traces the path of the lateral limb of the pentagon, dips behind the orbital septum, turns in direction above the supraorbital rim, and then exteriorizes through the central suprabrow incision. The surgeon's nondominant index finger can be used to palpate the needle as it is being advanced. The two ends of the silicone rod are threaded through the silicone sleeve, and the lid margin and contour are adjusted according to the amount of correction required and for maximal cosmesis. The two ends of the silicone rods are also knotted together, and a 6-0 silk suture is tied between the knots to prevent late slippage. The sleeve with the knots is then buried into the subperiosteal pocket. If needed, one may also hitch the silicone tube knot to the underlying periosteum. The single suprabrow stab incision is closed with silk suture or fibrin

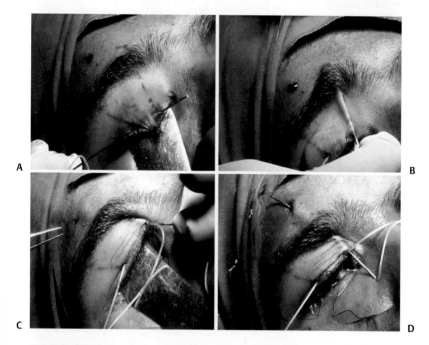

A

B

C

D

Fig. 2.6 **(A)** The needle is passed through the superficial tarsal tissue between the marks made on the upper eyelid. **(B)** The medial end of the tube is advanced through the medial needle exit point on the eyelid and advanced upward, dipping behind the septum, to the mark made on the medial eyebrow. **(C)** When the upper medial corner of the pentagon is reached, the needle is then turned and guided in the same surgical plane (without exteriorizing) using a combination of visualization and palpation. **(D)** The needle is brought out through the central suprabrow incision. The same is repeated on the other side. (All images courtesy of Soosan Jacob, Dr. Agarwal's Eye Hospital, Chennai, India)

glue to minimize scar formation. The Other needle puncture sites need not be sutured (**Fig. 2.7**).

The advantage of the technique is that with minimal skin incisions and less surgical time, the clinical outcome of a conventional frontalis sling procedure is obtained. Postoperative lid and brow edema, ecchymosis, pain, suture-related complications, and scarring due to multiple incisions and sutures can be avoided. The technique can be performed in all eyes with ptosis and poor levator function that necessitate a frontalis sling. The stab incision used is only ~2.5 to 3.0 mm. It is thus advantageous over the conventional procedure that involves five stab incisions, which creates more bleeding and edema in the immediate postoperative period and more scarring in the late postoperative period. Mild immediate postoperative edema may occur, but it generally resolves spontaneously within 24 hours. Though silicone material for frontalis sling suspension has been tried successfully, the guided sling procedure with a silicone sling has not been reported. There have been reports in the past of sling procedures using a minimum or no incision. The Jacob-Agarwal technique differs from these procedures in that the ends of the sling material are united in the central forehead incision (rather than in the eyelid incision as previously described by other authors), which provides an upward direction of traction for better lid height and contour. Also, the material used for the sling is the commonly available Seiff silicone suspension set, which ptosis surgeons are more familiar and comfortable with than nonabsorbable suture. Lid closure is also better with silicone sling material rather than with nonabsorbable slings. This technique therefore provides better aesthetic and functional results in patients with poor levator function and congenital ptosis. It is also optimal for patients with myopathies, myasthenia, third nerve palsy, and similar conditions where silicone suspension is conventionally preferred over other sling materials because of its inherent elasticity. This technique is unique in its simple learning curve, good cosmesis, smaller number of sutures with better functional results while retaining the usual advantages of standard sling procedures.

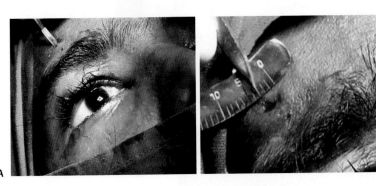

A   B

Fig. 2.7 **(A)** The two ends of the rod are passed through the silicone sleeve, and the lid margin and contour are adjusted according to the amount of correction required and for maximal cosmesis. **(B)** Measurement of the incision site is shown. (Both images courtesy of Soosan Jacob, Dr. Agarwal's Eye Hospital, Chennai, India)

◆ Dermatochalasis

This is a very common condition seen in elderly patients, usually presents bilaterally. It may be asymptomatic.

◆ Presentation

Patients present with redundant upper lid skin that can be associated with fat herniation through a weak septum. In moderate to severe cases, the excess lid can obstruct the superior visual field (**Fig. 2.8A,B,C**).

◆ Differential Diagnosis

Acquired or congenital ptosis, eyebrow ptosis, floppy eyelid syndrome, prolapsed lacrimal gland and eyelid edema.

A
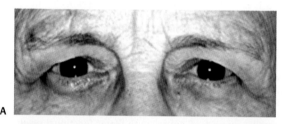

B
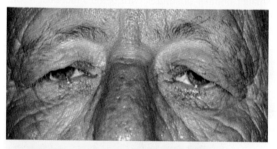

C
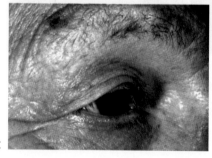

Fig. 2.8 **(A)** Bilateral dermatochalasis. **(B)** Dermatochalasis and brow ptosis. **(C)** Dermatochalasis with lash ptosis.

◆ Management

Includes blepharoplasty to remove excess skin. Patients often have a combined ptosis and need to be evaluated for this component. If so, they may benefit from ptosis surgery as well.

◆ Eyelid Retraction

Eyelid retraction occurs when the upper lids rest above or at the level of the superior limbus.

◆ Presentation

Patients often have other signs, including proptosis, inferior scleral show, lagophthalmos with resulting exposure keratopathy, and other signs of acute inflammation (conjunctivitis, chemosis). This is most commonly seen in thyroid eye disease (**Fig. 2.9**).

◆ Differential Diagnosis

Thyroid eye disease, as already mentioned. Other causes include contralateral ptosis with ipsilateral lid retraction secondary to Herring's law, aberrant third nerve regeneration, cicatricial changes or scarring of the upper lid, sympathetomimetic ophthalmic drops, overcorrection of ptosis surgery, chronic contact lens use, Parinaud syndrome, and Miller Fisher variant of Guillain-Barré syndrome.

◆ Management

When symptoms are mild, artificial lubrication of the ocular surface can often ameliorate the symptoms. Severe cases with little proptosis may require eyelid surgery. There have been a variety of techniques described to surgically correct eyelid retraction. Both posterior (transconjunctival) and anterior (cutaneous) approaches have been described. Both approaches involve a variable degree of levator muscle complex recession and/or mullerectomy to correct the retraction.

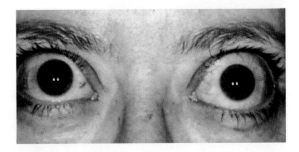

Fig. 2.9 Eyelid retraction and proptosis from thyroid eye disease.

◆ Floppy Eyelid Syndrome

This syndrome is a frequently misdiagnosed condition that can present unilaterally or bilaterally. It typically affects obese men who may also suffer from obstructive sleep apnea and is also associated with tobacco smoke.

◆ Presentation

The upper eyelids are loose and rubbery and tend to evert during sleep. The lax upper eyelid is everted easily when pulled superiorly toward the eyebrow during physical examination. The soft and rubbery tarsal plate can also be folded upon itself. This results in trauma to the exposed tarsal conjunctiva with subsequent chronic papillary conjunctivitis (**Fig. 2.10A,B,C**).

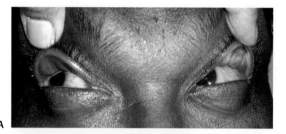

A

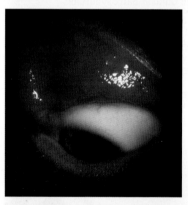

Fig. 2.10 **(A)** Floppy eyelid syndrome. **(B)** Floppy eyelid syndrome with papillary tarsal conjunctival changes. **(C)** Floppy eyelid syndrome. (Image **[A]** courtesy of Soosan Jacob, Dr. Agarwal's Eye Hospital, Chennai, India; Image **[C]** courtesy of Pablo Gili)

B

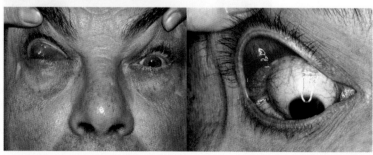

C

◆ **Differential Diagnosis**

Allergic conjunctivitis, giant papillary conjunctivitis, atopic keratoconjunctivitis, superior limbic keratitis, ectropion, dermatochalasis

◆ **Management**

In mild cases, taping of the eyelids or nocturnal eye shields can ameliorate symptoms. Severe cases may require horizontal lid shortening using full-thickness pentagonal wedge resection in the upper and lower eyelids.

◆ Chalazion

Chronic, lipogranulomatous inflammatory lesion located within the tarsus. These occur frequently and are caused by a buildup or blockage of secretion from meibomian gland orifices.

◆ **Presentation**

Can be seen in all ages, and presents with a gradually enlarging painless nodule. If large enough, upper eyelid lesions can induce astigmatism. The lesions can be multiple and bilateral. Make sure to evaluate the patient for blepharitis, ocular rosacea, and seborrheic dermatitis, which can predispose patients to chalazia (**Fig. 2.11A,B**).

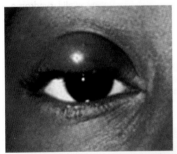

A

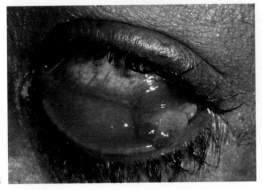

B

Fig. 2.11 **(A)** Upper eyelid chalazion. **(B)** Pyogenic granuloma. (Courtesy of Soosan Jacob, Dr. Agarwal's Eye Hospital, Chennai, India)

◆ Differential Diagnosis

Hordeolum (tender to palpation) and sebaceous cell carcinoma

◆ Management

Lesions that are new or small may resolve spontaneously. Warm compresses of 30 minutes, four times per day, may help relieve or reduce the inflammation. Topical antibiotics can also be used. Persistent lesions may be treated either by excision (posterior approach with the use of a chalazia clamp) or through intralesional steroid injection (0.5 to 2.0 mL triamcinolone acetonide, 5 mg/mL). Biopsy of recurrent lesions should be done to rule out a sebaceous cell carcinoma.

◆ Hordeolum

Painful nodules as a result of an acute bacterial infection, most commonly from *Staphylococcus aureus*. In contrast, chalazia are chronic lesions and typically not painful.

◆ Presentation

These can either present as an external hordeolum (margin of eyelid) or internal hordeolum (seen by everting eyelid). Internal hordeolums can cause severe conjunctivitis or chemosis. Usually associated with meibomian gland dysfunction and blepharitis (**Fig. 2.12**).

◆ Differential Diagnosis

Chalazion (not tender to palpation), blepharitis

◆ Management

Most cases are self-limited and will resolve within 5 to 7 days. Lid hygiene and warm compresses can help in their resolution. Some may persist and become cystlike, which may require surgical incision and curettage (see above treatment for

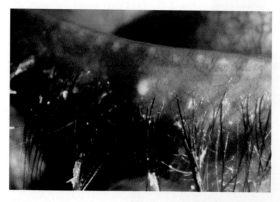

Fig. 2.12   External hordeolum.

chalazion). Treatment of accompanying blepharitis and meibomian gland dysfunction will help to prevent recurrences.

◆ Eyelid Edema

Swelling of eyelids due to fluid collection within the subcutaneous tissues

◆ Presentation

The thin skin and loose subcutaneous tissue are susceptible to water accumulation and edema, especially in the upper lids. Symptoms can be either inflammatory or noninflammatory. Inflammatory signs can include redness, sensation of heat and pain, and marked unilaterality. This can be secondary to infections such as cellulitis (preseptal or orbital), eczema, and abscess. In contrast, noninflammatory signs include pale skin color, cool skin, absence of pain, and bilaterality. This can be seen more commonly with systemic disorders (heart, kidneys, thyroid eye disease) and secondary to an allergic response. Recurrent episodes of persistent eyelid edema can result in stretching of the overlying thin skin and may result in blepharochalasis (**Fig. 2.13A,B**).

◆ Differential Diagnosis

Allergic response, hordeolum, abscess, eczema, dacryocystitis, cellulitis (preseptal or orbital), thyroid eye disease, dermatochalasis

◆ Management

Treat the underlying systemic or inflammatory disorder.

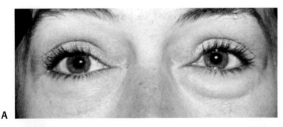

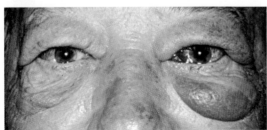

Fig. 2.13 **(A)** Left eyelid edema in a female with thyroid eye disease. **(B)** Left eyelid edema in a male with acute thyroid eye disease.

◆ Blepharoptosis and Blepharophimosis Syndrome

A rare, autosomal dominant, congenital syndrome

◆ Presentation

Moderate to severe ptosis (symmetrical) with poor levator function, shortened horizontal palpebral fissures, lateral ectropion of the lower lids, telecanthus (abnormally increased distance between the medial canthi of both eyelids), and epicanthal inversus (see the section on Epicanthus) (**Fig. 2.14**).

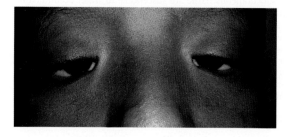

Fig. 2.14   Blepharophimosis syndrome. (Courtesy of Soosan Jacob, Dr. Agarwal's Eye Hospital, Chennai, India)

◆ Differential Diagnosis

Congenital or acquired ptosis, congenital fibrosis syndrome

◆ Management

Initially involves treatment of epicanthal folds and telecanthus followed later (usually a few months) by bilateral frontalis suspension. The patients need to be screened and followed up for amblyopia because it can develop in up to 50% of cases.

◆ Epiblepharon

An extra horizontal fold of skin extending across the anterior lid margin resulting in vertically oriented lashes

◆ Presentation

A common finding among eastern Asians, this should not be mistaken for congenital or acquired entropion. Unlike entropion, the lashes do not make contact with the cornea in primary gaze, but they often can in downgaze. The normal location of the lid becomes apparent when the fold of skin is pulled down (**Fig. 2.15**).

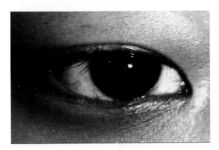

Fig. 2.15 Epiblepharon. (Courtesy of Soosan Jacob, Dr. Agarwal's Eye Hospital, Chennai, India)

◆ **Differential Diagnosis**

Congenital or acquired entropion

◆ **Management**

Management is usually not required because most cases spontaneously resolve with age. However, persistent cases or ones that cause symptoms (corneal epitheliopathy) are surgically managed by excising a strip of skin and orbicularis muscle (anterior lamellar resection) with or without fixation of the skin to the tarsus.

◆ Epicanthus

These are bilateral webs of skin that extend from the upper to lower eyelids toward the medial canthus. If large enough, they cause pseudoesotropia. They can be seen in syndromes such as blepharophimosis syndrome and trisomy 21.

◆ **Presentation**

Epicanthal folds can present in four various subtypes:

◆ *Epicanthus tarsalis*: The folds originate in the upper medial eyelid and extend into the medial canthus. This is the most common type seen in eastern Asians (**Fig. 2.16**).
◆ *Epicanthus inversus*: This type originates in the lower eyelid and extends into the medial canthus. This is associated with blepharophimosis syndrome.
◆ *Epicanthus palpebralis*: The folds extend from the upper to lower eyelids in a symmetric distribution.
◆ *Epicanthus superciliaris*: These are broad folds that extend from the eyebrow down to the lower orbital rim.

◆ **Differential Diagnosis**

Epiblepharon. Rule out syndromes associated with epicanthal folds such as blepharophimosis syndrome and trisomy 21.

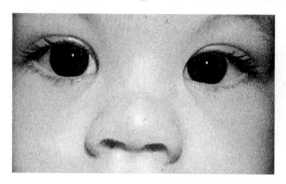

Fig. 2.16   Epicanthus tarsalis.

◆ Management

Epicanthus usually resolves by the age of 4. Several surgical procedures such as Z- or Y-V-plasties can be employed to repair persistent cases.

◆ Eyelid Coloboma

This is a partial- or full-thickness eyelid defect due to an embryonic cleft, usually triangular in shape, with its base at the margin.

◆ Presentation

These are rare defects, usually congenital and resulting from a lack of closure of the optic cup. They are most commonly seen in the upper lids (at the junction of the middle and outer thirds), either in isolation or with other syndromes. Keratinization or exposure keratopathy can occur depending on the severity of the coloboma. Colobomas can be accompanied by additional deformities such as microphthalmos or dermoid cysts (**Fig. 2.17**).

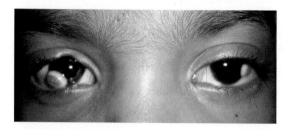

Fig. 2.17   Upper eyelid coloboma. (Courtesy of Soosan Jacob, Dr. Agarwal's Eye Hospital, Chennai, India)

◆ Differential Diagnosis

Ablepharon (congenital absence of eyelid), trauma. Rule out other syndromes associated with colobomas such as Goldenhar syndrome (oculoauriculovertebral dysplasia) and Franceschetti syndrome (mandibulofacial dystosis).

◆ Management

Conservative treatment with the use of lubricating drops and ointments if small and there is no risk of exposure keratopathy. However, defects usually need to be closed by primary, direct closure or, if large enough, will require the use of skin grafts or rotation flaps or both.

◆ Eyelid Tumors

Papilloma

The most common benign tumor of the eyelids.

◆ Presentation

These present as a pedunculated or sessile (broad-based) lesion. They are a benign tumor of epithelial origin (**Fig. 2.18A,B**).

◆ Differential Diagnosis

Molluscum contagiosum, chalazion, squamous cell carcinoma, basal cell carcinoma

◆ Management

Management can consist of observation or elective removal by excision. Shave biopsies can be performed if the diagnosis is uncertain.

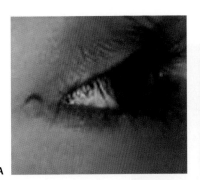
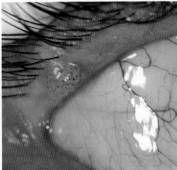

A   B

Fig. 2.18   **(A)** Papilloma. **(B)** Upper eyelid margin papilloma.

Seborrheic Keratosis

Slow-growing, discrete, greasy lesion with a friable surface

◆ Presentation

These often appear to be "stuck on" the skin. The lesion is usually brown and flat but can often be pedunculated (**Fig. 2.19A,B**).

◆ Differential Diagnosis

Nevus, melanoma, squamous cell carcinoma, acrochordon (skin tag), actinic keratosis

◆ Management

Curettage and excision are curative.

Actinic Keratosis

Also termed solar keratosis, this is a "premalignant" lesion seen in fair-skinned individuals who have been exposed to excessive sunlight.

◆ Presentation

Lesions can be scaly, flat, with hyperkeratotic features. They often begin as small, rough macules or papules (**Fig. 2.20**).

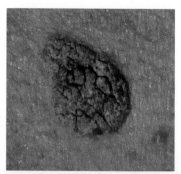

A

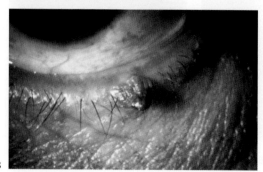

B

Fig. 2.19 (A) Seborrheic keratosis. **(B)** Seborrheic keratosis, lower eyelid.

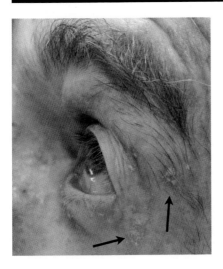

Fig. 2.20   Actinic keratosis (*arrows* depict lesions).

◆ Differential Diagnosis

Basal cell carcinoma, cutaneous horn, squamous cell carcinoma, seborrheic keratosis

◆ Management

These lesions should be biopsied for diagnosis and treated with complete excision or cryotherapy.

Keratoacanthoma

This is an uncommon but rapidly growing lesion with a central keratin mass.

◆ Presentation

They are often seen in fair-skinned individuals with excessive sunlight exposure. They can often regress spontaneously, leaving a central, sunken scar. They are histopathologically included in the spectrum of squamous cell carcinomas and clinically appear similar to squamous cell carcinomas (**Fig. 2.21**).

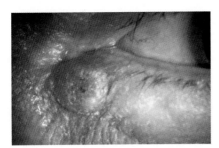

Fig. 2.21   Keratoacanthoma.

◆ Differential Diagnosis

Basal cell carcinoma, cutaneous horn, actinic keratosis, squamous cell carcinoma, and seborrheic keratosis

◆ Management

Biopsy suspicious lesions. Complete surgical excision with free margins is recommended. Laser or cryotherapy can be applied to small lesions.

Molluscum Contagiosum

These are virally transmitted lesions usually seen in younger patients (teenagers and children) or in immunocompromised patients.

◆ Presentation

They are noninflammatory, smooth, pearly, dome-shaped papules with central depressions often found near the upper and lower eyelids. They are transmitted by direct contact and are usually asymptomatic but can be associated with chronic conjunctivitis (**Fig. 2.22**).

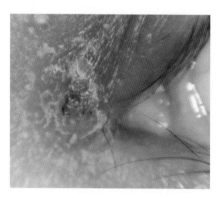

Fig. 2.22   Molluscum contagiosum.

◆ Differential Diagnosis

Basal cell carcinoma, squamous cell carcinoma, papilloma

◆ Management

Lesions can be excised by a curet or cryotherapy.

Nevi

Nevi are benign lesions that occur within the epithelium and dermis.

◆ Presentation

The lesions are derived from melanocytic cells and can be either pigmented or nonpigmented. Nevi can be histologically classified as junctional, compound, and intradermal. Intradermal nevi are confined within the dermal layer. They are usually nonpigmented and elevated. They have no malignant potential (**Fig. 2.23A**).

Junctional nevi are well circumscribed, flat, and uniformly brown. They are located at the junction of the epidermis and dermal layers and have a low potential for malignancy (**Fig. 2.23B**). Compound nevi have both junctional and intradermal involvement (**Fig. 2.23C**).

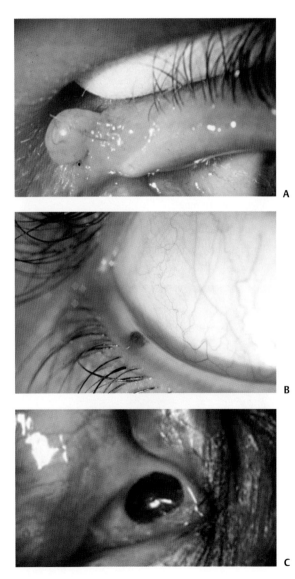

Fig. 2.23 **(A)** Intradermal nevi. **(B)** Junctional nevus. **(C)** Caruncular compound nevus.

◆ **Differential Diagnosis**

Malignant melanoma, basal cell carcinoma, benign lesions

◆ **Management**

Carefully document the size of the lesion with photographs. Surgically remove lesions that increase in size.

Nevus of Ota

Congenital oculodermal melanocytosis that involves both skin (dermis) and eye (episclera, sclera, and uveal tissues)

◆ **Presentation**

Patients present with deep, unilateral hyperpigmentation of the eyelid skin and ocular structures. These nevi are associated with iris hyperchromia and fundus hyperpigmentation. Patients are at an increased risk of glaucoma and, though rare, melanoma (**Fig. 2.24**).

◆ **Differential Diagnosis**

Malignant melanoma

◆ **Management**

Follow regularly for malignant change and glaucoma screening.

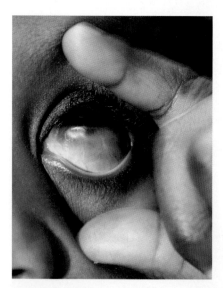

Fig. 2.24 Nevus of Ota. Note the relative sparing of dermal involvement.

Xanthelasma

Xanthelasma is a commonly seen condition that is frequently bilateral and often seen in elderly patients or those with hyperlipidemia. However, most patients with xanthelasma are normolipoproteinemic. These can rarely be the presenting sign of xanthogranulomatous disease.

◆ Presentation

Yellowish subcutaneous plaques are often found around the eyelids, especially around the medial canthal areas.

◆ Differential Diagnosis

Amyloidosis, eccrine hydrocystoma, atypical lymphoid infiltrate sarcoid

◆ Management

The lesions can be surgically removed electively; however, recurrences are common. Alternatively, excision or destruction by carbon dioxide, argon laser, cryotherapy, and chemical cauterization (chlorinated acetic acids) can be performed, though scarring and hyperpigmentation can occur.

◆ Cysts—Moll/Zeis/Sebaceous

Cysts of the glands can result in round, clear, and transilluminating lesions.

◆ Presentation

There are various types of ductal cysts. Cysts of Moll (apocrine sweat gland hydrocystoma) are usually found on the anterior lid margin and transilluminate well. They can be found in the medial canthal angle, and gravity can often result in ectropion. Eccrine sweat glands, though not confined to the lid margin, appear like apocrine cysts. Cysts of Zeis and sebaceous cysts contain oily secretions and therefore do not transilluminate (**Fig. 2.25A,B,C**).

◆ Differential Diagnosis

Benign and malignant lesions, chalazion, external hordeolum

◆ Management

Warm compresses and topical antibiotics are helpful. Marsupialization of the cysts is usually curative. Suspicious lesions should be sent for biopsy.

Syringoma

Syringomas are benign skin tumors of eccrine differentiation, more often found in women.

◆ Presentation

Skin-color papules are usually located on the eyelids and can increase in size and quantity.

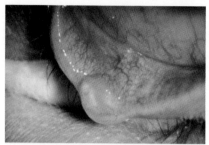

A

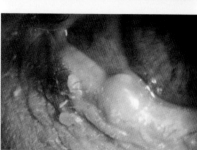

B

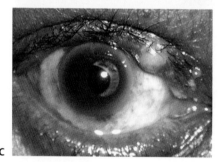

C

Fig. 2.25 **(A)** Apocrine hydrocystoma. **(B)** Eccrine hydrocystoma. **(C)** Sebaceous hydrocystoma.

◆ **Differential Diagnosis**

Verruca, xanthelasma, cylindroma

◆ **Management**

Papules can be electively removed by surgical excision or electrodissection and curettage. The lesions can recur.

Neurofibroma

Neurofibromas are infiltrative nerve cell tumors that are largely composed of Schwann cells.

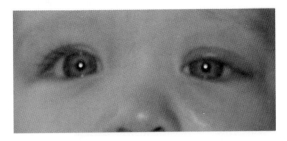

Fig. 2.26   Infiltrative neurofibroma of left orbit. (Courtesy of Deborah Alcorn, MD).

◆ Presentation

The tumors usually occur early in life and can be either nodular or plexiform. They can involve the upper lid (classic-shaped appearance) and frequently cause a mechanical ptosis (**Fig. 2.26**).

◆ Differential Diagnosis

Capillary hemangioma, lymphoma, rhabdomyosarcoma

◆ Management

Surgical excision can be attempted, but these lesions are very difficult to remove successfully.

◆ Tumors

Basal Cell Carcinoma

This is the most common eyelid malignancy. There is an increased risk in people with fair skin and in individuals with increased exposure to ultraviolet radiation (chronic skin damage).

◆ Presentation

These typically present as a firm lesion with raised margins. A central crater with superficial vascularization or ulceration can often be seen. Loss of eyelashes (madarosis) almost always suggests malignancy. Most commonly seen (in decreasing order of relative frequency) in the lower eyelids, medial canthus, upper eyelid, and lateral canthus (**Fig. 2.27A,B,C,D**).

◆ Differential Diagnosis

Nevus, papilloma, keratoaconthoma, malignant melanoma, squamous cell carcinoma

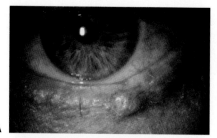

A

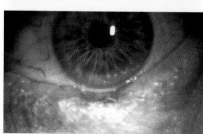

B

Fig. 2.27 **(A)** Basal cell carcinoma. **(B)** Ulcerating basal cell carcinoma. **(C)** Ulcerating basal cell carcinoma with necrosis of surrounding skin. **(D)** Ulcerating basal cell carcinoma with umbilicated, central crater.

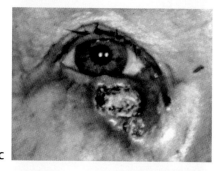

C

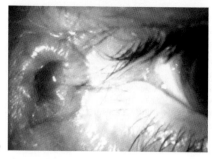

D

◆ Management

Biopsy suspicious lesions. Surgical excision with free margins (recommended 3 to 5 mm) of healthy tissue should be performed. Alternative treatment modalities include cryotherapy, electrodissection, curettage, Mohs micrographic surgery, and radiotherapy. These lesions have rare metastatic potential.

Squamous Cell Carcinoma

Squamous cell carcinomas comprise less than 5% of eyelid malignancies. Similar to basal cell carcinoma, the primary cause of most squamous cell carcinoma is cumulative lifetime sun exposure, especially in fair-skinned individuals.

◆ Presentation

Lesions can present as clinically similar to basal cell carcinomas, but they commonly grow rapidly with spread to regional lymph nodes. They can also extend into the intracranial cavity via perineural spread (**Fig. 2.28A,B,C**). Clinically these can present as three subtypes:

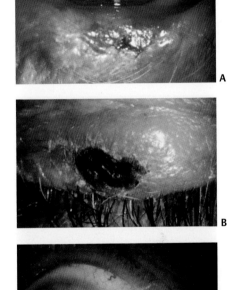

Fig. 2.28 **(A)** Squamous cell carcinoma. **(B)** Squamous cell carcinoma of upper eyelid. **(C)** Cystic squamous cell carcinoma.

- *Plaquelike*: Scaly, hyperkeratotic lesions at site of preexisting actinic keratosis
- *Nodular*: Hyperkeratotic nodule with crusting fissures
- *Ulcerating*: Well-defined everting borders with an erythematous and ulcerated base

◆ Differential Diagnosis

Basal cell carcinoma, keratoacanthoma, actinic keratosis

◆ Management

Surgical excision with free margins (recommended 3 to 5 mm) of healthy tissue or Mohs micrographic surgery should be performed. Lesions not completely resectable can be treated with adjunctive radiation or cryotherapy or both.

Sebaceous Cell Carcinoma

These are older-growing lesions frequently arising from the meibomian glands and usually seen in the upper eyelids. They are more commonly seen in older white women. They comprise approximately 5% of eyelid malignancies. There is often a delay in diagnosis given its insidious clinical appearance.

◆ Presentation

Can present either as a nodular or a pagetoid spreading meibomian gland carcinoma. The nodular type presents as a discrete nodule that often is mistaken for a chalazion. The pagetoid spreading subtype spreads into the dermis and epithelium in a diffuse pattern, often mimicking chronic conjunctivitis (**Fig. 2.29A,B**).

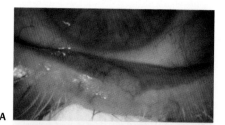

Fig. 2.29 **(A)** Sebaceous cell carcinoma of eyelid margin. **(B)** Sebaceous cell carcinoma involving most of the upper tarsal conjunctiva.

A

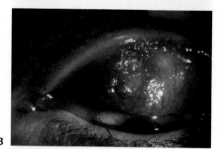

B

◆ **Differential Diagnosis**

Blepharitis, chalazion, superior limbic keratoconjunctivitis, chronic conjunctivitis, cicatricial pemphigoid

◆ **Management**

Surgical excision with wide surgical margins with frozen-section controls is often necessary. Conjunctival mapping helps evaluate pagetoid spreading. Evaluate local lymph nodes (preauricular and cervical), and perform a systemic evaluation for metastatic spread.

Cutaneous Malignant Melanoma

This is rarely seen on the eyelids but can manifest as potentially lethal skin lesions.

◆ **Presentation**

These often present as a slowly growing pigmented lesion, but almost half of lesions can be nonpigmented (**Fig. 2.30A,B,C**). They are clinically seen in three types:

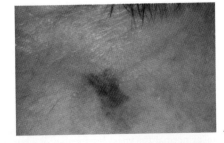

A

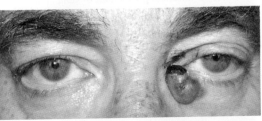

B

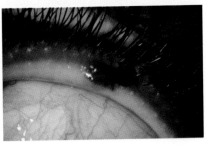

C

Fig. 2.30 (A) Lentigo maligna.
(B) Melanoma of medial canthus.
(C) Melanoma of upper eyelid.

◆ *Lentigo maligna (pre-melanoma lesion)*: A slow-growing pigmented lesion, often affecting elderly patients, which can develop into a melanoma
◆ *Superficial spreading*: Superficially spreading lesion with an irregular outline, variable pigmentation, and delay in penetration into deeper layers
◆ *Nodular*: A more aggressive lesion that has a tendency to invade deeper layers early in its growth

◆ Differential Diagnosis

Nevus, basal cell carcinoma, keratoaconthoma, seborrheic keratosis, squamous cell carcinoma

◆ Management

Excisional biopsy with 3- to 5-mm free margins is recommended for thin cutaneous periocular melanomas. Melanomas thicker (usually greater than 2mm in thickness) and located elsewhere may require 1 to 3 cm free margins depending on their thickness. The extent of surgical and adjunctive therapy is determined by tumor type, level, and clinical stage.

◆ Distichiasis and Trichiasis

Distichiasis can be either a congenital or an acquired condition of the eyelids and involves the abnormal growth of lashes from the orifices of the meibomian glands. Trichiasis is an acquired condition of eyelashes that are misdirected toward the globe.

◆ Presentation

Distichiasis can present in a variety of ways. The distichiatic lashes can be thin or of normal thickness, pigmented or nonpigmented, have normal orientation, or may be misdirected. Acquired cases of distichiasis can be seen in longstanding cicatrization associated with trachoma, chemical injury, Stevens-Johnson syndrome, and ocular pemphigoid. Trichiasis can be the result of scarring of the lid margin secondary to chronic trachoma, blepharitis, Stevens-Johnson syndrome, and herpes zoster ophthalmicus. In all cases, the lashes rub against the eye and can cause irritation, tearing, and corneal epitheliopathy. Longstanding cases can result in corneal ulceration and pannus (**Fig. 2.31A,B**).

◆ Differential Diagnosis

Entropion, epiblepharon, blepharitis, and topical prostaglandin analogue medications for glaucoma

◆ Management

Numerous approaches have been reported for treatment. Epilation is accomplished by lash removal with forceps (not a permanent solution) or more effectively with electrocautery, cryotherapy, or argon laser to individual lashes. Alternatively, they can be surgically approached in a variety of ways, including a combination of lamellar eyelid division with cryotherapy to the aberrant lashes or direct surgical excision by wedge resection.

Fig. 2.31 **(A)** Distichiasis. **(B)** Trichiasis (of upper lid). Note the cicatricial changes of both upper and lower lids.

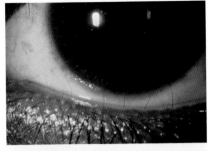

A

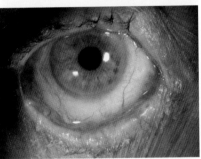

B

◆ Lacrimal System Disorders

Canaliculitis

Canaliculitis consists of either or both inflammation and infection of the upper or lower canaliculus.

◆ Presentation

The canalicular region is erythematous, indurated, and tender to palpation. Patients complain of epiphora with chronic mucopurulent discharge. The most common bacterial pathogen is *Actinomyces*, which produces granular-like concretions that are difficult to express from the puncti (**Fig. 2.32A, B**).

◆ Differential Diagnosis

Chronic dacryocystitis, ethmoidal mucocele

◆ Management

Local antibiotics should be used according to the pathogens identified on cultures and sensitivity (generally susceptible to penicillins and cephalosporins). Surgical incision (canaliculotomy) with drainage and curettage of the concretions is often used for successful treatment.

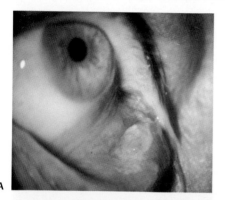

Fig. 2.32 **(A)** Chronic canaliculitis. **(B)** Eikenella canaliculitis.

A

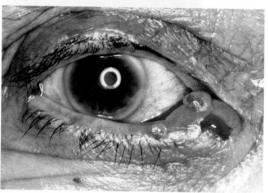

B

Dacryocystitis

This is an infection of the nasolacrimal sac; it is often unilateral and secondary to an acquired obstruction of the nasolacrimal duct.

◆ Presentation

Presentation can be acute or chronic. A stenosis or obstruction within the naso-lacrimal duct can lead to retention of tear fluid with subsequent superinfection. An acute course presents with a painful, localized erythema and inflammation around the lacrimal sac. An abscess can often develop with even a spontaneous rupture of the anterior skin leading to a draining fistula. Neonates can also present with dacryocystitis secondary to nasolacrimal duct obstruction. Chronic infection produces epiphora with associated conjunctivitis and minimal tenderness. Lacri-mal sac massage produces reflux of mucopurulent material from the puncti (**Fig. 2.33**).

◆ Differential Diagnosis

Nasolacrimal duct obstruction, orbital cellulitis, conjunctivitis, hordeolum

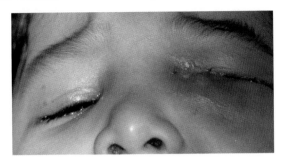

Fig. 2.33 Dacryocystitis, left lacrimal sac with associated preseptal cellulitis.

◆ **Management**

If mild, acute and chronic presentations can be initially treated with local and oral antibiotics, and once the acute symptoms have resolved, a dacryocystorhinostomy is often required. Severe dacryocystitis with secondary orbital cellulitis or abscess formation may require intravenous antibiotics. Abscess formations need to be treated with incision and drainage.

Nasolacrimal Duct Obstruction

This can be congenital or acquired. In congenital cases, there is a delay in the canaliculization of the lower portion of the nasolacrimal duct, which is seen in up to 20% of infants during the first year of life but is symptomatic in less than 4% of these children. Acquired cases can be secondary to trauma or infection.

◆ **Presentation**

Constant epiphora and wetting of the eyelashes. Mucopurulent material is often expressed from the lower puncti after lacrimal massage. Symptoms can worsen during an upper respiratory infection (**Fig. 2.34**).

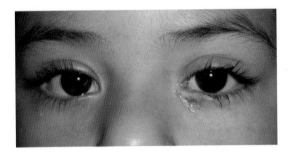

Fig. 2.34 Left nasolacrimal duct obstruction.

◆ Differential Diagnosis

Congenital glaucoma in infants, ethmoidal mucoceles, lacrimal sac tumors (benign or malignant), dacryocystitis, canaliculitis

◆ Management

Treatment should be delayed in infants until about 1 year of age because most (up to 95%) of cases self-resolve. Nasolacrimal duct probing and irrigation are usually curative in over 90% of infants. Recurrent failures often imply an anatomical problem and may require silicone intubation or balloon dilation. Persistent failures may need a dacryocystorhinostomy.

3 Orbital Infections, Inflammation, and Neoplasms

Praveen Saluja, Swati Ravani, Soosan Jacob, and Amar Agarwal

◆ Preseptal Cellulitis

Preseptal cellulitis is defined as a soft tissue infection anterior to the orbital septum. Infection posterior to this septum, anywhere in the orbit, is orbital cellulitis. Orbital cellulitis is a dangerous condition owing to the close proximity to the orbital apex, cavernous sinus, meninges, and brain. Bacterial infection of the eyelid anterior to the orbital septum typically affects children, usually secondary to lid infection such as severe acute hordeolum, skin laceration, an insect bite, or the spread of infection from the surrounding structures (paranasal sinuses, lacrimal sac, upper respiratory tract, including the middle ear). The infection does not penetrate the orbital septum, which separates the anterior structures from the orbit.

◆ Presentation

Symptoms include eyelid edema (which may lead to inability to open the eye), periorbital swelling, rubor, color, tenderness, without proptosis. Unlike orbital cellulitis, there is no pain with eye movements. Ocular motility, visual acuity, and pupillary reactions are all normal (**Fig. 3.1A,B,C**).

◆ Differential Diagnosis

- *Orbital cellulitis*: Decreased visual acuity, decreased sensation along the first division of the trigeminal nerve, eyelid edema, proptosis, chemosed conjunctiva, pain with eye movements, restricted eye movements, signs of ocular motility disorders
- *Cavernous sinus thrombosis*: Bilateral, decreased visual acuity, decreased sensation along the first and second division of the trigeminal nerve, proptosis and paresis of cranial nerves III, IV, and VI, chemosed conjunctiva
- *Chalazion*: Focal, usually without tenderness, gradually progressive chronic inflammation of the meibomian gland
- *Allergic edema of the eyelid*
- *Contact dermatitis*
- *Viral conjunctivitis associated with lid edema*: Watering, itching, stickiness of the eyelashes, conjunctival follicular reaction, with or without discharge and palpable preauricular lymph node
- *Erysipelas*: Acute streptococcal cellulitis (mostly has a clear-cut demarcation line) with signs of toxemia, including high-grade fever and chills
- *Others*: Insect bite, angioedema, trauma, osteomyelitis of paranasal sinuses, especially maxillary sinus

◆ Management

Check for a history of trauma, rapidity of onset, pain, fever, chills, cancer, diabetes, pulmonary diseases, and renal diseases. Chart the vitals (pulse, respiration, temperature, blood pressure). Examine for exophthalmometry, globe displacement, and resistance to retropulsion and examine the orbital rim. Record ocular movement and measure deviation with a prism bar. Pupils must be evaluated for light reflexes, including relative afferent pupillary defect (RAPD). Color vision, in-

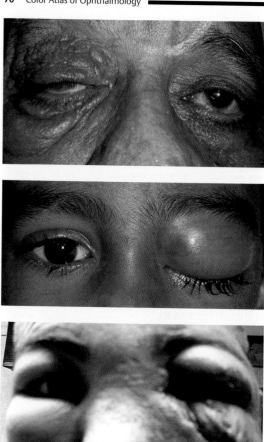

A

B

C

Fig. 3.1 **(A)** Preseptal cellulitis, allergic reaction. **(B)** Preseptal cellulitis, bacterial infection final. **(C)** Preseptal cellulitis, fungal infection.

traocular pressure (including the pressure in various gazes), and retinal evaluation should be recorded. Evaluate the cranial nerves (especially III, IV, V_1, V_2, VI,). Examine the head and neck for lymphadenitis. Gram staining and culture of any open wound and discharge should be performed at the earliest opportunity. A complete and differential blood count is performed if signs of toxemia exist.

Oral antibiotics are indicated in cases of mild inflammation, afebrile patient, age more than 5 years, good patient compliance. Drugs of choice include amoxicillin-clavulanate, or cefaclor, or cotrimoxazole, or erythromycin, clindamycin, amoxicillin-cloxacillin for a duration of 10 days. Intravenous antibiotics are indicated in moderate to severe inflammations. In cases of patient age less than 5 years, poor patient compliance, immunocompromised patients, no improvement with or worsening with oral antibiotics, drugs of choice include ceftriaxone with vancomycin. Supportive treatment includes hot fomentations, local antibiotics (polymyxin with bacitracin ointment), and nonsteroidal anti-inflammatory drugs (NSAIDs). Exploration of the wound is performed if needed.

◆ Orbital Inflammation

Orbital Cellulitis/Subperiosteal Abscess/Cavernous Sinus Syndrome

In orbital cellulites, infection occurs posterior to the orbital septum, usually secondary to the spread of infection from the surrounding structures (paranasal sinuses, lacrimal sac, upper respiratory tract including the middle ear) or lid infection, such as severe acute hordeolum, skin laceration, or an insect bite (**Fig. 3.2A,B,C**).

◆ Presentation

◆ *Orbital cellulitis*: Eyelid edema (*usually* leading to inability to open the eye), periorbital swelling, rubor, tenderness, proptosis, pain with eye movements, restricted ocular motility, decreased vision, retinal venous congestion, optic disk edema, purulent discharge, and decreased periorbital sensation. The following are main types:
  ◆ Sinus-related is the most common and is secondary to ethmoidal sinusitis; it affects children and young adults.
  ◆ Caused by adjacent structures like dacryocystitis, midfacial infection, or dental infection.
  ◆ Posttraumatic most commonly develops within 48 to 72 hours of an injury that penetrates the orbital septum.
◆ *Subperiosteal abscess*: Most frequently located along the medial wall of the orbit. Orbital abscess is relatively less common with sinusitis but is more common in posttraumatic or postoperative cases. Usually presents with medial mass, nonaxial proptosis, local tenderness, increased intraocular pressure, abscess (intraconal/extraconal).
◆ *Cavernous sinus thrombosis*: Bilateral, decreased visual acuity; decreased sensation along the first and second division of the trigeminal nerve; rapidly progressive proptosis; paresis of cranial nerves III, IV, and VI; congestion of the conjunctival veins; chemosed conjunctiva; dilated and sluggish pupil; signs of toxemia including high-grade fever, decreased level of consciousness, nausea, and vomiting.

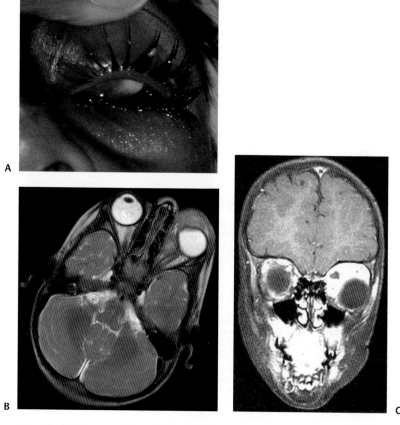

Fig. 3.2 **(A)** Ten-year-old boy with orbital abscess. **(B)** Magnetic resonance imaging (MRI) of an orbital abscess. **(C)** MRI, coronal section.

◆ Differential Diagnosis (Table 3.1)

- *Carotid cavernous fistula*: Spontaneous or posttraumatic, bruit on auscultation of globe; arterialized conjunctival vessels and conjunctival chemosis are not uncommon on computed tomographic scan. Enlarged superior ophthalmic vein (SOV), enlarged extraocular muscles, orbital color Doppler ultrasound shows reversed arterialized blood in SOV.
- *Erysipelas*: Acute streptococcal cellulitis. Mostly has a clear-cut demarcation line with signs of toxemia including high-grade fever, chills.
- *Others*: Insect bite, angioedema, trauma, osteomyelitis of paranasal sinuses (especially maxillary sinus), chalazion, allergic edema of the eyelid, contact dermatitis, viral conjunctivitis associated with lid edema.

Table 3.1 Differential Diagnosis of Orbital Inflammatory Conditions

Feature	Pseudotumor	Thyroid Exophthalmos	Orbital Cellulitis
1. Laterality	Unilateral	Bilateral	Unilateral
2. Age	20 to 50 years	Fourth to fifth decade	Children and young adults
3. Onset	Acute, subacute, chronic	Chronic	Acute
4. Clinical presentation	Proptosis, ptosis, chemosis with pain	Proptosis with lid signs	Periorbital swelling and tenderness
5. Laboratory findings	Increased ESR	Abnormal thyroid function tests	Increased WBC
6. Systemic symptoms	Malaise	Thyroid symptoms	Fever
7. Response to Steroids	Small doses	Higher doses	Responds to antibiotics

ESR, erythrocyte sedimentation rate; WBC, white blood cell count

◆ Management

The patient must be admitted to the hospital. Gram staining and culture of any open wound and discharge should be done at the earliest opportunity along with complete and differential blood count and blood cultures. Mucormycosis must be kept in mind, especially in diabetic and immunosuppressed patients. Lumbar puncture for suspected meningitis is performed under a physician's supervision. Neurologic opinion should be undertaken if the general condition of the patient dictates the same. Intravenous antibiotics such as ceftriaxone plus vancomycin, or vancomycin plus gentamicin, or vancomycin plus clindamycin with or without metronidazole are given initially followed by oral antibodies for 7 to 14 days. Hot fomentation is applied four to five times a day. Local antibiotics include polymyxin with bacitracin ointment. For corneal exposure, NSAIDs help combat pain and inflammation.

Monitor for the following warning signs:

◆ Dilated pupils
◆ Marked ophthalmoplegia
◆ Loss of vision
◆ Relative afferent pupillary defect
◆ Papilledema
◆ Perivasculitis
◆ Violaceous lids

Exploration of the wound is indicated if the patient is unresponsive to antibiotics, vision is decreasing, orbital abscess is present, and a diagnostic biopsy is needed. It is important to drain the orbital abscess as well as the infected sinuses. The following oral antibiotics are given only after the condition improves significantly: amoxicillin-clavulanic acid, or cefaclor, or cotrimoxazole, or erythromycin, clindamycin, amoxicillin-cloxacillin with or without metronidazole.

Thyroid-Related Ophthalmopathy

Graves' disease or diffuse toxic goiter, is an autoimmune process that includes one or more of the following: hyperthyroidism, ophthalmopathy, and infiltrative dermopathy.

◆ **Presentation**

Graves' disease usually occurs with hyperthyroidism, but normal thyroid function can also be noticed. It is five times more common in females (**Fig. 3.3A,B**). There are two types according to level of severity:

1. *Noninfiltrative (mild)*: Minimal inflammatory reaction leading to mild symptoms and signs.
2. *Infiltrative (severe)*: This type has a more fulminant course with inflammation, infiltration, and scarring. These patients have chemosis, proptosis, corneal exposure, myositis, and enlargement of muscles. It ultimately leads to corneal exposure, restricted movements, and diplopia.

Werner classification reflects the severity of the ophthalmopathy and is well known by the acronym of NO SPECS (as described below). Each grade is further subdivided as 0 to 4 and a to c:

◆ *Grade 0*: No signs or symptoms
◆ *Grade 1*: Only signs (lid retraction)
◆ *Grade 2*: Soft tissue involvement (e.g., chemosis)
◆ *Grade 3*: Proptosis (minimum)
◆ *Grade 4*: Extraocular muscle involvement
◆ *Grade 5*: Corneal involvement
◆ *Grade 6*: Sight loss

There are various signs in thyroid eye disease, which go by the discoverers' names (**Fig. 3.3C,D,E**) (**Table 3.2**).

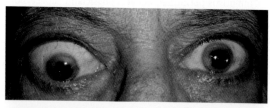

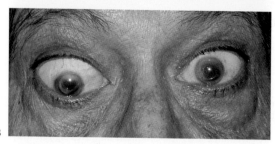

Fig. 3.3 **(A)** Thirty-five-year-old woman with dysthyroid orbitopathy with lid retraction. **(B)** Lid lags behind when patient looks down.

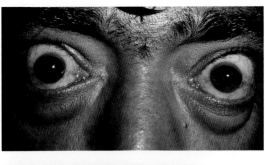

C

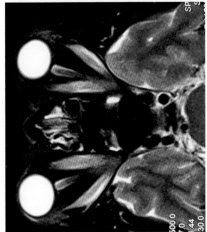

D

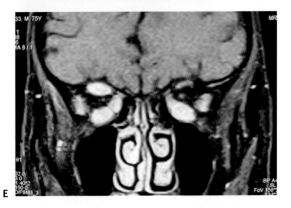

E

Fig. 3.3 (*Continued*) **(C)** Dysthyroid orbitopathy. **(D)** Computed tomographic (CT) scan, extraocular muscle enlargement sparing muscle tendons. **(E)** Coronal section CT scan.

Table 3.2   Ophthalmic Manifestations of Graves Disease

Most important signs
- Von Graefe: Upper lid lag on downgaze
- Dalrymple: Upper eye lid retraction

Upper eyelid signs
- Von Graefe: Upper lid lag on downgaze
- Dalrymple: Upper eyelid retraction
- Boston: Uneven jerky movement of upper lid on inferior movement
- Jellinek: Abnormal pigmentation of upper lid
- Kocher: Retraction of upper lid during fixation
- Gifford: Difficult eversion of upper eyelid

Pupillary signs
- Cowen: Extensive hippos of consensual papillary light reflex
- Lowey: Dilatation of pupil with 1:1000 epinephrine
- Knies' sign: Uneven difficult dilatation in dim light

Bruit signs
- Riesman: Bruit over eyelid
- Snellen sign: Bruit over the eye

Eye movement signs
- Ballet: Paralysis of one or more extraocular muscles (EOM)
- Möbius: Deficient convergence
- Suker: Inability to maintain fixation at extreme lateral gaze
- Wilder: Jerking of eyes on movement from abduction to adduction

Blinking signs
- Pochin: Reduced amplitude of blinking
- Stellwag: Incomplete or infrequent blinking

Lag signs
- Von Graefe: Upper eyelids lag on downgaze
- Griffith sign: Lower eyelid lag on upgaze

Conjunctival signs
- Goldzieher: Deep injection of temporal conjunctival vessels

◆ Differential Diagnosis

Orbital pseudotumor, cavernous sinus thrombosis, orbital cellulitis (see **Table 3.1**)

◆ Management

Management options for thyroid eye disease include observation, conservative interventions, oral corticosteroids, injected corticosteroids, external-beam radiotherapy, and surgery. Observation and conservative measures are appropriate for mild conjunctival injection and chemosis with normal cornea and optic nerve function. Advice to the patient includes sleeping with the head of the bed elevated and avoiding salt or monosodium glutamate to minimize fluid retention. Sunglasses are recommended to minimize photophobia. Nonpreserved artificial tears help decrease the ocular irritation. Glaucoma medications should be used only in patients with very high intraocular pressures and a family history of glaucoma. Surgical intervention should be performed in a stepped fashion: decompression first, strabismus surgery second, and eyelid surgery last. Patients should stop smoking and avoid secondhand smoke to limit the autoimmune exacerbation of thyroid eye disease.

Management of thyroid orbitopathy must take into account whether the disease is active or chronic and the degree to which the manifestations impact the patient's daily life or threaten sight. For example, mild eyelid retraction with minimal or no dry eye symptoms might be managed with conservative lubrication prior to elective eyelid surgery once the patient has stabilized. At the opposite end of the spectrum is the patient presenting with acute optic neuropathy resulting from apical crowding that requires urgent medical and/or surgical management.

Patients should be managed in close correspondence with an endocrinologist, who may elect to treat systemic hyperthyroidism via pharmacological suppression, surgical resection, or radioactive iodine. Recent studies suggest a benefit to steroid therapy in the peri-interventional period in minimizing the progression of orbitopathy.

General treatment options for the management of sequelae of thyroid orbitopathy include pharmacological therapy, radiation therapy, and surgical intervention. Mild cases with minimal ocular irritation or symptomatic diplopia may initially be managed conservatively with lubricating eyedrops and ointment, nocturnal taping, and Fresnel prisms.

Radiotherapy, generally 20 Gy delivered in 10 fractions over 2 weeks, has long been used as treatment for the orbital manifestations of thyroid disease as has been shown to be of benefit in improvement of motility. However, a recent prospective, randomized study by Gorman et al demonstrated no beneficial therapeutic effect of radiotherapy in moderate, symptomatic thyroid orbitopathy.

Surgical management can be divided into elective and urgent interventions. Elective surgery should proceed in the order of orbital decompression, strabismus surgery, and finally lid surgery, because each intervention as listed can influence the outcome of the subsequent interventions. There are a multitude of approaches to orbital decompression encompassing one to all walls, with or without endoscopic and transnasal exposure and with or without orbital fat decompression. Strabismus surgery should be utilized to maximize the field of binocular vision and generally includes recession of muscles on adjustable sutures. Eyelid procedures include blepharoplasty with or without removal of orbital fat, release of upper lid retraction via levator and or Muller muscle recession, and repair of lower lid retraction with spacer grafts.

Indications for urgent surgical intervention include optic neuropathy from apical crowding and corneal ulceration secondary to exposure. The management of these conditions can include many of the procedures outlined earlier in addition to urgent medical management with pulse corticosteroids, pharmacotherapy, and orbital irradiation.

Corticosteroids can provide short-term relief for symptoms and signs of thyroid eye disease, but hyperthyroid patients can suffer significant mood swings. In addition, tapering the steroids often results in rebound inflammation at least as severe as the original presentation. Other immunosuppressive agents have been used in the treatment of thyroid orbitopathy as steroid sparing agents, including cyclosporine, cytoxan, methotrexate, and azathioprine. Some favor combination therapy with cyclosporine and corticosteroids. Other treatment modalities include somatostatin analogues (octreotide), plasmapheresis, and intravenous immunoglobulin therapy.

Orbital Inflammatory Pseudotumor

Orbital inflammatory pseudotumor (OIP) consists of a spectrum of nongranulomatous inflammatory conditions of the orbit, with no known etiology or systemic associations, that produce proptosis due to a nonneoplastic inflammatory mass in the orbit. (Note: Some authors classify Tolosa-Hunt syndrome as a subtype of OIP.)

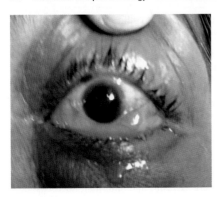

Fig. 3.4 Middle-aged woman with left eye pseudotumor.

◆ Presentation

OIP presents with abrupt onset of pain, proptosis (unilateral), conjunctival chemosis, epibulbar injection, visual loss, diplopia, and restricted ocular movements (**Fig. 3.4**). According to the different tissues involved, it is classified as one of the following:

◆ Myositis
◆ Dacryoadenitis
◆ Perioptic neuritis
◆ Posterior scleritis or tenonitis

Its clinical course is variable, and it may be regressed spontaneously without any treatment, or it may have prolonged inflammation or intermittent activity. A prolonged course may result in a frozen orbit secondary to fibrosis. Bilateral involvement is rare.

◆ Differential Diagnosis

Graves ophthalmopathy, orbital cellulitis, leukemia, cavernous sinus thrombosis, rhabdomyosarcoma (see **Table 3.1**)

◆ Management

Computed tomographic (CT) scans and magnetic resonance imaging (MRI) are essential in the workup of suspected OIP. Inflammatory signs predominate and may include involvement of the extraocular muscles (EOMs), orbital fat, lacrimal gland, choroid, and sclera. Orbital ultrasound may be of use in demonstrating thickening of the posterior Tenon capsule and in distinguishing the myositis of OIP from EOM involvement in thyroid orbitopathy because the muscular tendons will classically be involved in OIP and spared in thyroid disease.

The CT orbit shows extraocular muscle thickening involving tendinous insertion. Inflammation of the retrobulbar fat pad and contrast enhancement of the sclera due to tendonitis may produce a T sign or ring sign. Orbital ultrasound shows thickening of the posterior Tenon capsule along with muscle belly thickening (unlike thyroid related orbitopathy, which typically spares the tendons).

Systemic steroids (60 to 80 mg/day) are given. Rapid response is pathognomonic. Taper slowly over months to avoid recurrence. Pulsed intravenous steroids are given in severe vision-threatening cases. Radiotherapy is recommended in steroid-resistant cases. Chemotherapeutic agents such as cyclophosphamide, methotrexate, and cyclosporine are used for cases resistant to steroids and radiotherapy and in patients intolerant to steroids.

Orbital Lymphoma

Orbital lymphoma is a low-grade malignancy characterized by proliferation of monoclonal B cells (non-Hodgkin disease), which arises in lymph nodes or in extranodal sites such as the orbit.

◆ Presentation

The disease presents between the ages of 50 and 80 years with involvement of any part of the orbit. Bilateral involvement is rare. It occurs rarely in children. Most orbital lymphomas are low grade. Malignant lymphomas can produce a palpable mass that may be present in the anterior orbit. One can have painless progressive proptosis, accompanied by vision loss, occasional diplopia, lid edema, ptosis, and lacrimal gland involvement. A salmon-colored conjunctival tumor is characteristic (**Fig. 3.5A,B,C,D**).

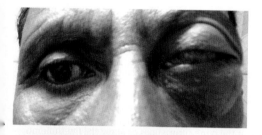

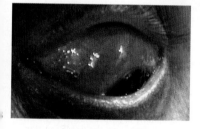

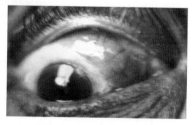

C

Fig. 3.5 **(A)** Fifty-five-year-old man with lymphoma. **(B)** Patient with lymphoma. **(C)** Salmon patch in conjunctiva.

◆ Differential Diagnosis

Metastasis, reactive lymphoid hyperplasia, pseudotumor, sarcoidosis

◆ Management

Computed tomographic scan shows a well-defined mass, located mostly in the anterior-superior lateral orbit, which molds to encompass adjacent structures. The lacrimal gland is frequently involved. Ultrasonography shows variable shape and borders of the lesion, which has low to medium internal reflectivity.

Radiotherapy (2500 to 3000 cGy) is the treatment of choice for less well-differentiated lesions. Chemotherapy can also be tried. A well-differentiated lesion without systemic involvement can be observed .Visual prognosis is excellent if the disease is confined to the orbit.

◆ Other Orbital Neoplasms

Dermoid Cyst

Dermoid cyst is a developmental, slow-growing choristoma (tumors with histologically normal cells in an abnormal location), lined with stratified squamous epithelium and filled with keratinized material and/or lipid. Most of these cysts are located in the eyelid and orbit, representing the single most common cause of periorbital neoplasm in children. They develop because of sequestration of the surface ectoderm pinched off at the bone suture lines or along the lines of embryonic closure. The cysts are lined with epidermis with dermal appendages such as hair follicles and sebaceous glands in the wall.

◆ Presentation

Dermoids are classified according to the anatomical site of presentation:

◆ Superficial dermoids (**Fig. 3.6A**)
  ◆ In front of the orbital septum and superotemporal or superonasal quadrants
  ◆ Presentation in infancy and childhood
  ◆ Palpable, firm, unilateral, localized mass, usually asymptomatic, may be mobile or fixed to the underlying structures and free from the overlying skin
◆ Deep dermoids (**Fig. 3.6B**)
  ◆ Posterior to the orbital septum, associated with bony sutures in the orbit but may extend across the bones in the frontal sinus, temporal fossa, or cranium
  ◆ Present in adolescence, may be seen in children and adults
  ◆ Proptosis, ocular displacement and bony defect, motility restriction, decreased vision. Spontaneous rupture produces severe orbital inflammation.

◆ Differential Diagnosis

Cavernous hemangioma, mucocele, optic nerve glioma, meningioma, neurilemmoma

◆ Management

◆ Superficial dermoids
  ◆ *CT scan of the orbit*: Round, well-defined lesions with enhancing rim and a lucent a center, which may contain calcium. There may be a well-corticated bone defect.
  ◆ *Echography*: A well-defined lesion with medium to high internal reflectivity, with an irregular acoustic structure; usually shows some compressibility
  ◆ *Complete surgical excision*: In one piece
  ◆ *Incomplete excision or capsular rupture*: May lead to recurrence with infiltration
◆ Deep dermoids
  ◆ *CT scan of the orbit*: Well-defined lesions with an enhancing rim. They may contain areas of calcification. The central lumen is nonenhancing, of variable density, and may show a fluid–fat interface. There may be a bone defect.
  ◆ *Echography*: A cystic mass with low to medium internal reflectivity is seen. Higher echoes occur only when the cyst is filled with keratin debris and fat.
  ◆ *Complete surgical excision*: In one piece, without rupture of capsule (**Fig. 3.6C–F**).

Capillary Hemangioma

Capillary hemangioma is a primary, unilateral, benign hamartoma of tightly packed capillaries, apparent at birth or within the first 8 weeks of life, strawberry red to purple. Most regress completely within 7 years of age. They are visible on the surface but may lie deep in the orbit. It is more commonly seen in the superonasal quadrant of the upper eyelid.

◆ Presentation

More common in girls. Involvement of superficial structures (dermis) results in a strawberry mark (strawberry nevus), single or multiple, usually elevated. Such patients may present with ptosis, sometimes associated with astigmatism and amblyopia. Involvement of the deep parts (and anterior orbit) appears as a bluish mass with a spongy texture. When the child cries or strains, the mass becomes more prominent and deepens in color. On examination, it is a circumscribed, soft red mass with a multinodular surface. Large feeding vessels are seen and can be the source of bleeding (**Fig. 3.7**).

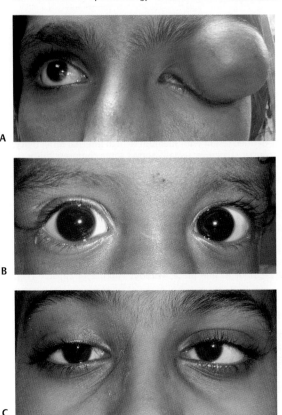

A

B

C

Fig. 3.6 (A) Young girl with a superficial dermoid. **(B)** A 4-year-old child with a dermoid involving the lateral canthal area. **(C)** A 9-year-old girl with a deep dermoid in the lateral orbit pushing the left eyeball medially.

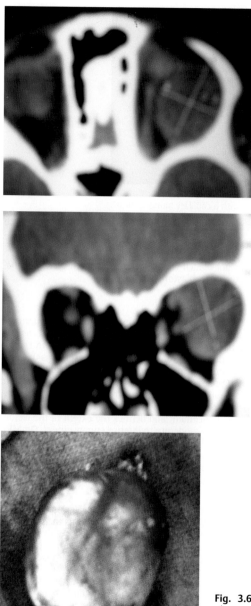

Fig. 3.6 (*Continued*) **(D)** Sagittal plane computed tomographic (CT) scan of a dermoid. **(E)** Coronal section CT scan. **(F)** Specimen of dermoid cyst excised, same patient specimen.

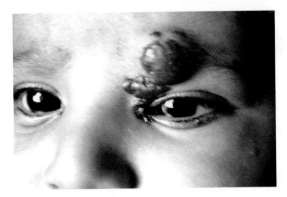

Fig. 3.7 Eight-month-old boy with a capillary hemangioma.

◆ Differential Diagnosis

Nevus flammeus (darker, does not blanch with pressure), dermoid cyst, encephalocele, lymphangioma, infection, neuroblastoma (**Table 3.3**)

◆ Management

Patient must be referred to a pediatrician for workup of systemic association(s) like high-output cardiac failure, Kasabach-Merritt syndrome (anemia, thrombocytopenia, low levels of coagulating factors due to their sequestration in the lesion), or Maffucci syndrome (endochordomatas and skin hemangiomas). Complete ophthalmologic examination must be done to rule out potential secondary events, namely, amblyopia, compressive optic neuropathy, and corneal exposure. Orbital ultrasound suggests a poorly outlined lesion, irregular in shape, high internal reflectivity, and an irregular acoustic structure with variable sound attenuation. CT scan shows contrast enhancement and defines the extent of the lesion. Deeper lesions are well defined with moderate to intense enhancement. On MRI, the lesion shows homogeneous and heterogeneous signals, being hypointense on T1 and hyperintense on T2 wedging. Flow voids appear as hyperintense regions. Gadolinium enhances the lesion moderately.

Observation is practiced in most of the cases because involution usually occurs in the following conditions:

◆ *Superficial conditions*: Severe cosmetic deformity and deprivation amblyopia are the major indications of intervention. The treatment options include intralesional (40 mg/mL triamcinolone plus 6 mg/mL betamethasone) or systemic (prednisolone 1 to 2 mg/kg/day) steroid. Other options include radiotherapy, yellow-dye laser, and topical corticosteroids. Surgery should be reserved for small, circumscribed lesions.

◆ *Deep conditions*: Large lesions or amblyopia usually warrant treatment with local radiotherapy (500 cGy) or systemic or local corticosteroids. Surgery may be attempted in small, circumscribed lesions. Prognosis is good for vision and for life.

Table 3.3 Vascular Lesions

Features	Capillary Hemangioma	Lymphangioma	Cavernous Hemangioma	Orbital Varices
Disease	Benign lid and orbital hamartoma	Benign lid and orbital tumor	Benign orbital tumor	Ectatic vascular channels
Onset	Soon after birth	Children	Adults	Young adults
Clinical features	Strawberry nevus and thrombo-cytopenia (Kasabach-Merritt syndrome)	Chocolate cysts	Axial proptosis	Exoph-thalmos or enoph-thalmos
Ultrasonography x-ray	High internal reflectivity	Cystic pattern	Well-defined round tumor with high internal echoes	Calcifica-tion
Computed tomographic scan	Irregular, poorly circum-scribed mass	Infiltrative, multilobulated lesions	Late enhance-ment with contrast	Enlarged vessels
Treatment	Observation, intralesional steroids, systemic steroids, la-ser, radiation	Observation, steroids, surgery	Observation, steroids	Conserva-tive

Lymphangioma

Lymphangioma is a rare vascular hamartoma of lymphatic channels that is he-modynamically isolated from the vascular system. Occurring predominantly in children and teenagers (most frequently in the first decade of life), the size of the lesion fluctuates with posture and Valsalva maneuver and with upper respiratory tract infections.

◆ Presentation

Superficial lesions occur in the conjunctiva or lid and are visible as cystic spaces with clear fluid partially filled with blood. Deep lymphangiomatous lesions clas-sically present with acute outset of painful proptosis resulting from spontaneous hemorrhage within the orbit. Such lesions are called chocolate cysts. The tumor mass may compress the globe or optic nerve, causing visual loss, refractive errors, secondary glaucoma, congestion of the optic nerve, and visual field defects (**Fig. 3.8A,B**).

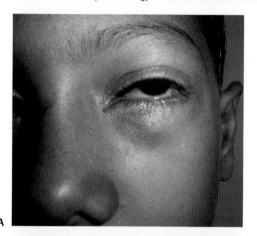

A

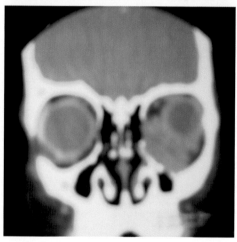

B

Fig. 3.8 **(A)** Ten-year-old boy with lymphangioma involving the lower nasal orbit. **(B)** Coronal section, computed tomographic scan.

◆ **Differential Diagnosis**

Optic nerve glioma, plexiform neurofibroma, capillary hemangioma, pseudotumor

◆ **Management**

The orbital lesion is seen as low-density cystic, intraconal and extraconal masses, with variable enhancement on magnetic resonance imaging. With T1 wedging they are hypointense, whereas T2 wedging response is variable, depending on the state of hemoglobin degeneration. Angiography shows no vascular component.

Management of lymphangiomas is challenging. Radiation and systemic steroids show limited sensitivity. Complete surgical excision is very difficult because of the infiltrative nature of the tumor. If acute hemorrhage causes symptoms, CO_2 laser or contact neodymium:yttrium-aluminum-garnet can be tried for homeostasis and obliteration of tumor as an alternative to evacuation, partial resection, or ligation. Amblyopia is common and is mostly from recurrent hemorrhage or globe compression.

Rhabdomyosarcoma

Rhabdomyosarcoma is the most common primary malignant orbital tumor in children (70% arise within the first decade of life). This soft tissue mesenchymal tumor accounts for up to 4% of all childhood malignancies. It arises from pleuripotent mesenchymal precursors that normally differentiate into striated muscle cells.

◆ Presentation

Presentation is usually in the first decade of life with a rapidly progressive proptosis, more commonly in boys. It frequently shows a mass in the upper part of the orbit, ptosis, and eyelid edema. The diagnosis is confirmed by biopsy. It can be grouped into four categories: embryonal, alveolar, pleomorphic, and botyroid in the orbit. The most common histological variant is embryonal followed by the alveolar type (**Fig. 3.9A,B,C,D**).

◆ Differential Diagnosis

Orbital cellulitis, pseudotumor, lymphangioma, metastatic neuroblastoma, ruptured dermoid cyst

◆ Management

In the past, patients with orbital rhabdomyosarcomas underwent orbital exenteration. Because of the malignant nature of the tumor, it was thought that radical resection provided the best chance for survival. Despite these measures, mortality remained as high as 70%. Over the past 30 years, with a combination of surgery, radiation, and chemotherapy, survival has approached 90%.

A staging classification was proposed by the Intergroup Rhabdomyosarcoma Study group in 1972. Complete resection of localized disease is categorized as group I. In general, microscopic residual disease or lymph node involvement is categorized as group II. Group III includes gross residual disease or incomplete resection. Group IV disease includes cases with metastasis at presentation. The stage of disease is dependent not only on the extent of the tumor but largely on the extent of resection. The same tumor can be a group I or II versus a group III depending on whether the surgeon performed an excision or incisional biopsy, respectively. The recommended regimen of radiation and chemotherapy is based on the stage of disease and is summarized following here.

Because of rhabdomyosarcomas' sensitivity to chemotherapy and radiation, an incisional biopsy followed by either chemotherapy, radiation, or both is preferred by most ophthalmologists. This approach is especially prudent with large tumors or tumors in which an excisional biopsy would likely harm the optic nerve, extraocular muscles, or other important orbital structures. The decision is more difficult for those smaller, more anterior tumors where complete excision without endangering other vital orbital structures is feasible. Most orbital rhabdomyosar-

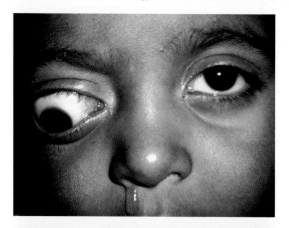

Fig. 3.9 (A) Three-year-old boy with rhabdomyosarcoma.
(B) Computed tomographic (CT) scan, sagittal section.

comas are located superonasally and in the extraconal space where excision would not violate the optic nerve or extraocular muscles. Such an approach may permit lower doses of radiation.

Judicious review of the CT and MRI scans is critical for surgical planning. Incisions directly overlying the tumor are the preferred approach to biopsy. For example, more posterior tumors are best approached via a cutaneous incision through the lid, whereas more anterior tumors that are visible in the conjunctival fornices may be approached via a transforniceal approach. For excisional biopsies, care should be taken to contain the tumor in its pseudocapsule and not to violate the periosteum to preserve the natural barrier to spread outside the orbit.

Irradiation for orbital rhabdomyosarcomas plays a secondary role to chemotherapy in management. Conventional fractionated doses totaling 4000 to 5000 cGy are usually sufficient to control tumor recurrence. However, at these doses, ocular complications of orbital irradiation, including radiation retinopathy, cataract, dry eyes, and radiation-associated keratopathy, are relatively common.

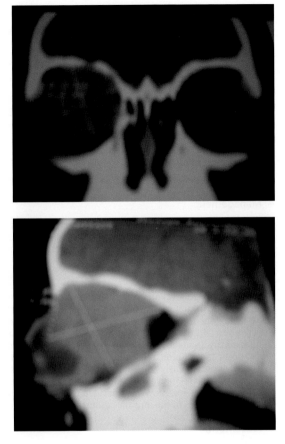

Fig. 3.9 (*Continued*) **(C)** CT scan, coronal section. **(D)** CT scan showing involvement of the eyeball.

With a combination of surgery, chemotherapy, and radiation, it is possible to control the tumor and salvage the eye in ~90% of cases of orbital rhabdomyosarcoma.

Supplemental chemotherapy has substantially improved survival rates of patients with orbital rhabdomyosarcomas. Patients who undergo surgery, radiation, and chemotherapy for rhabdomyosarcoma including but not limited to the orbit have been shown to have a 2-year disease-free survival rate of 82%, compared with 53% in those who undergo surgery and radiation alone.

Vincristine and actinomycin D have been the mainstays of chemotherapeutic agents employed in cases of orbital rhabdomyosarcoma. Newer agents such as ifosfamide and etoposide have been shown to produce a favorable response.

Cavernous Hemangioma

Cavernous hemangioma is usually seen in middle-aged women and is the most common benign intraorbital tumor in adults.

◆ Presentation

The tumor is unilateral, solitary, and typically located in the intraconal area. Proptosis is of the axial type. There is a predilection for middle-aged women, and the tumor may grow faster during pregnancy. The tumor may be associated with optic disk edema and retinal folds (striae). The vision may decrease by one or two lines. There may be restricted movements in extreme fields of gaze (**Fig. 3.10A–C**).

◆ Differential Diagnosis

Other intraorbital mass lesions such as dermoid cyst, lymphoma, schwannoma

◆ Management

Computed tomographic scan confirms the diagnosis. Most cavernous hemangiomas can be observed. If surgery is done, the tumor is seen to be a well-circumscribed, purple, encapsulated lesion with distinct vessels on its surface.

Carotid Cavernous Fistula

Orbital vascular abnormalities are a group of orbital disorders, congenital or acquired, arising from a variety of underlying conditions. Arteriovenous malformations, having feeder vessels from both internal and external carotid circulations, mostly occur after trauma (males, 15- to 30-year age range) but may also arise spontaneously (females, 30- to 60-year age range). Carotid cavernous fistulas (CCFs) occur mostly after basal skull fractures or penetrating orbital trauma and can occur spontaneously in persons with systemic hypertension. The high-flow CCFs arise when the internal carotid artery develops a defect within the cavernous sinus, whereas low-flow CCFs develop from the communication between the meningeal branches of the internal carotid artery and the cavernous sinus.

◆ Presentation

The patient notices a swishing noise in the head that is synchronous with the pulse. Because of the proximity of the ocular motor nerves to the cavernous sinus, impaired ocular motility and diplopia are early findings. Proptosis, lid and orbital edema, and dilated and tortuous conjunctival and episcleral veins develop later. Elevated episcleral venous pressure leads to ocular hypertension.

◆ *High-flow CCF*: Chemosis, corkscrew dilatation of the epibulbar vessels, orbital edema, proptosis, pulsatile exophthalmos, audible bruit, secondary glaucoma, retinal vascular dilatation, papilledema, rapid afferent papillary defect, decreased vision, occasional nerve palsies (III–VI are most common)
◆ *Low-flow CCF*: Chemosis, increased episcleral venous pressure, venous dilatation (**Fig. 3.11A,B,C**).

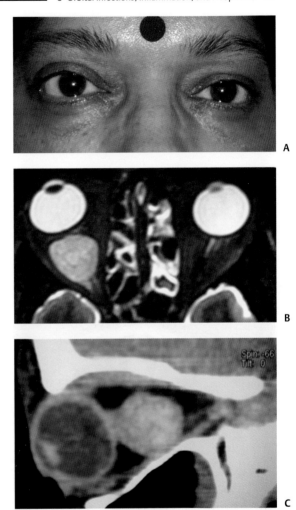

Fig. 3.10 **(A)** Young adult presenting with proptosis, a case of cavernous hemangioma. **(B)** Coronal section computed tomographic (CT) scan, cavernous hemangioma. **(C)** CT scan, cavernous hemangioma.

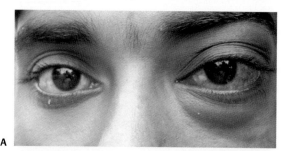

A

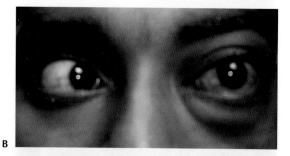

B

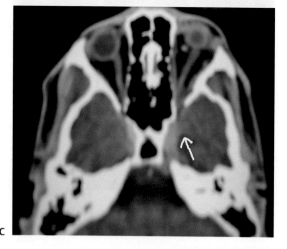

C

Fig. 3.11 **(A)** Carotid cavernous fistula with left eye propto-sis conjunctival congestion. **(B)** Restricted movements in the left eye. **(C)** Computed tomographic scan showing cavernous sinus involvement. Arrow marks cavernous sinus and also note prominent superior ophthalmic vein.

◆ Differential Diagnosis

Cavernous sinus thrombosis, pseudotumor, thyroid orbitopathy

◆ Management

Computed tomographic scan with contrast remains the initial procedure of choice. It shows dilated superior ophthalmic vein with enlargement of the superior orbital fissure and erosion of the anterior clinoid process. Ultrasonography of the orbit shows a dilated superior ophthalmic vein, mild thickening of the EOMs, and medium to high internal reflectivity from edema. MRI with gadolinium or magnetic resonance angiography is a useful tool to investigate further, supplementing the CT scan.

Small, spontaneous, low-flow fistulas resolve frequently (up to 40%) from thrombosis. Embolization is indicated only when vision loss, glaucoma, or severe pain is present. Traumatic high-flow fistulas rarely resolve on their own. With a high rate of visual loss in these patients intervention becomes the rule. The current trend involves interventional radiology with intravascular balloons or other embolization via catheter in the internal carotid artery.

Orbital Varices

Orbital varices may represent congenial foci of an abnormal vessel (the most common site is the upper nasal quadrant, and it is usually unilateral) or may be the late stage of other vascular abnormalities.

◆ Presentation

Intermittent proptosis, which is nonpulsatile and not associated with bruit. It can affect patients from early childhood to late middle age.

◆ Differential Diagnosis

Dermoid cyst, lymphangioma

◆ Management

Surgery is difficult because the lesions are friable and bleed easily, and in most cases, excision is incomplete. Indications for surgical intervention include repeated episodes of pain, thrombosis, severe proptosis, and optic nerve compression. Conservative treatment by CO_2 laser, yttrium-aluminum-garnet laser, or cautery is recommended. Embolization is possible if feeder vessels can be identified.

Mucocele

Mucoceles are cystic lesions originating from primary obstruction of a paranasal sinus (most commonly frontal or ethmoid sinuses) following trauma, sinusitis, or, rarely, a tumor, that slowly enlarge causing bone deformity with erosions of the orbit. Consisting of a cystic mass filled with mucus, mucoceles may be bound by an eggshell layer of bone and when infected are referred to as *pyoceles*.

◆ Presentation

Mucoceles most commonly arise from the frontal and ethmoidal sinus. Patients present with a combination of proptosis, a palpable fluctuant mass, headache, diplopia, ptosis, and epiphora or globe displacement. Swelling of the upper eyelid medially is common. Pain is not common in the absence of infection (**Fig. 3.12A–D**).

◆ Differential Diagnosis

Dermoid cyst, osteoma, pseudotumor

◆ Management

Computed tomographic scan shows an opacified frontal or ethmoidal sinus, loss of ethmoid septae, and a bony dehiscence. The cystic content shows variable density and is nonenhancing. Ultrasonography reveals a very well-defined mass with sharp surface spikes and low internal reflectivity. Mucocele is associated with a very large bony defect adjacent to a paranasal sinus. Treatment is surgical removal of the cyst lining and reestablishment of normal drainage. Obliteration of the sinus with fat or muscle may be necessary to treat recurrences.

Metastatic Orbital Lesions

These lesions represent 2 to 10% of all orbital tumors. In children, neuroblastoma, Ewing sarcoma, and acute myeloid leukemia are common. The most common primary sites in adults are the breast, bronchus, prostate, skin melanoma, gastrointestinal tract, and kidney.

◆ Presentation

A mass in the anterior orbit causing axial or nonaxial displacement of the globe is most common. Infiltration of orbital tissue characterized by ptosis, diplopia, and indurated skin surrounding the orbit is common. Inflammatory reaction is seen. It may be seen presenting either as proptosis with decreased visual acuity, diplopia, pain, paresthesia, increased intraocular pressure, and exposure keratopathy, or in cases of cicatrizing carcinomas such as certain secondaries from the breast, as enophthalmos (**Fig. 3.13A–D**).

◆ Differential Diagnosis

Orbital pseudotumor, rhabdomyosarcoma, leukemias

◆ Management

Treatment is aimed at preserving vision and relieving pain. The main options are radiotherapy and hormonal therapy (the latter in cases of breast and prostatic metastasis). Chemotherapy is often useful in controlling the systemic disease. A biopsy may sometimes be required to establish the nature of the primary. Generally, only palliative therapy can be offered.

Fig. 3.12 **(A)** Orbital abscess from frontal sinus with pansinusitis. **(B)** CT scan axial section showing the orbital abscess. **(C)** CT scan sagittal section showing spread of infection behind the orbital septum. **(D)** The patient also has ethmoidal and maxillary sinusitis.

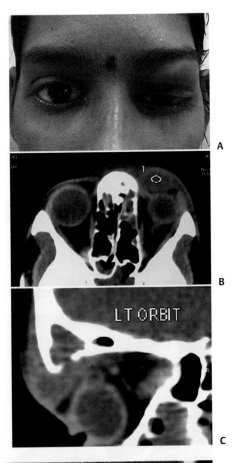

A

B

C

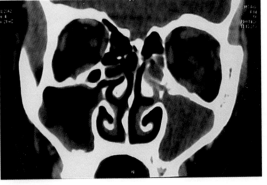

D

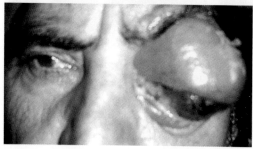

Fig. 3.13 **(A)** Eight-year-old girl suffering from leukemia. **(B)** Computed tomographic scan, leukemia involving the orbit. **(C)** Neuroblastoma. **(D)** Secondaries in orbit.

◆ Lacrimal Gland Enlargement

Lacrimal Gland Inflammation

Inflammatory causes, which are not uncommon, include dacryoadenitis, sarcoidosis, and orbital inflammatory pseudotumor. A decreased Schirmer test suggests an inflammatory lesion.

Lacrimal Gland Tumors

Benign Mixed Tumor (Pleomorphic Adenoma)

These are slowly growing lesions usually seen in the fourth to fifth decades of life.

◆ Presentation

A long history of more than 1 to 2 years is generally obtained, and it usually presents as a noninfiltrating lesion in the lacrimal gland area with fullness of the superotemporal lid and orbit and painless inferonasal proptosis. The upper lid contour may take an ~ shape (**Fig. 3.14**).

◆ Differential Diagnosis

Inflammatory lesions, tumors of the lacrimal gland, dermoids

◆ Management

Computed tomographic scan shows a well-circumscribed, pseudoencapsulated lesion in the lacrimal fossa.

◆ Patients with a long-standing, painless, slowly growing mass with a well-circumscribed appearance on imaging studies are presumed to have a pleomorphic adenoma.
◆ Treatment is extirpation, consisting of a lateral orbitotomy with intracapsular removal of all lesional tissue with careful attention to prevent violation of the pseudocapsule.

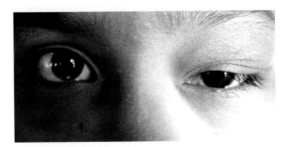

Fig. 3.14 Mass in upper orbital region in young girl.

◆ Incisional biopsy of these lesions is contraindicated because, although histologically benign, incomplete excision often leads to repeated recurrences (as high as 30% in some studies) and malignant transformation.
◆ Small, fingerlike protuberances outside the main tumor bulk with subsequent seeding of the residual tumor are believed to be responsible for this phenomenon.
◆ For pleomorphic adenomas, long-term studies reveal an increased incidence of malignant transformation (10% at 20 years and 20% at 30 years) associated with multiple recurrences for lesions that had frequent incisional biopsies and incomplete removal of the primary tumor.

Adenoid Cystic Carcinoma

Adenoid cystic carcinoma is the most common malignant lacrimal gland tumor, representing 50% of malignant tumors of the lacrimal gland and 25% of all lacrimal gland tumors.

◆ Presentation

Most cases are seen in the third decade of life with a second bimodal peak in the teenage years. Adenoid cystic carcinomas and other malignancies can also present with pain secondary to perineural or bony involvement. Diplopia and diminished visual acuity can be seen with rapidly progressive lesions. Adenoid cystic carcinoma usually presents as an irregular mass, producing bony erosion (70%) and occasional calcification (20%).

◆ Differential Diagnosis

Inflammatory lesions, tumors of the lacrimal gland, dermoids

◆ Management

Adenoid cystic carcinomas carry a poorer prognosis because of bony extension and perineural infiltration. These patients have a 50% at 5-year and 75% at 15-year mortality rate. Death is commonly due to intracranial spread and pulmonary metastasis. Histological pattern is also of prognostic significance, with a cribriform pattern having a 70% at 5-year survival compared with a 20% at 5-year survival with a basaloid pattern. CT scan, along with clinical appearance, helps in preoperative diagnosis. Treatment consists of en bloc complete surgical excision of the orbit and its contents (**Fig. 3.15A–D**).

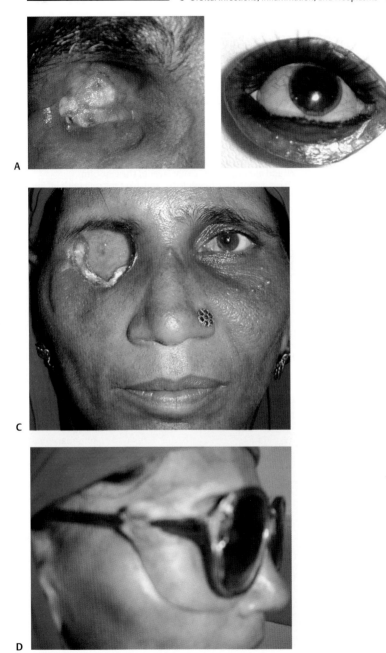

Fig. 3.15 **(A)** Exenteration done in a 35-year-old woman with adenoid cystic carcinoma. **(B)** Spectacle prosthesis. **(C)** Exenteration done in a 35-year-old woman with adenoid cystic carcinoma. **(D)** Same patient, spectacle prosthesis.

4 External Diseases

Guillermo Simón-Castellví, Pablo Gili-Manzanaro, Sarabel Simón-Castellví,
José María Simón-Castellví, Cristina Simón-Castellví, and
José María Simón-Tor

◆ Blepharitis and Ocular Rosacea

Anterior blepharitis is a bilateral chronic inflammatory process of the eyelids, which may secondarily result in corneal and conjunctival changes, with severe dry eye. It may result in corneal and conjunctival irritation due to the secretion into the eye of inflammatory substances and alteration of the oily layer of the tear film.

Staphylococcal blepharitis, seborrheic blepharitis, and acne rosacea with lid and ocular involvement are commonly found in patients with blepharitis. Hordeolum and chalazion formation is also commonly seen.

◆ Presentation

Presentation includes itching, irritation, tearing, foreign body sensation, crusting on the lid margins, lash loss (madarosis) or lash misdirection (trichiasis), ulceration of the lid margin (tilosis), red and thickened eyelids, and chronic conjunctivitis. Meibomitis (sebaceous gland dysfunction) may also be present (**Fig. 4.1A–D**).

- ◆ *Infectious*: Fibrin collarettes on the lashes
- ◆ *Seborrheic*: Seborrheic dermatitis, tear film instability
- ◆ *Ocular rosacea*: Greasy skin; facial telangiectasia; erythema of the cheeks, forehead; and nose; rhinophyma. Commonly, peripheral corneal immune infiltrates (aseptic, due to staphylococcal type IV hypersensitivity)

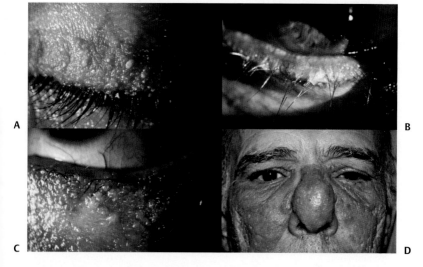

Fig. 4.1 **(A)** Fibrin collarettes; **(B,C)** lid margin telangiectasia; **(D)** erythema of the cheeks in a patient with ocular rosacea.

◆ Differential Diagnosis

Other kinds of conjunctivitis (infectious, allergic, or toxic), and dry eye. Rule out sebaceous gland carcinoma in unilateral cases.

◆ Management

◆ *Lid hygiene*: Commercially available ready-for-use lid scrubs or warm-water soaks with diluted neutral baby shampoo in the morning and at night, tear supplements, antibiotic gels (e.g., fusidic acid) or ointment (e.g., erythromycin or bacitracin)
◆ *Diet*: Vitamin and omega-3 supplementation, salmon intake, olive oil intake
◆ *Flax oil*: The best source is ground flax seeds so ligin and fiber are included
◆ *Tapered topical steroids*: For severe inflammation or corneal infiltrates or phlyctenules. Dual-action topical antiallergic medication provides relief (e.g., ketotifen fumarate 0.025%, azelastine hydrochloride 0.05%, olopatadine hydrochloride 0.1%.)
◆ *Oral systemic tetracyclines*: For acne rosacea in adults (oral doxycycline, 500 mg 1 g/every 6 hours for 1 month of treatment)
◆ *Abundant artificial tears and topical lubricants*: For dry-eye symptoms (e.g., topical sodium hyaluronate 0.18%)
◆ Treatment is tapered according to symptoms

◆ Conjunctivitis

Any inflammation of the conjunctiva is referred to as conjunctivitis.

Adenoviral Conjunctivitis (Epidemic Keratoconjunctivitis, Pharyngoconjunctival Fever)

Adenoviral infections predominate in summer months. Most textbooks refer to viral conjunctivitis as infections produced by adenoviruses (epidemic conjunctivitis, adenoviral conjunctivitis). But different viruses are responsible for different types of conjunctivitis. Picornavirus (mainly enterovirus 70 and Coxsackievirus A24) are responsible for acute hemorrhagic conjunctivitis, which is clinically similar to adenoviral conjunctivitis but more severe. It is highly contagious and occurs in epidemics.

◆ *Epidemic keratoconjunctivitis*: Caused by adenoviruses 8 and 19 with characteristic preauricular lymph node, pharyngitis, and subepithelial infiltrates 5 to 10 days after the initial symptoms
◆ *Pharyngoconjunctival fever*: Caused by adenoviruses 3 and 7, with fever and pharyngitis; associated with public swimming pools in summer

◆ Presentation

Classic signs include red eye (unilateral or bilateral), ciliary injection (mild iritis), and epiphora. In cases of adenoviral conjunctivitis, the patient refers to recent exposure to an individual with red eyes at home, school, or work or has a history of recent symptoms of an upper respiratory tract infection. The incubation period is 5 to 12 days. Acute follicular conjunctival reaction mainly in the inferior tarsal conjunctiva, chemosis, preauricular adenopathy, subconjunctival petechiae (very small hemorrhages), and sometimes early, nonspecific mild punctate keratopathy may be seen. Subepithelial infiltrates develop 5 to 12 days after the initial symptoms (suggest adenovirus serotypes 8 and 19). Corneal opacities can persist for a few weeks to months (we have seen up to 2 years). They can decrease visual acuity and cause glare symptoms. Epithelial ulceration (partial or total) may occur. Eyelid edema and sub-conjunctival hemorrhage suggests acute hemorrhagic conjunctivitis. In severe cases, membranes and pseudomembranes can lead to conjunctival scarring and symblepharon.

Symptoms include photophobia and eye pain if there is corneal involvement (adenovirus), intense watery discharge (serous), and itchy eye(s). It is usually benign and self-limited and generally has a longer course than acute bacterial conjunctivitis, lasting for ~2 to 4 weeks (**Fig. 4.2A,B**).

◆ Differential Diagnosis

Other epidemic keratoconjunctivitis, herpes simplex infection, herpes zoster infection, infectious mononucleosis (with eye involvement), Epstein-Barr virus infection, Dimmer keratitis, brucellosis

◆ Management

Most cases are self-limited, with no morbidity, and require no specific treatment. Highly contagious cases require strict hygiene measures. Instruct your patient that

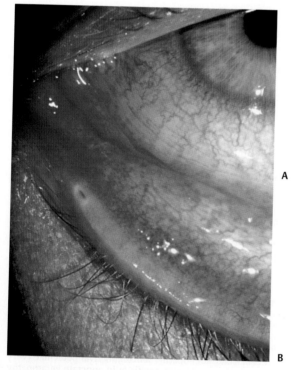

A

B

Fig. 4.2 (A, B) Adenoviral conjunctivitis.

despite symptomatic treatment the condition may worsen. Cool compresses and artificial refreshed tears provide relief (four to eight times daily for 2 to 4 weeks). Dark glasses can help. Provide relief for flulike symptoms with oral antihistamines and decongestants. Low-dose topical steroids (e.g., fluorometholone) combined with vasoconstrictors and dual-action topical antiallergic medication provide comfort (e.g., ketotifen fumarate 0.025%, azelastine hydrochloride 0.05%, olopatadine hydrochloride 0.1%.). Topical gel of ganciclovir has clearly proven effective in shortening disease course. Topical broad-spectrum antibiotics may help to prevent secondary bacterial infection. Topical steroids are used for pseudomembranes or when subepithelial infiltrates impair vision. They dramatically suppress conjunctival inflammatory signs, relieve symptoms, and are associated with resolution of the corneal subepithelial infiltrates when present. We always prescribe topical steroids after ruling out herpes simplex infection. We have never seen recurrence of subepithelial infiltrates after gradually tapering steroids. Be careful: topical steroids may worsen an underlying herpes simplex virus infection!

Acute Hemorrhagic Conjunctivitis (Epidemic Hemorrhagic Keratoconjunctivitis)

This type of conjunctivitis is also known as Apollo 11 conjunctivitis and is due to picornavirus (coxsackievirus A24 or enterovirus group 70). Acute hemorrhagic conjunctivitis affects mostly children and young adults in the lower socioeconomic classes.

◆ Presentation

It begins with an initial period of catarrhal inflammation, followed, in a day or two, by the appearance of conjunctival petechiae that coalesce to form subconjunctival hemorrhages. The explosive onset is a painful, rapidly progressive follicular conjunctivitis. It is self-limited in a couple of weeks and starts with subconjunctival diffuse hemorrhage, more frequent in the upper bulbar, and symptoms of viral conjunctivitis such as preauricular lymphatic node and anterior segment inflammation together with flulike symptoms. There is periorbital pain. The lids often become swollen and indurate (lid edema). Chemosis, seromucous discharge, photophobia, and tearing are also seen (**Fig. 4.3**).

◆ Differential Diagnosis

Adenoviral or bacterial infection, subconjunctival hemorrhage, keratitis

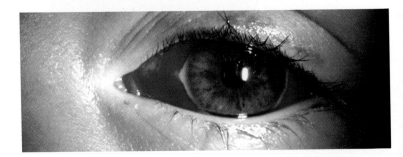

Fig. 4.3   Acute hemorrhagic conjunctivitis.

◆ Management

No treatment is usually necessary. Bed rest, dark glasses, cold compresses, and analgesics (e.g., paracetamol 500 mg every 8 hours) are helpful. Given that this is highly contagious, strict hygiene measures should be observed. Provide relief of flulike symptoms with oral antihistamines and decongestants. Low-dose topical steroids combined with vasoconstrictors and dual-action topical antiallergic medication provide comfort (e.g., ketotifen fumarate 0.025%, azelastine hydrochloride 0.05%, olopatadine hydrochloride 0.1%.). Topical gel of ganciclovir has proven efficacy in shortening disease course. Topical broad-spectrum antibiotics may help to prevent secondary bacterial infection.

Herpes Simplex Keratoconjunctivitis

Most textbooks refer to viral conjunctivitis as that produced by adenoviruses (epidemic conjunctivitis, adenoviral conjunctivitis), but different viruses are responsible for different types of conjunctivitis or keratoconjunctivitis. Herpes simplex virus (HSV) is the most dangerous cause, especially HSV type 1 (mouth, genital). HSV type 2 may also be a cause, especially in children and neonates. HSV affects a variety of ocular tissues and may cause ocular dermatitis, epithelial and stromal keratitis, and even iridocyclitis (**Fig. 4.4A,B**).

◆ Presentation

Red painful eye (unilateral or bilateral, usually unilateral), photophobia-epiphora, acute follicular conjunctival reaction mainly in the inferior tarsal conjunctiva,

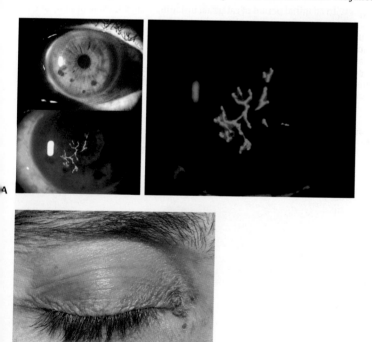

Fig. 4.4 **(A)** Herpetic dendritic corneal ulcer. **(B)** Associated skin lesions.

chemosis, sometimes early nonspecific mild punctate keratopathy, classic dendrite-like corneal ulceration with terminal bulbs. Fluorescein stains the ulcer base, whereas rose bengal stains the ulcer edges. Usually occurs in sexually active adults. In cases left untreated or in late diagnosis or inmunocompromised patients it can lead to disciform keratitis, interstitial keratitis, and iridocyclitis.

◆ Differential Diagnosis

Epidemic keratoconjunctivitis, varicella-zoster herpetic infection, corneal abrasion

◆ Management

◆ *Ophthalmic ganciclovir gel (preferred) or acyclovir ointment* (five times daily, 7 to 10 days is usually enough). Ganciclovir gel is much less toxic for the corneal epithelium than acyclovir. Use in children may not be approved for herpes simplex in some countries. Alternatives include 3% vidarabine ointment (five times daily, until reepithelialization or 7 days), 1% trifluridine drops (1 drop every 2 hours, maximum 9 drops), or 0.5% idoxuridine drops (one drop, five times per day, 7 days).
◆ *Epithelial debridement and patching*: Use ganciclovir and antibiotic ointment.
◆ *Add topical antibiotic drops, gel, or ointment to avoid superinfection*: Dark glasses, antihistamines (e.g., levocabastine every 8 to 12 hours) and vasoconstricting drops provide relief. Oral famciclovir reduces duration and the risk of recurrence.
◆ *Concomitant use of topical ganciclovir, steroids, and oral famciclovir*: Required for disciform keratitis, interstitial keratitis, and iridocyclitis. In the case of iridocyclitis, prescribe cycloplegia.

Acute Bacterial Conjunctivitis

Because of the excellent defense systems of the eye, acute bacterial conjunctivitis is uncommon, but it is still the most common eye disease. In most cases self-limited and benign, it is characterized by the presence of abundant mucopurulent discharge in a patient with red eye. There is considerable overlap in the presenting findings from different bacteria. Only expert clinicians may be able to recognize the probable infective agent at a clinical level.

◆ *Epidemiology/transmission*: Infectious for the first 48 hours of treatment

◆ Presentation

◆ *Signs*: Redness with variable conjunctival injection (hyperemia), palpebral conjunctiva being more affected than bulbar, lid swelling (marked lid edema characteristic of *Haemophilus influenzae* and *Corynebacterium diphtheriae*), membranes that are commonly seen with *Streptococcus pyogenes* and *Corynebacterium diphtheriae*, and chemosis (bulbar conjunctiva and forniceal). There is usually no preauricular adenopathy or skin involvement, the cornea is usually clear (possible corneal ulceration if untreated), and the pupil reacts normally.
◆ *Symptoms*: Unilateral, sudden onset of red eye with significant irritation and foreign body or gritty sensation (no outstanding pain), which progresses to the other eye in 2 to 5 days. It is usual for symptoms to be present for several days or weeks at the time of presentation. An uncommonly long duration or frequent recurrences suggest that other factors or conditions may be present (e.g., chronic dacryocystitis, urethritis). The patient has sticky lids or matting of eyelashes, especially in the morning, with seromucoid (at the beginning) or mucopurulent copious grayish, yellow, or green discharge (later). White discharge is due to abundant mucus and suggests allergic reaction. Visual acuity is preserved except for the expected mild blur due to the discharge and debris in the tear film. Consider gonococcal conjunctivitis if there is excessive purulent discharge.

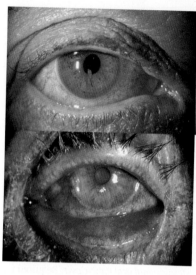

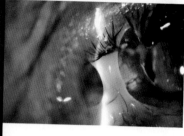

A

B

C

Fig. 4.5 **(A)** Conjunctival congestion. **(B)** Mucopurulent discharge. **(C)** Conjunctival congestion and lid edema.

- *Complications*: *Staphylococcus aureus* blepharitis is seen in chronic bacterial conjunctivitis and external hordeolum (stye). Gonococcus can penetrate the intact corneal epithelium leading to perforation (**Fig. 4.5A–C**).

Differential Diagnosis

Any cause of red eye (e.g., viral conjunctivitis, allergic conjunctivitis, any keratitis, uveitis, acute angle closure glaucoma)

Management

- *Lid cleansing*: It is important to keep the lids clean and remove all discharge.
- *Broad-spectrum topical antibiotic*: Most cases of bacterial conjunctivitis clear in 48 to 72 hours with a low dose of any broad-spectrum antibiotic applied topically. Continue treatment for at least 7 days. Highly responsive to empirical treatment (e.g., tobramycin, norfloxacin, levofloxacin). Two drops in affected eyes, every 3 to 4 hours, for 1 week.
- *Ointments and gels*: Very useful with children (day and night) or for overnight use in adults
- *Cultures*: Consider for cases refractory to topical treatment

Chlamydia Trachoma

Chlamydial organisms are responsible for neonatal conjunctivitis, adult inclusion conjunctivitis, trachoma, and lymphogranuloma venereum (Nicolas-Favre disease, in tropical regions, rarely affects the eye). Chlamydial (inclusion) conjunctivitis typically affects sexually active teens and young adults, and *Chlamydia* is the most frequent infectious cause of neonatal conjunctivitis in the United States. Adult inclusion conjunctivitis, also called paratrachoma, is due to *Chlamydia trachomatis* serotypes D to K, whereas true trachoma is due to *Chlamydia trachomatis* serotypes A to C (**Fig. 4.6A,B**).

- **Presentation** (Table 4.1)

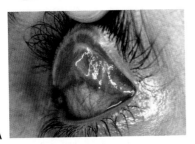
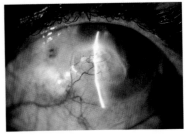

A

B

Fig. 4.6 **(A)** Trachoma, cicatricial ptosis, lid everted following trachoma. **(B)** Trachoma corneal ulceration.

Table 4.1   Presentation of Chlamydia Trachoma

	Adult Inclusion Conjunctivitis (Paratrachoma or Oculogenital Syndrome)	Trachoma
Transmission	Oculogenital (venereal)	Ocular
Epidemiology	Sporadic	Endemic
		Flies and other fomites ease spreading
Endemic region	Developed countries (Europe, United States)	Underdeveloped countries (Africa, Asia, Middle East); hot, dry climates
Reservoir	Eye and nose	Eye and nose
	Genital tract in males and females	
Age of infection	Young adults (men and women, 15–30 years)	Children (100% are infected in endemic areas before age 2)
	Sexually active	
Incubation period	8–10 days	5–8 days
	6 days in children	
Presentation	Acute or chronic	Acute or chronic
Laterality	Uni-/bilateral (may be asymmetric)	Almost always bilateral
First signs	Follicular conjunctivitis	Red eye and mucopurulent discharge (acute or chronic)
	Mucopurulent discharge	Follicular conjunctivitis (superior tarsal follicles and papillae)
		Very slow evolution (in years)
		No membranes
		Conjunctival injection, punctate keratitis, superior corneal pannus, follicles (most dense in the inferior cul-de-sac) may be present
		A palpable preauricular node is almost always present (prominent lymphoid reaction)

(Continued on page 108)

Table 4.1 (*Continued*) **Presentation of Chlamydia Trachoma**

	Adult Inclusion Conjunctivitis (Paratrachoma or Oculogenital Syndrome)	Trachoma
Complications	No scarring of the conjunctiva	Ocular signs and symptoms include the chief complaint that an eye infection has persisted longer than 3 weeks despite treatment with topical antibiotics
		Conjunctival scarring (limbal Herbert pits, von Arlt lines in superior and sometimes inferior tarsal conjunctiva)
		Epithelial superficial keratopathy, pannus: superficial corneal vascularization
		Dry eye
		Bacterial superinfection
		Blindness
Course	Weeks (may have acute start)	Chronic (years)
	Rule out other venereal infections (gonorrhea and syphilis)	May have acute start
Prognosis	Good	Poor in chronic untreated cases or reinfection (common)
		Reinfection with other pathogens is frequent

◆ **Management**

- ◆ Saline rinsing clears the mucopurulent debris from the lids and conjunctiva.
- ◆ Azithromycin (Zithromax) 1 g by mouth is the drug of choice. One dose has been documented as being as effective as doxycycline for the treatment of genital chlamydial infection. For greater safety we prescribe 500 mg, once every day for 3 days.
- ◆ Alternatives:
  - ◆ Oral amoxicillin or erythromycin 250 to 500 mg, orally, four times daily, for 3 or 4 weeks
  - ◆ Oral doxycycline 100 mg, orally, twice daily, for 1 week (be alert for pregnancy or lactation)
  - ◆ Oral tetracycline 250 to 500 mg, orally, four times daily, for 1 week (contraindicated in pregnant or lactating women and children under age 8)
  - ◆ Topical antibiotics are relatively ineffective (but useful). Topical therapy is adjunctive but not essential: rifampicin (drops or ointment), or erythromycin ointment (drug of choice for pregnant women), or tetracycline drops or ointment, three times daily, for 7 days. We always prescribe adjunctive topical therapy.
  - ◆ In children use oral erythromycin suspension, 40 mg/kg/day, in four divided doses for 2 weeks.

- ◆ In pregnant women use erythromycin 250 to 500 mg, orally, four times daily, for 3 weeks.
- ◆ Topical fluoroquinolone (ofloxacin or ciprofloxacin) if there is a corneal infection
- ◆ Topical steroids can give temporary relief (start a few days after topical antibiotics).
- ◆ Treat sexual partners. A condom does not protect against chlamydial conjunctivitis.

Chlamydia/Adult Inclusion Conjunctivitis

This condition is sexually transmitted and typically found in young adults. It presents as chronic follicular conjunctivitis caused by *Chlamydia trachomatis* serotypes D to K. A history of vaginitis, cervicitis, or urethritis may or may not be present.

◆ Presentation

Presentation includes chronic, bilateral, red, and irritated eye. Inferior tarsal or bulbar conjunctival follicles, superior corneal pannus, palpable preauricular node, or tiny, gray-white peripheral subepithelial infiltrates may be present. A stringlike, mucous discharge is typical.

◆ Differential Diagnosis

All other forms of chronic conjunctivitis

◆ Management

- ◆ Diagnostic tests include slit-lamp examination, direct chlamydial immunoflourescence test, or *Chlamydia* culture of the conjunctiva. Conjunctival scraping with Giemsa stain shows basophilic intracytoplasmic inclusion bodies in epithelial cells, polymorphonuclear leukocytes, and lymphocytes in newborns.
- ◆ Azithromycin 1 g by mouth single dose, doxycycline 100 mg by mouth twice a day, or erythromycin 500 mg by mouth four times a day for 7 days is given to the patient and sexual partners.
- ◆ Topical erythromycin and tetracycline two to three times a day for 2 to 3 weeks are other treatment options.

Chronic Conjunctivitis and Recurrent Corneal Abrasions

Chronic conjunctivitis and recurrent corneal abrasions may have their origins in a lid disease (e.g., blepharitis), a lid malposition (e.g., entropion), or a lacrimal way dysfunction (e.g., dacryocystitis). Left untreated, these conditions can result in severe damage to the ocular surface as a result of different corneal and conjunctival complications. Determining the cause is essential to indicate adequate treatment.

◆ Presentation

Symptoms include recurrent or chronic conjunctivitis (red eye, discharge, etc.), spasmodic inversion of the eyelid margin (spasmodic entropion), foreign body sensation, ocular surface irritation, corneal abrasions, and scars. In advanced cases there can be vision problems (astigmatism, leukomas in the visual axis), restric-

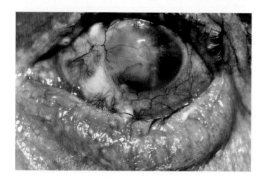

Fig. 4.7 Spasmodic entropion with corneal ulceration sequelae.

tion of ocular motility (pseudopterygium, symblepharon), and blindness (in underdeveloped countries where surgery is unavailable) (**Fig. 4.7**).

◆ Differential Diagnosis

Trichiasis, distichiasis, dacryocystitis, trachoma, chemical burns, autoimmune disorders (e.g., pemphigoid)

◆ Management

Treatment varies with the cause of recurrent conjunctivitis. Until surgery can be performed, botulinum toxin injections provide immediate temporary relief of spastic entropion by weakening the pretarsal orbicularis oculi muscle. Dacryocystorrhinostomy is performed in complete obstruction of lacrimal pathways. Treat complications when necessary (e.g., topical antibiotic drops and ointments for infectious conjunctivitis). Provide extraocular lubrication with gels and ointments to reduce the risk of abrasions.

Giant Papillary Conjunctivitis

Papillae may be present in an otherwise healthy person. Papillae are generally present in the superior lid tarsal conjunctiva, most often papillae are due to an intense allergic response, either contact (contact lens users, as part of a Gell-Coombs type 1 immunoglobulin E–mediated hypersensitivity reaction) or spring allergy (vernal keratoconjunctivitis). Giant papillary conjunctivitis is a chronic reversible inflammatory condition. In the presence of giant papillae consider the following:

◆ Vernal conjunctivitis
◆ Atopic keratoconjunctivitis
◆ Giant papillary conjunctivitis of contact lenses
◆ Giant papillae of prostheses, corneal scleral shields
◆ Ends of nylon sutures, cyanoacrylate glue, extruded scleral buckles

◆ Presentation

Patients present with itching, red eyes, foreign body sensation, mucous discharge, and the presence of giant papillae at slit-lamp examination (cobblestone aspect), usually in prostheses or contact lenses wearers (associated with use of all types

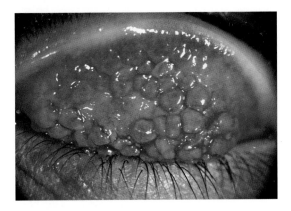

Fig. 4.8   Giant papillae. Vernal conjunctivitis.

of contact lenses—hard, hydrogel, scleral, prosthetic, etc.). The condition can be more aggressive in children, with lid swelling and pseudoptosis of the superior lid (**Fig. 4.8**).

◆ **Differential Diagnosis**

Atopic conjunctivitis, vernal conjunctivitis

◆ **Management**

Discontinue contact lens or prosthesis wear for at least 3 to 4 weeks. Most patients do not require more aggressive treatment. Topical mast cell–stabilizing solutions, antihistamines, and topical steroids (drops and ointments) can be used. Exceptionally, giant papillae may require steroid depot injection at the tarsus. Silver nitrate or radiosurgery surgical curettage of large/giant papillae may be useful in some cases (e.g., corneal ulceration). Plasmapheresis has been successfully used as adjunct therapy for patients with high immunoglobulin E levels (e.g., vernal conjunctivitis). Encouraging the patient to replace contact lenses frequently, use preservative-free lens solution, and increase lens hygiene all are good preventive measures.

◆ **Cicatrizing Disorders**

Ocular Cicatricial Pemphigoid

Cicatricial pemphigoid is an autoimmune disorder of unknown etiology, where circulating antibodies and complement bind to the basement membrane of mucosal tissues. It is a chronic, bilateral, papillary cicatrizing conjunctivitis (**Fig. 4.9**).

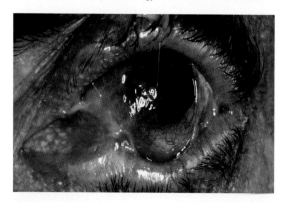

Fig. 4.9 Benign pemphigoid.

◆ **Presentation**

◆ *Age of presentation*: Aged adults (rarely seen in children)
◆ *Sex*: Women are affected twice as frequently as men.
◆ *Main early feature*: Chronic bilateral papillary cicatrizing conjunctivitis
◆ *Ocular findings*:
  ◆ Conjunctival hyperemia with dry eye symptoms, tearing, itching, photophobia, foreign body sensations
  ◆ Discharge (i.e., catarrhal, mucous, membranous)
  ◆ Eyelids manifest trichiasis, distichiasis, meibomian gland dysfunction, blepharitis
  ◆ Conjunctiva manifests papillae, follicles, keratinization, subepithelial fibrosis, conjunctival keratinization with foreshortening of the fornices and symblepharon and/or ankyloblepharon (end stage, immobilizes the eye)
  ◆ Cornea manifests superficial punctate keratitis, epithelial defect, ulcerations, neovascularization, keratinization, stromal opacities, perforation (pseudotrachoma)

◆ **Differential Diagnosis**

Chlamydial infections (trachoma, inclusion conjunctivitis), atopic keratoconjunctivitis, adenoviral conjunctivitis, long-term ocular medication (old antiglaucoma medications, e.g., epinephrine), chemical (alkali) or thermal burns, radiation exposure (therapeutic or not), Sjögren syndrome, sarcoidosis, dermatobullous disorders (toxic epidermal necrolysis, congenital ichthyosiform erythroderma, epidermolysis bullosa), erythema multiforme, *Corynebacterium diphtheriae* conjunctivitis, epithelioma

◆ **Management**

◆ No topical agent is really effective in stopping activity (dexamethasone ointment may help). Best controlled with systemic therapy.
◆ To slow disease progression try the following:
  ◆ Subconjunctival steroid injections such as triamcinolone (Trigon, Bristol-Myers Squibb, New York) or betamethasone (Celestone, Schering Corp., Kenilworth, NJ). We use prolonged-release betamethasone, injecting as much as possible, subconjunctivally (Celestone-Cronodose, Schering Corp., Kenilworth, NJ the strongest "depot" steroid).

◆ Abundant artificial tears and topical lubricants in patients with dry eye symptoms
◆ Steroid ointments (e.g., dexamethasone ointment, two to four times daily)
◆ Systemic immunosuppressive therapy, usually continued for 9 to 12 months. Must be controlled by a specialist in immunosuppressive therapy (e.g., diaminodiphenylsulfone or cyclophosphamide + systemic prednisone)
◆ Systemic corticosteroids for severely inflamed eyes that do not respond to immunosuppression alone
◆ Treat complications such as epilation of an aberrant lash (mechanical, laser, cryodestruction), punctal occlusion for dry eye, or lid surgery for entropion.

Stevens-Johnson Syndrome

Stevens-Johnson syndrome is an acute hypersensitivity reaction consisting of an inflammatory vesiculobullous reaction of the skin and mucous membrane. Immune complex deposition is incited by medications, including sulfonamides, anticonvulsants, aspirin, penicillin, isoniazid, diamox (acetazolamide), and many more, and sometimes infectious organisms (herpes simplex virus, streptococci, adenovirus, mycoplasma).

◆ Presentation

There is an acute onset of fever, rash, red eyes, malaise, arthralgias, and respiratory tract symptoms. Classic "target" skin lesions (maculopapules with a red center and a white surround on an erythematous base) are concentrated on the hands and feet. Other symptoms include ulcerative stomatitis and hemorrhagic lip crusting. The mortality rate is 10 to 33%.

Ocular signs include mucopurulent or pseudomembranous conjunctivitis, episcleritis, and iritis in the acute phase. Late complications include conjunctival scarring or symblepharon, trichiasis, eyelid deformities, tear deficiency, corneal neovascularization, ulcer, perforation, or scarring.

◆ *Erythema multiforme major (Stevens-Johnson syndrome)*: Immune complex deposition in the dermis with subepithelial vesiculobullous reaction of the skin and mucous membranes
◆ *Erythema multiforme minor*: Only skin involvement
◆ *Toxic epidermal necrolysis*: The most severe form, causing extensive intraepithelial vesiculobullous eruptions and epidermal necrosis; more common in children and immunosuppressed patients

◆ Differential Diagnosis

Ocular cicatricial pemphigoid, chemical burns, radiation, squamous cell carcinoma

◆ Management

Taking a history to rule out a precipitating factor is important. Slit-lamp examination, including eyelid eversion with examination of the fornices, conjunctival or corneal cultures, and consultation with internal medicine, is a must. Hospitalize the patient, remove the initiating factor, and provide supportive care as the mainstays of treatment.

Ocular management includes management of associated dry eye, iritis, topical steroids for ocular surface inflammation, daily pseudomembrane peel, and symblepharon lysis with a glass rod or moistened cotton swab, systemic or topical vitamin A, and intravenous immunoglobulin. To manage the late complications penetrating keratoplasty with stem cell transplant, and amniotic membrane transplant, or permanent keratoprosthesis may be required.

Dry-Eye Syndrome

Most dry eyes are multifactorial. The eye can be dry as a result of defective production of tears (e.g., age-related dry eye in menopausal women) or excessive evaporation (e.g., exophthalmos).

◆ **Presentation**

◆ *Symptoms*: Foreign body sensation, sensation of ocular dryness and grittiness (initially at the end of the day and later throughout the whole day), hyperemia and ocular irritation (exacerbated by smoky or dry environments, indoor heating systems, prolonged reading, or use of computers), mucous discharge, excessive tearing (secondary to reflex secretion)
◆ *Signs*: Red eyes, conjunctival hyperemia, decreased tear meniscus, increased debris in the tear film, superficial punctate keratopathy (with fluorescein, lissamine green, and/or rose bengal positive staining), mucous plaques and discharge, corneal filaments (severe cases), corneal epithelial defects or ulcers (in more severe cases) (**Fig. 4.10**).

◆ **Differential Diagnosis**

Any conjunctivitis (especially toxic forms, which are more difficult to differentiate). Careful history and workup should help to establish the origin of the dry eye (e.g., air conditioning, Sjögren syndrome)

◆ **Management**

True dry eye cannot be cured, but eye sensitivity can be lessened and measures taken so the eyes remain healthy by means of artificial tears or tear substitutes. No contact lens patient or glaucoma trabeculectomized patient should be out of artificial tear lubrication or tear substitutes!

◆ *First step*: Supplemental lubrication (mild and moderate keratitis sicca)
    ◆ *Artificial tears*: Preferably preservative-free artificial tears (drops 4 to 14 times a day, depending on the severity of the case). Our preferred ocular lubricant is sodium hyaluronate (0.18 to 0.4%).

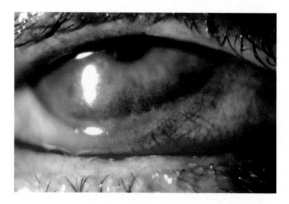

Fig. 4.10 Dry eye, lagophthalmos, corneal and conjunctival rose bengal staining.

◆ *Viscous artificial tear drops or gels*: However, they temporarily blur the vision.
◆ *Lubricating ointments*: For more severe cases (generally reserved to bedtime, because vision blur lasts minutes or hours). Not to be used with contact lenses.
◆ *In severe cases*: Use a patch with lubricating ointment at night.
◆ *In case of abundant mucus*: Remove the mucous and add 10% N-acetylcysteine, three to four times daily.
◆ *Artificial tear insert (e.g., Lacrisert, Aton Pharma, Inc., Lawrenceville, NJ)*: Place into the inferior cul-de-sac every morning.
◆ *Special goggles, moisture chamber glasses*: To reduce evaporation and retain humidity around the globe.
◆ *In case of suspected inflammation or in case of unsatisfactory results*: Try topical steroids (before cyclosporine).
◆ *Treat any associated abnormalities*: (e.g., in blepharitis, suppress inflammation with topical steroids and local antibiotics, and/or systemic tetracyclines)
◆ *Intermediate step*:
  ◆ *Temporary punctal occlusion*: With collagen (dissolvable) or silicone (permanent) plugs in case of severe aqueous tear deficiency (to preserve endogenous water)
  ◆ *In-office cauterization of the inferior lacrimal puncti*: If the patient is satisfied with temporal occlusion results
  ◆ *Minimize exposure*: Consider tarsorrhaphy or botulinum-toxin-induced ptosis.
◆ *Last step*: Surgical treatment (only for very severe cases, with ulceration or corneal perforation)
  ◆ *Closure of perforation or descemetocele*: Cyanoacrylate tissue adhesive
  ◆ *Corneal or corneoscleral patch*: For an impending or frank perforation (amniotic membrane, fascia lata)
  ◆ *Lateral temporary tarsorrhaphy*: For example, after facial nerve paralysis, after trigeminal nerve lesions, or for severe exophthalmos secondary to thyroid disease
  ◆ *Conjunctival flap:* Aids in preventing corneal melt and perforation by covering the cornea with conjunctiva

Several varieties of contact lenses can aid in the treatment of dry eye. Hard contacts may stimulate reflex tearing and thus increase the volume of tears. Some hard scleral contact lenses may be beneficial by preventing evaporation from a large portion of the ocular surface. The U.S. Food and Drug Administration has approved one type of contact lens (Proclear Toric XR lens, CooperVision, Fairport, NY) with an indication for dry eyes. This is a soft lens that has some unique properties. It has a high water content like other soft lenses, but it also has a component that retains water better than most other soft lenses. This reduces the dehydration that occurs with most soft contact lenses. Clinical studies have demonstrated improvement in comfort and signs of dryness on the surface of the eye with this contact lens when compared with a group of other lenses with which it was tested. Nevertheless, contact lenses alone have no place in the treatment of dry eyes; concomitant use of artificial teardrops (and periodic checkups) is essential.

◆ In some cases, small punctal plugs may be inserted in the inferior lacrimal punctum to slow drainage and loss of tears.
◆ *Cyclosporine 0.05% ophthalmic emulsion (Restasis, Allergan, Inc., Irvine, CA)*: Can be used to relieve dry eyes caused by suppressed tear production secondary to ocular inflammation. Safety for use in children and during pregnancy has not been established.
◆ *Autologous serum*: It has a beneficial effect on corneal epithelium (20% autologous serum diluted in normal saline).

◆ *Tetracyclines*: Traditionally used as antibiotics, they also have important antiinflammatory properties. Very useful (doxycycline) in treating acne rosacea dry eye. Tetracyclines are also effective against recurrent corneal erosions and phlyctenular keratoconjunctivitis.
◆ *Oral pilocarpine (Salagen, Novartis Pharmaceuticals UK Ltd., Surrey, UK)*: Initially used in xerostomia (salivary gland dysfunction, common after irradiation of the neck in oncology), it has been found useful in severe xerophthalmia by stimulating tear secretion (5 to 10 mg/8 h). Good results are seen in Sjögren syndrome after a few weeks of treatment.
◆ *Salivary gland transplantation into the inferior tarsal conjunctiva*: Has been reported to be useful in dry-eye conditions with severe permanent lacrimal gland dysfunctions (not useful in Sjögren syndrome). Technically complex.

◆ Symblepharon

Symblepharon is an adhesion between the palpebral conjunctiva and the bulbar conjunctiva or cornea. Symblepharon is usually the result of a trauma (surgery, chemical or radiation burns) or superficial eye inflammation (erythema multiforme, trachoma, burns, pemphigoid, Stevens-Johnson syndrome).

◆ Presentation

Symptoms include adhesion between the palpebral conjunctiva and the bulbar conjunctiva or cornea, lid deformities, functional lacrimal occlusion and tearing, entropion, and distichiasis (**Fig. 4.11**).

◆ Differential Diagnosis

Diagnosis is apparently clinical and is seldom confused with other disease entities.

◆ Management

Treatment is often frustrating, and progressive scarring cannot be completely controlled or reversed. Growth prevention includes breaking early adhesions with a rectal thermometer twice a day and steroid ointments. Conformers can be tried. Surgical Z-plasty with amniotic membrane or mucosal graft can be tried. The use of

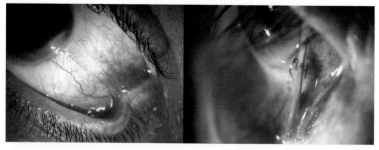

A   B

Fig. 4.11 Symblepharon: **(A)** between bulbar and palpebral conjunctiva; **(B)** at the lateral canthal angle.

amniotic membrane can be beneficial in that it facilitates epithelialization, maintains normal epithelial phenotype (with goblet cells when performed on the conjunctiva), and effectively helps in reducing inflammation, vascularization, and scarring. Immunosuppressant therapies (methotrexate, cyclophosphamide, cyclosporine, azathioprine, etc.) can help in the acute episodes of the illness. In late cicatricial stages, treat collateral effects such as dry eye syndrome, and punctal occlusion.

◆ Pinguecula, Pterygium, and Lipoid Degeneration

Pinguecula

Pingueculae are the most common benign conjunctival tumors. They usually affect middle-aged individuals but can also be found in children and young people, especially those with dyslipidemia. Pingueculae have no sex or racial predilection. They seem related to chronic exposure to the sun.

◆ Presentation

Pingueculae are usually asymptomatic, yellowish/whitish, slightly raised, interpalpebral lipid-like deposits in the nasal (more frequent) and temporal limbal conjunctiva. Uni- or bilateral (usually bilateral and asymmetrical), they may become vascularized and inflamed (pingueculitis). In a case of inflammation, patients experience foreign body sensation and conjunctival redness around the pinguecula, corneal punctate epitheliopathy, and corneal thinning secondary to dryness (dellen ulceration). These patients may complain of dry-eye symptoms and foreign body sensation (**Fig. 4.12A,B**).

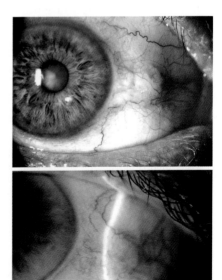

Fig. 4.12 **(A)** Pingueculae.
(*Continued on page 118*)

A

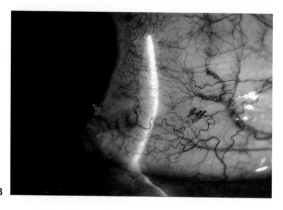

B

Fig. 4.12 (*Continued*) (**B**) Pinguecula and melanoma.

◆ Differential Diagnosis

Pterygium, conjunctival dermoid, conjunctival neoplasia (a unilateral, white, vascularized mass), phlyctenule, pannus, conjunctival retention cyst (a clear, fluid-filled sac), limbal follicles

◆ Management

- ◆ No treatment is necessary in cases with good lubrication results, which have a lower risk of pingueculae formation (preservative-free tear substitutes are preferable).
- ◆ Consider surgical partial or total resection under local anesthesia in the following:
  - ◆ Severe cases (giant pingueculae) where pterygium is present and interfering with vision
  - ◆ Chronically inflamed severe cases
  - ◆ Uncomfortable contact lens wear
  - ◆ Bad corneal lubrication with dellen formation
  - ◆ Cosmetic problems
- ◆ In the case of inflammation, use ocular lubrication and mild topical steroids (e.g., fluorometholone), with decongestants (e.g., naphazoline).
- ◆ Prevention is possible for people with occupations or hobbies that increase the risk of pinguecula (sailing, fishing, skiing, gardening, outdoor construction work). Sun goggles, ultraviolet-blocking coatings, or goggles that limit dust exposure are helpful.

Pterygia

Like pingueculae, pterygia have been related to exposure to ultraviolet light (both ultraviolet A [UV-A] and UV-B). Risk factors include living in subtropical and tropical climates, outdoor activities (e.g., golf, sailing, fishing), dry windy climates, dust, and fumes. A genetic predisposition has been described. There are two groups of pterygium patients: pterygia with minimal proliferation and atrophic appearance

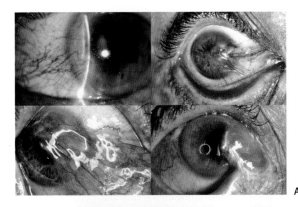

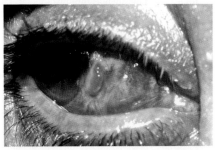

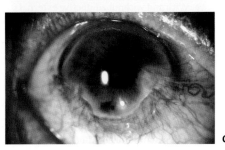

Fig. 4.13   **(A)** Pterygium. **(B)** Pterygium postsurgical papilloma. **(C)** Terrien's marginal degeneration.

(slow-growing pterygia, with low incidence of recurrence after excision) and elevated fibrovascular pterygia (rapid growth, aggressive clinical course, and high rate of recurrence after excision) (**Fig. 4.13A,B,C**)..

There is a predilection for males, and occurrence is more frequent in the nasal conjunctiva.

◆ Presentation

A triangular, fleshy, elevated mass of bulbar conjunctiva grows over the cornea within the interpalpebral fissure. Small pterygia are asymptomatic. They can become inflamed, with redness, foreign body sensation, and ocular irritation (dry-eye symptoms). In advanced cases, patients experience vision problems (astigmatism, progression over the visual axis), restriction of ocular motility, and blindness (in underdeveloped countries where surgery is unavailable).

◆ Differential Diagnosis

Pingueculae, amyloidal degeneration of the conjunctiva, pseudopterygium, neoplasia (e.g., carcinoma in situ, squamous cell carcinoma)

◆ Management

◆ Good intensive lubrication is essential.
◆ Topical steroids such as prednisolone acetate (Pred Forte, Allergan, Inc., Irvine, CA) 1%, three to four times daily and antihistamines provide relief of inflammation.
◆ Indications for surgery include the following:
  ◆ Cosmetic reasons
  ◆ Discomfort due to recurrent inflammation
  ◆ Before it encroaches on the pupillary area
◆ Multiple different surgical procedures work in the first group of pterygium patients (atrophic, slow growing), but none can be said to work satisfactorily in the second group of patients (fast growing, aggressive clinical course):
  ◆ Simple excision
  ◆ Simple excision and repair with conjunctiva autoplasty
  ◆ Simple excision and sliding flaps of conjunctiva
  ◆ With and without adjunctive external β radiation therapy (1000 to 2000 reps at limbus or thiotepa 1:2000 solution) and/or intraoperative topical mitomycin-C or postoperative 5-fluorouracil
  ◆ Primary excision plus free grafts of conjunctiva and limbal tissue (limbal autograft) or amniotic membrane: for aggressive or recurrent pterygia

Lipoid/Lipid Degeneration of the Cornea and Conjunctiva

Lipid degeneration of the cornea and conjunctiva may occur in primary or secondary form. The primary form is usually bilateral and more diffuse and is caused by lipid serum dyscrasias such as Tangier familial high-density lipoprotein deficiency or lecithin cholesterol acyltransferase deficiency. The secondary form is by far the most common form of this rare disease, is more localized, and is due to the presence of corneal blood vessels after ocular trauma or interstitial or herpetic keratitis.

◆ Presentation

White, yellow, or cream-colored dense opacification of the corneal stroma is seen in a diffuse or localized manner. Cholesterol crystals occur in the corneal or conjunctival stroma surrounding aberrant blood vessels. The conjunctival feeder vessels are dilated, and there are symptoms of dry eye (**Fig. 4.14**).

◆ Differential Diagnosis

Aspect at slit lamp is diagnostic. Rule out degenerated epithelioma.

Fig. 4.14 Cornea conjunctival lipoid degeneration.

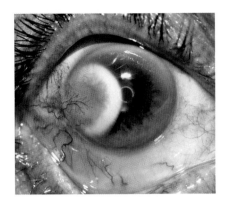

◆ Management

Treat the underlying condition to reduce the risk of progression (reduce fat serum levels). Attempt closing the feeder vessels with argon laser photocoagulation. Severe cases with affected pupillary area may require penetrating keratoplasty, although this degeneration may recur in the graft.

◆ Conjunctival Retention Cysts

Conjunctival lymphatic cysts are soft, translucent, and mobile. Large cysts may give dry eye or foreign body sensation (eye discomfort or tearing). A conjunctival cyst may reveal different possible origins and can be due to parasitic infestation (e.g., cisticercosis), which has to be ruled out when the patient has traveled to endemic regions, or it may be an accessory lacrimal gland, a posttraumatic inclusion cyst (of conjunctival epithelium), or simply a lymphatic cyst (the most common).

◆ Presentation

Soft, translucent, and mobile fluid-filled mass within the conjunctiva, alone or in groups, found at slit-lamp examination. More frequent in the bulbar conjunctiva and in the inferior tarsus or inferior cul-de-sac (**Fig. 4.15**).

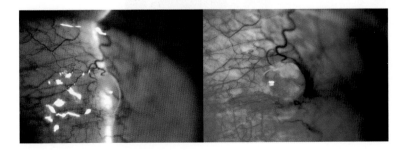

Fig. 4.15 Conjunctival lymphatic retention cyst.

◆ Differential Diagnosis

Cyst of malignant origin (rule out parasitic infestation and hematic dyscrasia)

◆ Management

These cysts need no treatment unless they cause persistent dry eye or foreign body sensation. Topical lubricants provide relief. Their wall can be easily broken inferiorly with a few shots of neodymium:yttrium-aluminum-garnet laser applied inferiorly on the cyst walls, with care to avoid conjunctival vessels. Postsurgical cyst can be excised.

◆ Superior Limbic Keratoconjunctivitis

This condition is of unknown etiology and associated with thyroid disease. In superior limbic keratoconjunctivitis, conjunctival laxity might induce inflammatory changes from mechanical trauma of hypertrophic papillae of the upper tarsal conjunctiva. It affects mainly adult women. A similar condition is found in soft contact lens wearers using thimerosal-preserved solutions.

◆ Presentation

Symptoms include tearing, burning, superior hyperemia, and foreign body sensation. Patients with filaments are extremely symptomatic. Inflammation of the superior bulbar conjunctiva results in edema with redundant conjunctiva. There is predominant involvement of the superior limbus, adjacent epithelial keratitis, and papillary hypertrophy of the upper tarsal conjunctiva. The inferior conjunctiva and cornea appear normal. The age range is 20 to 70 years. Occurrence is predominantly in females, is usually bilateral, and may be asymmetrical, with remissions and exacerbations. Dry eye is often present (**Fig. 4.16**).

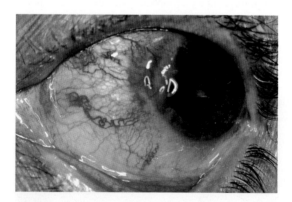

Fig. 4.16   Superior limbal keratoconjunctivitis.

◆ **Differential Diagnosis**

Clinical findings are diagnostic (inflammation of the superior bulbar conjunctiva with absolutely normal appearance of the inferior conjunctiva and cornea).

◆ **Management**

Conservative treatment offers only temporary relief of symptoms (pressure patching, Plano T bandage contact lens, Baush & Lomb Inc., St. Louis, MO). Silver nitrate (0.5 to 1.0% solution) is applied with a saturated cotton swab. It usually relieves symptoms for 1 month and can be repeated safely. Topical antihistamines and mast cell stabilizers (e.g., olopatadine hydrochloride 0.1%, ketotifen fumarate 0.025%, azelastine hydrochloride 0.05%) are helpful. Moisturizing drops and ointments provide only minimal relief. Cryotherapy and a surgical approach can be taken in recalcitrant cases involving resection or recession of the superior bulbar conjunctiva or in-office thermocauterization of the superior bulbar conjunctiva with a disposable ophthalmic cautery under topical anesthesia. The use of topical steroids is usually ineffective.

◆ Episcleritis

Episcleritis is a transient, self-limited inflammatory process of the episclera. Most episcleritis is idiopathic, but it can also be associated with systemic disorders such as rheumatoid arthritis, acne rosacea, and atopy.

◆ **Presentation**

There is an acute onset and diffuse or nodular ocular redness without irritation or pain. Inflamed episcleral vessels radiate posteriorly from the limbus (**Fig. 4.17A,B**).

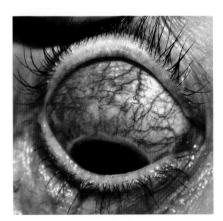

Fig. 4.17 **(A)** Episcleritis. (*Continued on page 124*)

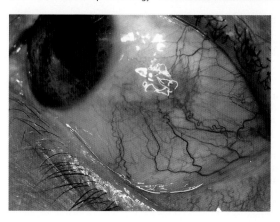

Fig. 4.17 *(Continued)* **(B)** Nodular episcleritis.

◆ Differential Diagnosis

Scleritis, uveitis, conjunctivitis

◆ Management

The condition is self-limited; no treatment is needed. Topical steroids or nonsteroidal antiinflammatory drugs (NSAIDs) or a combination of these can accelerate recovery. Vasoconstrictors and refrigerated artificial tears provide relief.

◆ Scleritis

Scleritis is a granulomatous inflammation of the sclera that may present in association with systemic diseases such as rheumatoid arthritis, systemic lupus erythematosus, polyarteritis nodosa, or Wegener granulomatosis. Scleritis can be self-limiting or can progress to a potentially blinding necrotizing process. Possible complications include scleral thinning (especially in recurrent scleritis), scleromalacia perforans, sclerosing keratitis, peripheral corneal melting, uveitis, cataract, macula edema, choroidal granulomas, and retinal detachment. Posterior scleritis occurs much less frequently than anterior scleritis and may extend into the anterior segment of the eye. In cases of necrotizing scleritis, infection has to be ruled out.

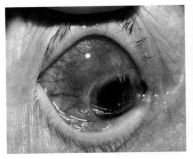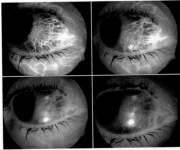

Fig. 4.18   Scleritis table.

◆ Presentation

There is severe ocular pain with or without decreased vision (suspect posterior involvement if vision is compromised). Onset of scleritis is more gradual than is seen in episcleritis and is accompanied by uni- or bilateral red eye, lacrimation, and photophobia (**Fig. 4.18**).

◆ Differential Diagnosis

Conjunctivitis, uveitis, episcleritis

◆ Management

Management includes systemic NSAIDs (e.g., indomethacin, ibuprofen, naproxen), topical steroids (e.g., betamethasone, dexamethasone) and systemic oral steroids (oral steroids preferred over topical), and immunosuppressant therapies (e.g., methotrexate, cyclophosphamide, cyclosporine, azathioprine). Systemic treatment works better than topical, which has to be considered accessory to a systemic antiinflammatory regimen.

◆ Dilated Vessels

Dilated Vessels and Ocular Vein Varicosities

Dilated vessels are commonly seen in healthy patients, especially women with venous insufficiency. They may be a sign of venous congestion or raised episcleral pressure, either due to carotid cavernous fistula or to any orbit expansive process or inflammatory disease of the eye. Dilated episcleral sentinel vessels can be present in cases of malignant melanoma of the choroid or ciliary body.

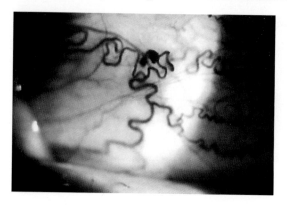

Fig. 4.19 Dilated vessels.

◆ Presentation

Presentation is asymptomatic. Foreign body sensation occurs in the case of varicosities. Other signs and symptoms of red eye or orbit expansive process may also be seen. Thyroid disease presents with dilated vessels, mainly over the external rectus muscles (**Fig. 4.19**).

◆ Differential Diagnosis

Any cause of red eye (conjunctivitis, idiopathic raised episcleral pressure, venous insufficiency, carotid cavernous sinus fistula, episcleritis, scleritis, chronic irritation, glaucoma surgery)

◆ Management

No treatment is needed if the condition is idiopathic. Varicosities can be successfully reduced using argon laser photocoagulation. The occasional use of vasoconstrictors improves cosmetics but there is no definitive treatment. Treat the concomitant illness.

Dilated Episcleral Vessels in Sturge-Weber Syndrome

Sturge-Weber syndrome is a rare neurological disorder present at birth, characterized by a birthmark (usually on the face) known as a port-wine stain caused by an overabundance of capillaries around the trigeminal nerve beneath the surface of the face. Neurological problems arise due to a loss of nerve cells and calcification of tissue in the cerebral cortex of the brain on the same side of the body as the birthmark (angiomatosis of the central nervous system). Neurological symptoms include seizures that begin in infancy and may worsen with age. Convulsions usually happen on the side of the body opposite the birthmark and vary in severity. There may be muscle weakness on the same side. Some children will have developmental delays and mental retardation. Sturge-Weber syndrome rarely affects other body organs.

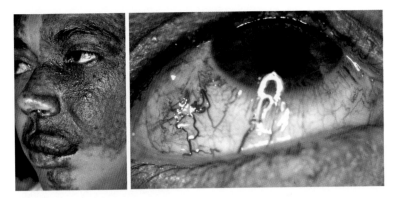

Fig. 4.20   Sturge-Weber syndrome table.

◆ Presentation

Characteristic facial birthmark (can vary in color from light pink to deep purple). Most patients with angioma that affects the superior lid have glaucoma at birth or will develop it later. Dilated episcleral vessels are seen, along with buphthalmos, seizures, convulsions, muscle weakness, mental retardation or learning disabilities, and possible developmental delay (**Fig. 4.20**).

◆ Differential Diagnosis

Facial angioma without neurological manifestations, other causes of elevated episcleral pressure (e.g., thyroid ophthalmopathy, thrombosis of the cavernous sinus, carotid-cavernous fistula)

◆ Management

Treat the symptoms. Treat increased intraocular pressure with eyedrops (avoid miotics). Surgery can be performed on serious cases of glaucoma. Laser treatment can lighten or remove the facial birthmark. Anticonvulsant medicines are used to control seizures. Physical therapy is helpful in children with muscle weakness.

Carotid Cavernous Sinus Fistula

Carotid cavernous fistulas are uni- or bilateral abnormal communications (shunts) of the carotid arteries directly or indirectly into the veins of the cavernous sinus. They are frequently caused by trauma, although they can be spontaneous in menopausal women. Depending on the amount of blood injected into the sinuses, they can produce different amounts of neuro-ophthalmological manifestations.

◆ Presentation

Patients present with arterialized dilated vessels of the conjunctiva and orbit, unilateral or bilateral, proptosis, lid edema, papilledema, retinal edema with hemorrhages, uveitis, secondary glaucoma associated with elevated venous pressure, anterior segment ischemia, and iris atrophy. There can also be visual loss and dysfunction of the extraocular muscles. Pulsating exophthalmia occurs in advanced (i.e., high-flow) cases. Patient refers to an audible sound that follows the heart rate. Cavernous sinus syndrome (cranial nerve II, IV, and VI palsy) and Tolosa-Hunt syndrome may also present (**Fig. 4.21A,B**).

◆ **Differential Diagnosis**

Cavernous sinus thrombosis, dural sinus arteriovenous fistula, cavernous sinus arteriovenous malformations, orbital pseudotumor, thyroid orbitopathy, orbital amyloidosis, orbital tumor, orbital cellulitis, mucormycosis

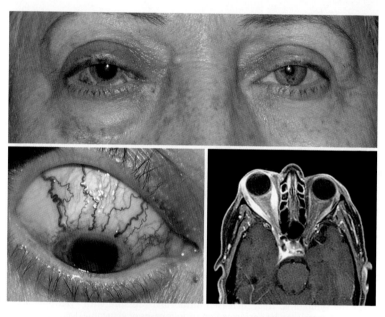

A

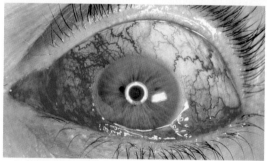

B

Fig. 4.21 **(A)** Carotid cavernous fistula. **(B)** Carotid cavernous fistula.

◆ Management

Neurosurgery by a neuroradiologist (detachable balloon or metallic coil embolization) accomplishes reversal of ocular manifestations in patients with vision at risk or patients with intolerable symptoms (high-flow shunts). Low-flow shunts (mainly traumatic) spontaneously occlude with time. The gamma knife can be used where available.

◆ Pigmented Conjunctival Lesions

Ocular or Oculodermal Melanocytosis (Congenital Melanosis Oculi)

Ocular Melanocytosis

This nonheritable congenital hyperpigmentation of the eye has increased frequency in whites. Pathology shows an increased number of melanocytes in the affected tissues. The condition can progress with the use of topical prostaglandin analogues (e.g., latanoprost) used to treat glaucoma.

◆ Presentation

Presentation includes increased gray or bluish pigmentation of the globe (sclera and episclera) that is usually unilateral (**Fig. 4.22**).

◆ Differential Diagnosis

Primary acquired melanosis (affects the conjunctiva only and other mucoses), oculodermal melanocytosis (nevus of Ota), nevus, melanomas, pigmented deposits, foreign body iron deposits

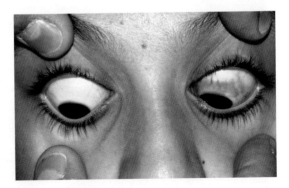

Fig. 4.22 Ocular melanocytosis.

◆ Management

No treatment is needed. Careful periodic ocular examinations are required because of the increased risk of uveal melanomas in affected individuals.

Oculodermal Melanocytosis

This condition is caused by diffuse distribution of proliferated melanocytes and is more common in Asians and blacks. It is associated with ipsilateral glaucoma.

◆ Presentation

Asymptomatic. Unilateral facial and/or blue-gray pigmentation of the globe, usually following the ipsilateral distribution of the trigeminal nerve (V1 and V2) (**Fig. 4.23**).

◆ Differential Diagnosis

Primary acquired melanosis, nevus, melanomas, pigmented deposits, foreign body iron deposits, facial angioma

◆ Management

No treatment is needed. Rule out glaucoma, retinitis pigmentosa, and congenital cataract. Oculodermal melanocytosis rarely undergoes malignant transformation.

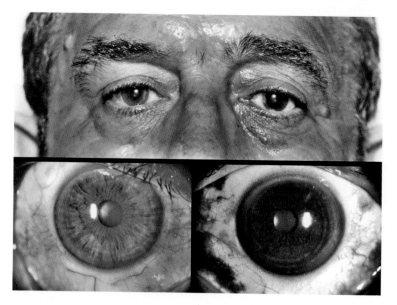

Fig. 4.23 Oculodermal melanocytosis. Heterochromia.

Conjunctival Pigmentations[1]

Melanocytic benign conjunctival lesions are very common, especially in darker-skinned individuals, including blacks or African Americans, Hispanics, and Gitanos, in the limbal area or caruncle. Presentation greatly differs from one patient to another. The lesions have no malignant potential, although nevi very rarely give rise to malignancy (junctional and compound nevi). Chronic use of topical epinephrine (as a cosmetic), silver-containing compounds (argyrosis), retained iron foreign body, atabrine, tetracyclines, clofamicine, imbibed mascara granules, radiation, hormones (pregnancy, Addison disease), chemicals (arsenic, thorazine), and some chronic disorders (like trachoma or xeroderma pigmentosum) are potential causes of pigmentation increase (darkening of the lesions). Nevertheless, the most common cause of pigmentation increase is the topical use of prostaglandin analogues to lower intraocular pressure. Conjunctival pigmentation is no sign of malignancy.

◆ Presentation

Conjunctival benign epithelial melanosis presents as a flat brownish pigmentation seen especially in blacks or African Americans, in the limbal area or caruncle. Conjunctival pigmented lesions close to the lacrimal gland can be benign, but always consider malignancy because malignancy may be more extensive than is clinically apparent. Suspect malignancy if pigmentation increases in parallel to surface growth (**Fig. 4.24A–D**).

◆ Differential Diagnosis

Conjunctival melanoma

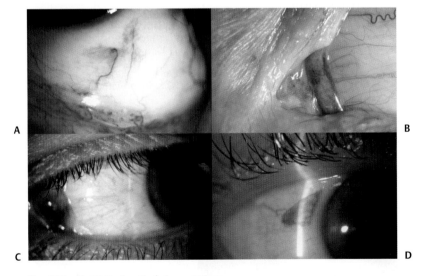

A B C D

Fig. 4.24 **(A–D)** Conjunctival pigmentations.

---

[1]Nomenclature may be confusing, and classification is often controversial: we have used the most widely accepted names.

◆ Management

Use close observation and follow-up with photographic documentation. Fluorescein angiography may help to visualize feeder vessels in melanomas. In case of doubt, excisional biopsy should be performed.

Malignant Melanoma of the Conjunctiva

Malignant melanoma of the conjunctiva is rare, but it is the most common pigmented malignancy of the conjunctiva and accounts for 2% of all ocular malignancies. It is far less common than intraocular choroidal melanoma. It can appear in a previously healthy part of the conjunctiva (de novo, from melanocytic cells of the basal layer of conjunctiva, in ~20 to 25% of cases), from a preexisting conjunctival junctional or compound nevus (~20% of cases), from a primary acquired conjunctival melanosis (~60% of cases). The incidence of conjunctival melanoma is increasing among white men in a trend similar to that of skin melanoma. Conjunctival melanoma is probably related to sun exposure (**Fig. 4.25**).

◆ Presentation

Clinical presentation is variable, with a raised, pigmented or nonpigmented lesion (some have little or no pigment, which is rare) that grows and/or bleeds and/or fixates to the underlying tissues. Peripheral corneal infiltration is possible. Some grow around the limbus. Sometimes there is pigmentation of the lid margins or lid skin (rare, poor prognosis). Regional lymph nodes (parotid, preauricular, submandibular, and cervical) may be affected. Distant metastases are possible, with spread by the lymphatic vessels and bloodstream. Direct extension to the eyeball and orbit is possible if there is late diagnosis.

Suspect melanoma if

◆ a preexisting nevus grows or has increased vascularity
◆ a preexisting conjunctival nevus at the limbus has rapid vertical growth
◆ a preexisting nevus grows or has increasing nodularity or changes in pigmentation or bleeds, or develops inflammation
◆ a previously flat area of pigmentation develops nodular thickening
◆ there is local conjunctival increased vascularity (with or without a pigmented lesion)

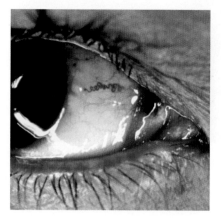

Fig. 4.25　Semilunar fold melanoma.

◆ the conjunctiva fixates to the sclera
◆ you observe hemorrhage in a pigmented lesion
◆ you observe an ulcerative area in the conjunctiva that does not heal with topical medication

◆ Differential Diagnosis

Benign pigmented lesions [nevus, melanosis, foreign body, pigmented deposits (chemicals, mascara granules)]. Suspect malignant melanoma in the case of a growing pigmented lesion. Not all conjunctival melanomas are pigmented; they can look like a squamous or sebaceous gland carcinoma, a papilloma, lymphoid hyperplasia, and even a pterygium. Metastatic tumor to the conjunctiva (extremely rare, e.g., secondary melanoma from cutaneous tumor).

◆ Management

Management depends on pathological staging [varies in different countries: clinical tumor, node, metastases (TNM) classification, pathological classification, and histopathological type and grade].

◆ Can be treated conservatively with the proton accelerator.
◆ Complete resection of tumor (with care to avoid tissue dissemination). Pathological examination is required at the time of excision.
  ◆ Conjunctival melanomas at the limbus: Absolute alcohol epitheliectomy + wide local resection (partial lamellar scleroconjunctivotenonectomy with a 2–3 mm clear zone) + cryotherapy of the bed and borders of excision
  ◆ Palpebral conjunctival melanomas (or fornical): Surgical resection with absolute alcohol treatment to the scleral base and cryotherapy to the surrounding conjunctiva
  ◆ Large invasive melanomas: Orbital exenteration? (almost always metastases have already occurred at the time of treatment). We prefer the proton accelerator.
◆ A conservative approach with topical mitomycin-C is under research.
◆ Adjunctive radiotherapy and/or chemotherapy may be needed.
◆ Life-long close observation follow-up with palpation of lymph nodes (three to four times yearly)

◆ Blue Sclera and Scleral Staphyloma

Blue Sclera in Osteogenesis Imperfecta

Blue sclerae in infancy and childhood reflect either an abnormal thinness of the sclera or an increased scleral transparency. The underlying uveal pigment produces the blue-gray appearance. Slight blue sclerae are common in neonates, particularly if they are premature. It can be considered a normal variant in the first several months of life. In case of persisting pronounced blueness, ophthalmological evaluation is needed to rule out the presence of elevated intraocular pressure (IOP). Pediatric and orthopedic evaluation is needed to rule out inherited diseases responsible for the blue-tinted sclerae, such as osteogenesis imperfecta.

Osteogenesis imperfecta is a rare inherited congenital disorder with extreme bone fragility, caused by mutations in the genes that codify for type I procollagen (*COL1A1* and *COL1A2*). At least four types of osteogenesis imperfecta have been

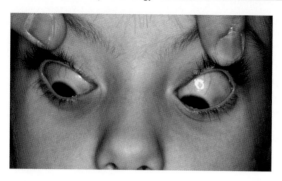

Fig. 4.26 Osteogenesis imperfecta. Blue sclera.

described. The age when fractures begin varies widely. Patients with mild forms may present with fractures in infancy or may not have fractures until adulthood. The more severe cases may have fractures in utero.

◆ Presentation

Presentation is asymptomatic; there are no ocular symptoms. In patients with osteogenesis imperfecta, the sclera can be blue or white (**Fig. 4.26**).

◆ Differential Diagnosis

Blue sclera also may occur in other disorders, such asalkaptonuria, progeria, cleidocranial dysplasia, cutis laxa (pseudoxanthoma elasticum), Ehlers-Danlos syndrome, Marfan syndrome, Cheney syndrome, Menkes syndrome, and pyknodysostosis. Some high or extreme myopes may present with "blue-sclera" due to scleral thinning.

◆ Management

No ocular treatment is needed. Other systemic investigations and treatment are to be done. Genetic counseling is helpful.

Blue Sclera and Scleral Staphylomas

Congenital glaucoma in an infant or a young child is characterized by three main symptoms: excessive tearing (epiphora), sensitivity to light (photophobia), and spasms or squeezing of the eyelids (blepharospasm). There are both primary (maldevelopment of anterior chamber angle) and secondary forms with diverse causes. The condition is more frequently bilateral. Its severity is variable (**Fig. 4.27**).

Whether enlargement of the eye occurs or not depends on the age of onset of the glaucoma. The eye being distensible in infancy, elevated intraocular pressure may result in eye enlargement (buphthalmos). Corneal enlargement can also occur in the early first years, and the sclera can expand during the first decade. Scleral thinning (ectasia) and bulging bluish areas of thinned sclera lined by uveal tract (staphyloma) can also be seen in advanced cases. The corneal horizontal diameter also increases. Corneal enlargement results in ruptures in the Descemet membrane (Haab striae).

Fig. 4.27 Staphylomas in congenital glaucoma buphthalmos.

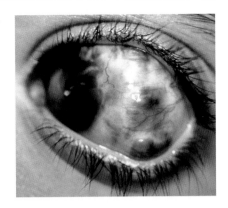

◆ Presentation

Epiphora, photophobia, and blepharospasm are seen in a newborn or young infant. Buphthalmos, ectasia, staphylomas, and increased corneal diameter may also be present. Corneal edema or Haab striae may be seen at slit-lamp examination, (which may not always easy to perform in babies).

◆ Differential Diagnosis

With causes of blue sclera (e.g., osteogenesis imperfecta), neoplasias, and causes of congenital glaucoma:

- ◆ Dysgenesis of the iris, angle, and peripheral cornea with or without systemic abnormalities (e.g., Rieger anomaly syndrome, Axenfeld anomaly syndrome, Peter anomaly, aniridia, Marfan syndrome, Weill-Marchesani syndrome)
- ◆ Phakomatoses (e.g., neurofibromatosis, Sturge-Weber syndrome)
- ◆ Metabolic disease (e.g., oculocerebrorenal syndrome or Lowe disease, homocystinuria)
- ◆ Inflammatory (e.g., rubella, juvenile xanthogranuloma)
- ◆ Chromosomal deletion/duplication (e.g., Turner syndrome, trisomy 13–15)

◆ Management

Topical medical treatment is used to reduce IOP until surgery can be safely performed. Beta-blockers and miotics rarely work (though they may help). Carbonic anhydrase inhibitors can be used to help reduce corneal edema and allow a better inspection of anterior chamber structures. Modern drugs (e.g., prostaglandin analogues, brimonidine tartrate) can be tried, although their use in infantile glaucoma is not currently accepted.

Surgery aims at reduction of complications of IOP increase (e.g., amblyopia, staphylomas, optic nerve atrophy). We use our own surgical technique, called Simon's pectinotomy (surgical ablation of trabeculodysgenetic tissue–iridopectineal tissue by means of an instrument of our own design), combined, or not, with a goniotomy, trabeculotomy, or trabeculectomy. Glaucomatous cupping in infants has proven to be reversible when successful surgery is performed early.

◆ Conjunctivalization of the Cornea

Dense leukomas, severe scarring, and conjunctivalization of the cornea can be found after bone marrow transplantation, severe corneal or intraocular infections, or ocular radiation therapy. A similar condition can be the result of severe chemical burns or autoimmune disorders.

◆ Presentation

Severe scarring, leukoma, and conjunctivalization of the globe are seen (**Fig. 4.28**).

◆ Differential Diagnosis

Phthisis bulbi, atrofia bulbi, endophthalmitis sequelae, Stevens-Johnson syndrome, erythema multiforme, chemical burns

◆ Management

Palliative treatment to alleviate discomfort consists of surface lubrication with nonpreservative artificial tears or ointments, punctal occlusion, and humidifiers or moisture chambers to decrease tear film evaporation. Surgical tarsorrhaphy is used for intractable dry eye. Mydriatics and covering the globe with amniotic membrane can provide relief. Cosmetic prosthesis after enucleation is performed if needed.

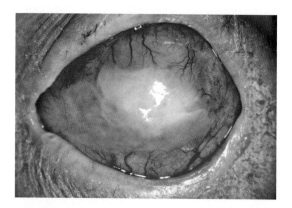

Fig. 4.28 Massive corneal neovascularization and opacification following radiotherapy.

◆ Conjunctival Metaplasia in Ectropion

Metaplasia of the conjunctiva is an uncommon disease where the conjunctival mucosa changes into a skinlike surface due to chronic exposure of the conjunctiva to air and light. We also describe keratinization of the conjunctiva.

◆ Presentation

Conjunctival hyperemia and lacrimation are seen in a patient suffering from intense chronic lid eversion (ectropion). There is also foreign body sensation (**Fig. 4.29**).

◆ Differential Diagnosis

Squamous cell carcinoma of the conjunctiva

◆ Management

Intense lubrication with eye drops, gels, and ointments until surgery of ectropion is performed.

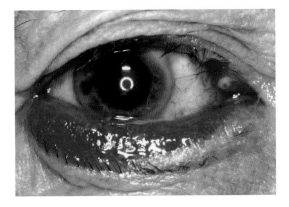

Fig. 4.29   Conjunctival metaplasia in ectropion.

◆ Chemosis

Chemosis consists of conjunctival and subconjunctival edema. In general, chemosis is a nonspecific sign of eye irritation.

◆ Presentation

Liquid collection is seen under the conjunctiva. Sometimes the conjunctiva becomes so swollen that the eyes cannot close properly. Other signs and symptoms depend on the cause of chemosis (**Table 4.2**) (**Fig. 4.30A–C**).

◆ Differential Diagnosis

Any cause of chemosis (**Table 4.2**)

Table 4.2   Common Causes of Chemosis

Severe local inflammation:
  Gonococcus, viral or chlamydial conjunctivitis
  Allergic or hypersensitivity reaction
  Endophthalmitis
  Panophthalmia
  Local irritation
Trauma:
  Ruptured globe
  Posttrabeculectomy
  Postsurgical after scleral or vitreoretinal surgery
Generalized edema:
  Nephropathy (of any origin)
  Heart disease (congestive)
  Quincke edema
  Urticaria
  Myxedema
Venous congestion
  Cavernous sinus
  Orbital tumor
  Orbital cysts
Orbital inflammation:
  Orbital cellulitis
  Endocrine thyroid disease (thyrotoxicosis)
Drugs:
  Atropine
  Epinephrine
  Glaucoma medications
  Trifluridine
Parasites:
  Trichinella spiralis dissemination

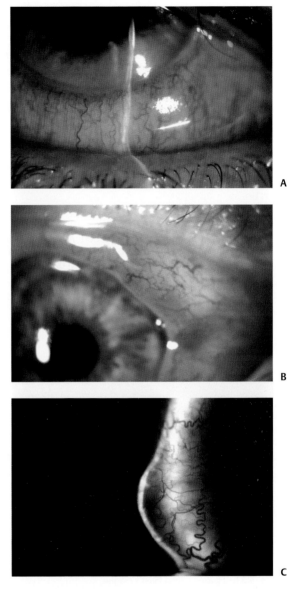

Fig. 4.30   **(A)** Mild chemosis. **(B)** Massive chemosis. **(C)** Massive chemosis.

◆ Management

Treat the underlying condition (e.g., treat allergic conjunctivitis if chemosis is due to an allergic reaction). Chemosis after trabeculectomy is highly desirable and does not need to be treated: the novice may be tempted to perform early surgical revision of the filtering bleb, which is only necessary if atalamia with corneal edema is present.

◆ Hyaline Pillat Scleral Plaque

Pillat scleral plaque is an involutive thinning of the sclera, with hyaline degeneration, resulting from traction forces of extraocular muscles, especially the lateral rectus.

◆ Presentation

A grayish punched-out area is seen anterior to the insertion of the lateral rectus muscles. Slit-lamp examination is diagnostic. There is no clinical manifestation, but the plaques are visible in older patients (**Fig. 4.31**).

◆ Differential Diagnosis

Scleromalacia, melanosis bulbi, scleral ectasia, staphylomas

◆ Management

No treatment is needed.

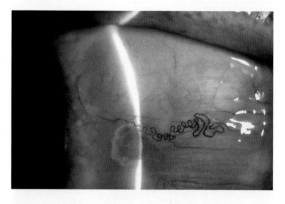

Fig. 4.31   Hyaline scleral Pillat's plaque.

5 Cornea

W. Barry Lee and Ivan R. Schwab

◆ Cornea Infections

Herpes Simplex Virus

Herpes simplex virus (HSV) is a DNA virus that involves various stages of infection, including a primary systemic infection, an inactive latent stage, and a recurrent infectious stage following reactivation of the latent viral state. Unilateral infection is most common, but bilateral infection can occur in up to 10% of cases (more likely in atopic individuals) (**Fig. 5.1A,B**).

◆ Presentation

◆ *Primary infection stage*: Upper respiratory infection symptoms with or without prodromal signs of fever, malaise, and fatigue. Associated preauricular lymphadenopathy is not uncommon. Ocular involvement in the primary stage most commonly involves vesicles on the periorbital skin with or without a follicular blepharoconjunctivitis. Infection may rarely present in the conjunctiva or cornea with a follicular conjunctivitis and punctate keratitis or dendritic keratitis. In the latent stage, the virus remains dormant in the sensory nerve ganglia.

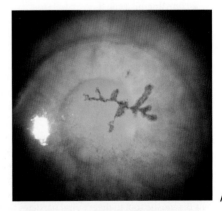

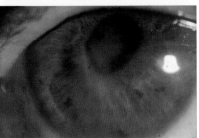

Fig. 5.1 **(A)** Corneal dendrite highlighted by rose bengal from herpes simplex virus (HSV) intraepithelial keratitis. **(B)** Corneal scar and iris atrophy from HSV stromal keratitis.

- *Recurrent infection stage*: The virus travels down nerve axons to sensory nerve endings to infect the ocular surface. Corneal findings include the following:
    - Punctate epithelial keratopathy
    - *Dendritic intraepithelial keratitis*: An ulcer of the epithelium with thin, branching figures and terminal bulbs at the end of each branch with swollen borders
    - *Immune stromal keratitis*: Ground-glass–like corneal haze, scarring, and potential thinning with late neovascularization and lipid deposition. The epithelium is often intact but may break down in severe cases with progression to necrotizing keratitis.
    - *Necrotizing stromal keratitis*: A corneal ulcer with an epithelial defect, stromal infiltration, thinning, and necrosis. There is a high risk for perforation.
    - *Marginal ulcer*: A perilimbal epithelial lesion with stromal infiltration, pannus, and thinning
    - *Neurotrophic ulcer*: A corneal ulcer resulting from corneal anesthesia from viral damage to sensory corneal nerves. Impaired corneal innervation leads to an ulcer with an epithelial defect containing smooth, rolled borders.
    - *Endothelitis*: Focal or disciform corneal stromal edema with endothelial keratic precipitate and anterior chamber cellular reaction

- **Differential Diagnosis**

- Differential diagnosis of dendritic epithelial keratitis:
    - Other viruses [herpes zoster virus, Epstein-Barr virus, epidemic keratoconjunctivitis (EKC)]
    - Healing epithelial defects
    - Soft contact lens wear
    - Tyrosinemia type II
    - *Acanthamoeba*
    - Rosacea
    - Superficial hypertrophic dendriform epitheliopathy (SHDE)
- Differential diagnosis of stromal keratitis
    - Herpes zoster
    - Bacterial keratitis
    - *Acanthamoeba*
    - Staphylococcal marginal keratitis (marginal ulcer cases)
    - Rosacea
    - Collagen vascular disease
    - Mooren ulcer (marginal ulcer cases)

- **Management**

Diagnosis is usually clinical, but scrapings can be performed with Giemsa stain or Papanicolaou smear. Polymerase chain reaction or antigen detection can be used as a diagnostic tool to detect viral particles from scrapings or culture.

- *Dendritic intraepithelial keratitis*: Debridement of dendrite may or may not be performed. Begin trifluridine 1%, one drop every 2 hours (nine times daily) or vidarabine ointment five times daily for 10 to 14 days. The Herpetic Eye Disease Studies (HEDS) found oral antivirals do not prevent the subsequent risk of stromal keratitis. Consider cycloplegic agents and avoid corticosteroids.
- *Immune stromal keratitis*: Antivirals with either oral agents (acyclovir, valacyclovir, or famciclovir) or topical trifluridine can be used in conjunction with topical corticosteroids in cases with severe stromal scarring and decreased visual acuity; however, topical antivirals do not penetrate intact epithelium

well; thus for deep stromal keratitis cases, oral agents may work best. The HEDS trial showed that topical corticosteroid together with antivirals reduced persistence and progression of stromal inflammation and shortened the duration of stromal keratitis. Oral antivirals (valacyclovir 500 mg once daily or acyclovir 400 mg twice a day) can be used for long-term suppression and avoid corneal toxicity. Long-term suppression is especially helpful for patients with multiple recurrences of stromal keratitis. Higher doses should be used for active disease. Corticosteroids should be tapered to the lowest dose that controls inflammation.

◆ *Neurotrophic keratitis*: Preservative-free lubricant drops and ointments can be beneficial with or without bland antibiotic ointment use to prevent secondary bacterial infection (i.e., erythromycin ointment). Persistent epithelial defects can be treated with tarsorrhaphy or autologous serum drops. Therapeutic bandage lens wear can be used temporarily with close observation and consideration of prophylactic antibiotic treatment. Emergent surgical treatment may include lamellar or penetrating keratoplasty, cyanoacrylate glue patching, amniotic membrane grafting, or conjunctival flaps in situations where visual rehabilitation is poor.

Herpes Zoster Virus

Herpes zoster virus (HZV) is a DNA virus also known as varicella virus. It has a primary infection manifested as a self-limited infection of childhood (chicken pox) followed by a period of latency in which the virus is dormant in the neural ganglia. Reactivation causes herpes zoster (shingles) in ~20% of individuals. Herpes zoster cases include 15% that affect the ophthalmic nerve distribution of the trigeminal nerve (cranial nerve V1 division). Infection always involves a single dermatome, making it unilateral.

◆ **Presentation**

◆ *Primary infection stage*: Chicken pox. Occurs as a self-limited infection in children. Symptoms include a maculopapular rash, along with prodromal symptoms of fever, malaise, and upper respiratory infection symptoms. A vaccine is now available for children typically at 12 months of age to prevent chicken pox. A vaccine is also available for immunocompetent individuals over the age of 65. Can be life threatening if a primary infection develops in adulthood or in immunosuppressed patients.
◆ *Latent stage*: Virus is dormant in the neural ganglia.
◆ *Recurrent or reactivation stage*: Virus travels down a single dermatome with pain, paresthesias, and dysesthesia, followed by a unilateral maculopapular rash along the involved dermatome. Ocular involvement occurs in more than 70% of patients with cranial nerve V1 involvement. Corneal findings include a punctate or dendritic epithelial keratitis, nummular subepithelial infiltrates, stromal keratitis, disciform keratitis, and granulomatous keratic precipitate from uveitis. Neurotrophic keratopathy, corneal scarring, corneal neovascularization, interstitial keratitis, lipid keratopathy, and keratolysis can also occur (**Fig. 5.2A,B,C**).

◆ **Differential Diagnosis**

HSV, bacterial, or fungal infection; collagen vascular disease or immune-related corneal ulcers; exposure-related corneal ulcers

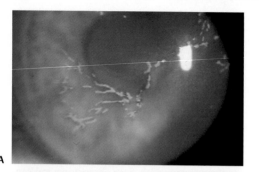

A

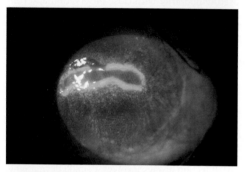

B

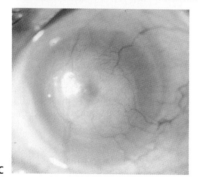

C

Fig. 5.2 (**A**) Dendrite from primary herpes zoster virus (HZV) infection. (**B**) Neurotrophic ulcer following herpes zoster ophthalmicus. (**C**) Corneal melt after HZV necrotizing stromal keratitis.

◆ Management

Oral antivirals (acyclovir, valacyclovir, or famciclovir) reduce viral shedding from lesions and decrease the incidence and severity of the most common ocular complications for herpes zoster ophthalmicus. Oral therapy, if begun within 72 hours of symptom onset, may reduce the incidence and duration of postherpetic neuralgia. Treatment is typically used for 7 to 10 days (valacyclovir, 1 g three times a day; acyclovir, 800 mg five times daily; or famciclovir, 500 mg three times a day. Topical antivirals are not effective in herpes zoster. Intravenous antivirals are indicated for patients at risk for systemic dissemination due to severe immunosuppression.

Topical cycloplegia and topical corticosteroids can be beneficial for severe stromal scarring and uveitis.

Epstein-Barr Virus

Epstein-Barr virus (EBV) is a DNA virus in the herpesvirus family. Typically transmitted from saliva with a subclinical infection most commonly occurring in the first decade of life. In the latent period the virus is dormant in B lymphocytes and mucosal epithelial cells of the pharynx. Ocular disease is uncommon but can occur. Infection later in life causes mononucleosis.

◆ Presentation

Pain, redness, and decreased vision along with an acute follicular conjunctivitis can occur with enlargement of the lacrimal glands and lymphadenopathy. Corneal findings include epithelial dendrites or punctate keratitis, corneal neovascularization, and interstitial and/or stromal keratitis. A nummular keratitis as seen with HZV or HSV can occur (**Fig. 5.3**).

◆ Differential Diagnosis

See the differential for dendritic keratitis and stromal keratitis listed earlier.

◆ Management

Diagnosis is dependent on the detection of EBV antibodies to various viral components. Viral capsid antigens appear in acute infection with immunoglobulin M (IgM) antibodies appearing first followed by IgG antibodies. Antibodies to early antigens also occur in acute infectious stages and decrease to low or undetectable after initial infection. Antibodies to EBV nuclear antigens appear weeks to months after infection and can be used as a marker of previous EBV infection. Supportive treatment with topical lubricant drops, gels, or ointments can improve epithelial keratitis. Oral antivirals remain unstudied with EBV stromal keratitis. Topical corticosteroids may reduce subepithelial infiltrates, nummular keratitis, and corneal neovascularization.

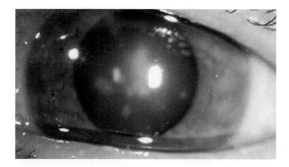

Fig. 5.3 Multiple cornea stromal opacities from Epstein-Barr virus stromal keratitis.

Bacterial Corneal Ulcer

An infectious infiltrate of the cornea, bacterial corneal ulcer is also known as a bacterial corneal ulcer. Risk factors include contact lens wear (most common cause), corneal trauma, and an altered corneal surface such as a corneal abrasion or punctate keratopathy. Any disorder compromising the corneal epithelial integrity can lead to a bacterial infection. Common gram-positive bacterial causes include *Staphylococcus* species, *Streptococcus* species, and *Bacillus* species (common after trauma). More common gram-negative bacterial causes include *Pseudomonas aeruginosa*, *Proteus*, *Enterobacter*, and *Serratia*.

◆ Presentation

Often acute pain, redness, photophobia, tearing, and discharge. A white spot may be visible to the patient that may represent either the infiltrate within the cornea or a layered hypopyon if in the lower portion of the cornea. Bacterial keratitis may present with concurrent corneal edema, corneal stromal thinning, necrosis, purulent debris within the ulcer, and white blood cell infiltration within the cornea or the anterior chamber (**Fig. 5.4**).

◆ Differential Diagnosis

Viral cause (particularly HSV or HZV), fungal cause, *Acanthamoeba*, shield ulcer from vernal keratoconjunctivitis, immune-mediated corneal ulcer, sterile marginal ulcer, staphylococcal marginal keratitis

◆ Management

- ◆ Obtain a history of contact lens wear, trauma, or foreign body.
- ◆ Obtain an ocular history of systemic disease or previous eye conditions that may predispose to breakdown or instability of the corneal epithelium (exposure keratopathy, recurrent erosion, dry-eye disease, corneal abrasions, eyelid abnormalities).
- ◆ Obtain a corneal scraping for various culture media and a Gram stain or potassium hydroxide prep on glass slides. Consider culturing contact lenses, cases, and solution when available.

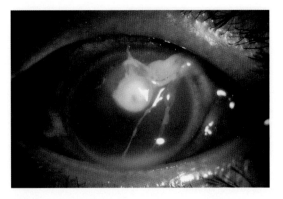

Fig. 5.4 Central bacterial corneal ulcer, epithelial/mucous debris, and hypopyon from *Pseudomonas aeruginosa*.

◆ Large central ulcers should be placed on broad-spectrum fortified topical antibiotics using either cefazolin (50 mg/mL) or vancomycin (25 or 50 mg/mL), one drop every 30 minutes for gram-positive coverage along with a topical aminoglycoside for gram-negative coverage. A common agent is tobramycin (14 mg/mL), one drop every 30 minutes. Small peripheral ulcers can be treated with monotherapy with a fluoroquinolone used one drop every 30 minutes. Treatment can be adjusted with close follow-up examinations and by utilization of bacterial culture results, including identification and medication sensitivities/susceptibilities. Some physicians may also use a loading dose of antibiotics every 15 minutes for the first 2 hours.
◆ Cycloplegia (homatropine or scopolamine, one drop twice a day) is helpful for pain relief from ciliary spasm and prevention of posterior synechiae.
◆ Contact lens wear should be discontinued when applicable.
◆ Hospitalization should be considered if compliance is an issue with medication use.

Acanthamoeba

Acanthamoeba keratitis is a corneal infection or ulceration caused by a ubiquitous protozoan found in fresh water and soil. It exists as a dormant cyst or an active mobile form known as a trophozoite. Most cases occur in association with poor contact lens hygiene, contact lens wear in fresh water sources, or cleaning contact lenses in fresh water, well water, or homemade saline solutions.

◆ Presentation

Patients experience acute, severe pain, often out of proportion to corneal findings. Associated redness, photophobia, tearing, and blurred vision progress over the course of several weeks. Seek a contact lens history or fresh water exposure in association with contact lens wear or cleaning. Findings begin with a punctate epithelial keratitis followed by subepithelial haze and infiltration. A radial perineuritis may be seen along with pseudodendritic keratitis. A late and ominous finding is stromal ulceration, necrosis, and subsequent ring ulceration with keratolysis (**Fig. 5.5A,B,C**).

◆ Differential Diagnosis

HSV, HZA, bacterial keratitis, fungal keratitis, immune-related ulcer

◆ Management

◆ Obtain a corneal scraping or corneal biopsy. Utilize calcofluor white, Giemsa, H&E, or Gram stain to identify cysts of trophozoites. Corneal culture on nonnutrient agar with *Escherichia coli* overlay can detect infection. Consider culturing the contact lens or case.
◆ Confocal microscopy when available can be beneficial for identification of these structures in the absence of severe stromal ulceration.
◆ Discontinue contact lens wear.
◆ Combination therapy is most effective, but early diagnosis is the most critical factor for successful treatment:
  ◆ Diamidines (propamidine, hexamidine)
  ◆ Biguanides (chlorhexidine digluconate, polyhexamethylene biguanide, alexidine)

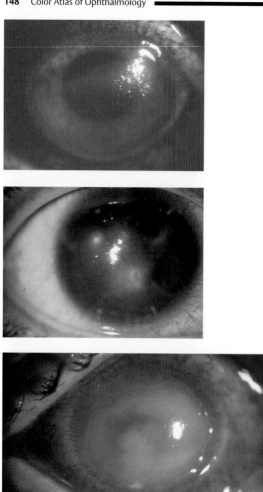

Fig. 5.5 **(A)** *Acanthamoeba* keratitis with severe punctate keratopathy and early central corneal haze. **(B)** Central corneal ulcer and radial perineuritis from *Acanthamoeba*. **(C)** Ring ulcer and stromal necrosis from late *Acanthamoeba* keratitis.

◆ Aminoglycosides (paromomycin, neomycin)
◆ Imidazoles/triazoles (clotrimazole, itraconazole, ketoconazole, miconazole, metronidazole)

- ◆ Biguanides have become first-line therapy because of cysticidal activity, and they can be used alone or in combination plus a diamidine and/or a topical or oral aminoglycoside agent.
- ◆ Treatment is often needed for many months.
- ◆ Corticosteroids should be avoided if possible unless severe inflammation and pain do not improve. Careful observation must occur if corticosteroids are used because of potential reactivation of trophozoites from dormant cysts.
- ◆ Keratoplasty techniques may be needed, but outcomes improve if surgery can be delayed after several months of antiamoeba treatment.

Fungal Keratitis

Fungal infection involving the cornea. Risk factors most commonly include trauma involving breakdown of the corneal epithelium from plant or vegetable matter. Trauma from contact lens wear is another risk factor, although a relatively new risk factor from contact lens wear includes cleaning solutions, as seen with the now discontinued ReNu with MoistureLoc solution (formerly manufactured by Bausch & Lomb, Rochester, NY), and the development of a *Fusarium* keratitis outbreak worldwide. Systemic and topical corticosteroids are additional risk factors to fungal infection and can incite dramatic progression of a fungal keratitis or ulceration. Common fungal agents may include *Candida*, *Fusarium*, *Paecilomyces*, and *Aspergillus* species among others.

◆ Presentation

Fungal keratitis infections are more indolent than bacterial or viral corneal infections unless topical corticosteroids have been used. Symptoms include eye pain, redness, tearing, photophobia, and decreased vision. The history can be an important factor in assessing the risk of fungal infections. A white spot over the cornea is commonly seen from either the stromal ulcer or hypopyon. Anterior uveitis, corneal edema, posterior corneal plaques, and a layered hypopyon are common (**Fig. 5.6**).

◆ Differential Diagnosis

Bacterial, viral, or *Acanthamoeba* keratitis

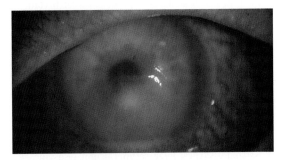

Fig. 5.6 Fungal corneal ulcer and hypopyon from *Candida albicans* in immunosuppressed patient.

◆ Management

All corneal ulcers should be treated as with bacterial keratitis initially and started on broad-spectrum topical antibacterial medications until culture-proven fungal infection is identified from corneal scrapings or culture media. Scrapings with Giemsa, periodic acid–Schiff, or Grocott-Gomori methenamine-silver nitrate stains can identify fungal elements. Culture media should include either Sabouraud agar or brain–heart infusion broth. Natamycin 5% is the treatment of choice for filamentous *Fusarium* infections, whereas topical miconazole 1% is the treatment of choice for *Paecilomyces*. Amphotericin B 0.15% or topical voriconazole is the treatment of choice for yeast keratitis and *Aspergillus* infection. Drops are typically started every 1 to 2 hours and often supplemented with oral antifungal imidazoles or voriconazole. Corneal debridement may be needed in subsequent visits to improve topical medication penetration. Surgical keratoplasty techniques may be needed in severe cases with keratolysis or significant nonresponsive posterior corneal plaques. Treatment is often needed for several months, and corticosteroids should be avoided during this time. Cycloplegia may be beneficial in cases with significant uveitis or hypopyon to prevent posterior synechiae formation.

◆ Corneal Inflammation and Surface Disorders

Interstitial Keratitis

This is a nonsuppurative inflammation of the corneal stroma that typically involves corneal neovascularization and eventual lipid deposition and scarring. Most cases result from a hypersensitivity reaction to infectious microbes or associated antigen within the cornea. Several viral, bacterial, and helminth infections are associated with this condition.

◆ Presentation

Initial symptoms include pain, tearing, photophobia, and perilimbal injection. Keratic precipitate and anterior uveitis may develop. With progression, deep stromal neovascularization develops with central spread. Corneal scarring and edema may ensue. A salmon-pink patch may appear within the cornea from severe stromal neovascularization cases. Ghost vessels eventually develop with lipid and scar formation. Stromal scarring and opacification can become severe. (**Fig. 5.7A,B**).

◆ Differential Diagnosis

- ◆ Congenital syphilis (usually bilateral and develops late in the first decade of life)
- ◆ Acquired syphilis (rare and usually unilateral with occurrence in adulthood)
- ◆ Viral corneal infections (HSV, HZV, EBV, mumps, rubeola)
- ◆ Tuberculosis (confirm with Tb skin test)
- ◆ Leprosy
- ◆ *Chlamydia trachomatis* (history of sexual contact)
- ◆ Helminth infections [*Onchocerca volvulus* (onchocerciasis) from foreign travel in endemic region]
- ◆ Lyme disease (history of tick exposure; check Lyme titers)
- ◆ Sarcoidosis (chest x-ray, serum calcium, lysozyme, and angiotensin-converting enzyme level)
- ◆ Cogan syndrome (autoimmune disorder with interstitial keratitis, vertigo, and hearing loss)

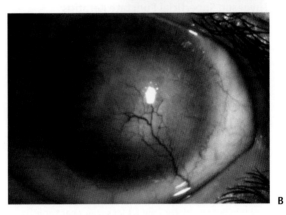

A

B

Fig. 5.7 **(A)** Interstitial keratitis from congenital syphilis with ghost vessels on retroillumination. **(B)** Herpes simplex virus interstitial keratitis and corneal scarring.

◆ Management

Treatment begins with identification of the cause. Serological testing is very important in making a diagnosis. A screening test such as a Rapid Plasma Reagin (RPR) or a treponeme-specific test such as Fluorescent Troponemal Antibody (FTA-ABS) or microhemagglutination assay (MHA-TP) can detect syphilis. Systemic treatment is indicated depending on the underlying cause (e.g., systemic antibiotics with syphilis, tuberculosis, Lyme disease). Inflammation in interstitial keratitis cases is controlled with topical corticosteroids and cycloplegic agents once an infectious cause is elicited. See the section on HSV and HZV for treatment.

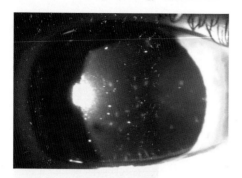

Fig. 5.8 Punctate keratitis and multiple corneal opacities typical of Thygeson superficial punctate keratitis.

Thygeson Superficial Punctate Keratitis

This nonspecific superficial punctate keratitis typically occurs in young children to older adults. The cause is unknown, although speculation exists as to whether a virus is the underlying agent. Multiple corneal lesions develop but typically respond rapidly to corticosteroids, suggesting an immunological basis for keratitis.

◆ Presentation

Symptoms include recurrent episodes of tearing, photophobia, foreign body sensation, and mild blurred vision. Conjunctival injection is usually minimal or absent. Corneal findings include multiple raised epithelial lesions that are gray to white granular opacities that wax and wane in location and number and are usually bilateral with potential asymmetry (**Fig. 5.8**).

◆ Differential Diagnosis

Subepithelial infiltrates with epidemic keratoconjunctivitis (EKC), EBV, staphylococcal hypersensitivity, contact lens overwear keratitis

◆ Management

Supportive treatment with topical lubricant tears or gels with or without bandage contact lens wear can be useful in milder cases. Low-dose topical corticosteroids can promote rapid resolution of corneal lesions; however, lesions typically recur with discontinuation of drops. Long-term corticosteroid treatment with fluorometholone 0.1% or loteprednol 0.5% can work well at varying dose regimens with slowly tapering doses from an initial dosing of four times a day. Topical cyclosporine and topical trifluridine have also been used with anecdotal success. The lesions eventually resolve, but this may take months to years for permanent resolution of recurrent episodes.

Shield Ulcer

Shield ulcer is a noninfectious corneal ulcer in the setting of vernal keratoconjunctivitis that is often bilateral and seasonal (more common in spring). A history of atopy is common. The condition more often presents in males.

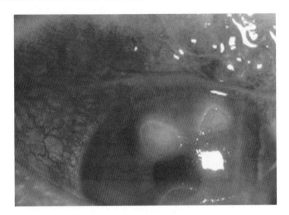

Fig. 5.9 Peripheral vernal shield ulcers seen in vernal kerato-conjunctivitis.

◆ **Presentation**

Presentation includes itching, photophobia, foreign body sensation, blurred vision, redness, and mucous discharge. Shield ulcer can be associated with giant papillary conjunctivitis and limbal follicles known as Horner-Trantas dots (collections of degenerated eosinophils and epithelial cells). A superior punctate keratopathy typically develops followed by a breakdown of epithelium and eventual oval-shaped ulcers (shield ulcers) with underlying stromal opacification. Association can occur with keratoconus and floppy eyelid syndrome (**Fig. 5.9**).

◆ **Differential Diagnosis**

Atopic keratoconjunctivitis, infectious ulcer, immune-mediated ulcer

◆ **Management**

Patients should avoid potential allergens and use cool compresses, preservative-free lubricants, topical and/or systemic antihistamine or mast cell stabilizers, and topical or systemic corticosteroids. Alternative topical or systemic immunosuppressant agents such as cyclosporine A may provide benefit with close follow-up.

◆ **Exposure Keratopathy**

Exposure keratopathy is also referred to as neuroparalytic keratopathy. Causes include facial nerve palsy, severe proptosis, and scarring of the lids. The condition may be associated with weak Bell phenomenon. It is the result of improper wetting of the ocular surface by the tear film.

◆ Presentation

Symptoms range from mild inferior punctate epithelial changes to severe corneal melting with corneal perforation.

◆ Differential Diagnosis

Neurotrophic keratopathy, recurrent erosions, infectious keratopathy, dry eye, autoimmune diseases

◆ Management

Frequent instillations of lubricants and taping the lids form the mainstay of the treatment. Lid surgeries to correct the lid abnormalities may be required.

◆ Filamentary Keratitis

An ocular surface inflammatory condition characterized by mucous plaques and strands of the corneal surface. Filaments represent strands of epithelial cells attached to the corneal surface over a core of mucus with firm attachment to the adjacent corneal nerves.

Common conditions associated with this finding include eyelid malposition such as lagophthalmia and poor eyelid blink, contact lens overwear keratitis, atopic conditions, and chronic ocular surface inflammatory conditions such as superior limbic keratoconjunctivitis, aqueous tear deficiency, and dry-eye syndrome.

◆ Presentation

Patients experience pain, foreign body sensation, redness, dryness, and photophobia. Mucous plaques in strands or globules are visualized entrapped within the corneal epithelium. The filaments stain with fluorescein dye. Conjunctivochalasis, punctate corneal staining between filaments, and a low tear meniscus are common associated findings (**Fig. 5.10**).

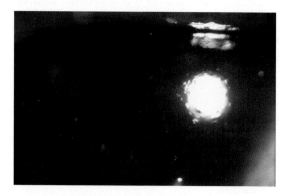

Fig. 5.10   Filamentary keratitis.

◆ **Differential Diagnosis**

Recurrent erosions, epithelial defects

◆ **Management**

Debridement of the filaments can be performed with a cotton-tipped applicator following a topical anesthetic. Lubricant drops, gels, or ointments can be beneficial from four times a day to hourly dosing. Sodium chloride drops or acetylcysteine drops can also be used four times a day. Additional treatments may include a therapeutic bandage lens and autologous serum drops. Punctal plugging should be avoided until filament recurrence is prevented.

◆ **Neurotrophic Keratopathy**

Neurotrophic keratopathy is a chronic surface disorder resulting from hypoesthesia or anesthesia of the trigeminal nerve. A variety of factors, including HSV, HZV, radiation therapy, previous brain tumor resection, or trauma to the trigeminal nerve, as well as diabetes, topical anesthetic or preservative abuse, chemical burns, and leprosy are associated with this condition.

◆ **Presentation**

Blurred vision, redness, and chronic epithelial defects or ulceration are seen at presentation, along with punctate corneal staining in the central or inferior cornea with or without associated epithelial defects. Corneal thinning, filamentary keratitis, scarring, corneal surface asperity, and an elevated hyperplastic epitheliopathy can be associated findings (**Fig. 5.11**).

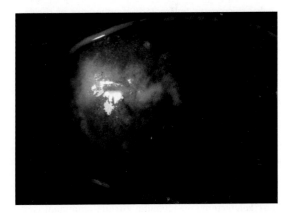

Fig. 5.11 Neurotrophic keratopathy.

◆ Differential Diagnosis

Corneal abrasion, recurrent erosion, infectious ulcer, dry-eye syndrome, and autoimmune disease

◆ Management

Identify the underlying cause. Lubricant drops, gels, and ointments can protect the corneal surface from further breakdown. Temporary or permanent punctal closure can also benefit. A tarsorrhaphy is often needed to decrease the amount of exposed surface area to the cornea. Therapeutic bandage lens wear should be used cautiously with close follow-up. A conjunctival or amniotic membrane graft can be used in severe situations, with lamellar or penetrating keratoplasty used in cases of severe corneal melting or perforation. Autologous serum drops can also be a useful adjunct to treatment.

◆ Recurrent Erosion

Recurrent corneal erosion (RCE) syndrome is characterized by a disturbance at the level of the corneal epithelial basement membrane, resulting in defective adhesions and recurrent breakdowns of the epithelium. Common causes of recurrent erosions include epithelial basement membrane dystrophy, corneal injuries, alkali burns, foreign bodies, postinfectious ulcers from herpes simplex, Cockayne syndrome, Reis-Bücklers dystrophy, postvitrectomy, photocoagulation, and contact lenses, among others.

◆ Presentation

Many patients (80 to 90%) are asymptomatic. Some can present with pain, blurred vision, astigmatism, epithelial blebs, and foreign body sensation with recurrent erosion. Patients can present with a variety of signs such as epithelial loss, epithelial microcysts, bullae, lack of adherence of sheets of epithelium, epithelial filament formation, corneal abrasion, brownish granular edema (brawny edema), and areas of healed epithelium, which may even resemble a dendritic figure, a pseudodendrite.

◆ Differential Diagnosis

Corneal abrasion, corneal dystrophy, corneal foreign bodies, dry eye, and infective keratitis

◆ Management

Management of RCE syndrome is usually aimed at regenerating or repairing the epithelial basement membrane to restore the adhesion between the epithelium and the anterior stroma. Recurrent corneal erosions respond to topical lubrication therapy, bandage soft contact lenses, debridement, antibiotic ointment, and patching. Surgical options include anterior stromal puncture, excimer laser diamond burr keratectomy, neodymium:yttrium-aluminum-garnet (Nd:yAG) laser treatment, and superficial phototherapeutic keratectomy.

◆ Congenital Anomalies

Microcornea

The normal corneal diameter is normally 9.5–10mm at birth and 10–12.5mm at adulthood.

◆ Presentation

The term microcornea is given to an adult cornea with less than 10mm diameter. Most cases occur sporadically. Microcornea may occur in isolation or part of a generally small eye (microphthalmos). If it occurs as an isolated entity, the normal lens size causes a disparity with the small cornea resulting in angle-closure glaucoma.

◆ Differential Diagnosis

Nanophthalmos, microphthalmos, sclerocornea

◆ Management

Treatment is directed at any associated ocular abnormalities

Megalocornea

◆ Presentation

Megalocornea is the term given to the condition in which the corneal diameter exceeds 11mm at birth, or 12mm after 2 years of age. It has been associated with ectopia lentis, iris transillumination, pigment dispersion, arcus and mental retardation.

◆ Differential Diagnosis

Buphthalmos, anterior chamber dysgenesis syndromes. As compared to buphthalmos, the size of the globe and the intraocular pressure are normal.

◆ Management

Treatment is directed at any associated ocular abnormalities

Anterior Embryotoxon

It is a congenital anomaly of the cornea which is not visually significant.

◆ Presentation

Anterior embryotoxon refers to a congenital broad superior limbus with an otherwise normal anterior chamber. It is also used to describe a congenital arcus, arcus juvenilis, similar to the arcus senilis that occurs in old individuals.

◆ Differential Diagnosis

Posterior embryotoxon, Arcus senilis, Axenfeld Reiger syndrome.

◆ Management

Observation and follow-up.

Posterior Embryotoxon

It represents a thickened and anteriorly displaced Schwalbe's line that is easily visible.

◆ Presentation

Posterior embryotoxon is the most common anomaly of the cornea. It may be seen as a white ring near the limbus on slit-lamp examination and as a prominent, anteriorly displaced Schwalbe's line on gonioscopy.

◆ Differential Diagnosis

Anterior embryotoxon, Arcus senilis, Axenfeld Reiger syndrome.

◆ Management

Observation and follow-up.

Sclerocornea

It is a congenital anomaly of the cornea resulting in decreased vision.

◆ Presentation

Sclerocornea refers to a sclera-like appearance of the cornea, which may be peripheral or involve the whole cornea. It is associated with corneal flattening and other anomalies of anterior chamber development.

◆ Differential Diagnosis

Microphthalmos, buphthalmos, and other causes of opaque cornea.

◆ Management

Visual prognosis in severe cases is very poor.

◆ Dystrophies

Anterior Corneal Dystrophies

Epithelial Basement Membrane Dystrophy (EBMD)

Also known as Cogan microcystic edema or map-dot-fingerprint corneal dystrophy, this is perhaps the most common of all corneal dystrophies. Bilateral (but may be asymmetrical) with autosomal dominant inheritance, but most cases are sporadic. The condition results from abnormal epithelial turnover and redundant basement membrane.

◆ Presentation

Patients may remain asymptomatic or may develop decreased vision, foreign body sensation, photophobia, tearing, and potentially painful corneal erosions. Slit-lamp examination of EBMD shows gray-white subepithelial patches (maps), gray-white

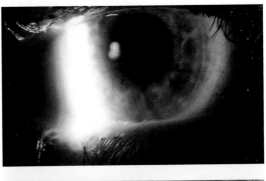

A

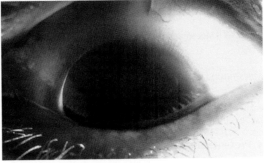

B

Fig. 5.12 **(A)** Fingerprint pattern seen with epithelial basement membrane dystrophy (EBMD). **(B)** Map pattern seen with EBMD.

parallel lines (fingerprints), or subepithelial microcysts (dots). The findings are best seen on retroillumination (**Fig. 5.12A,B**).

◆ Differential Diagnosis

Traumatic corneal erosion, Meesmann dystrophy, early Reis-Bücklers dystrophy, corneal intraepithelial neoplasia (CIN)

◆ Management

No treatment is required for asymptomatic cases. For symptomatic cases, sodium chloride drops or ointment can be beneficial. Patients with concurrent dry-eye disease should use additional preservative-free artificial tears or gels. Therapeutic bandage lenses can provide temporary relief. Surgical options include anterior stromal puncture, Na:Yag stromal puncture, epithelial debridement, phototherapeutic keratectomy, or diamond burr keratectomy.

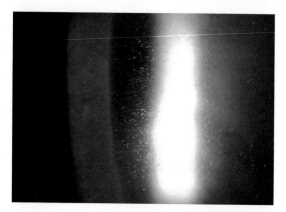

Fig. 5.13   Meesmann dystrophy.

Meesmann Dystrophy

Meesmann dystrophy is a rare bilateral autosomal dominant condition occurring early in life that results from a thickened basement membrane with a fibrogranular "peculiar substance" (possibly hyaline) within the epithelial cells.

◆ Presentation

Patients may present with pain, blurred vision, photophobia, tearing, and redness from recurrent erosions. Tiny epithelial vesicles are seen from limbus to limbus, most clearly on retroillumination (**Fig. 5.13**).

◆ Differential Diagnosis

Cystinosis, corneal guttae, epithelial basement membrane dystrophy (EBMD), traumatic recurrent erosion

◆ Management

No treatment is required unless recurrent erosions develop. Similar treatments may be performed as with EBMD, although a deep anterior lamellar keratoplasty can also be useful in cases recalcitrant to recurrent erosion treatment options.

Reis-Bücklers Dystrophy

Reis-Bücklers dystrophy is a progressive bilateral autosomal dominant dystrophy that develops early in life. Genetic linkage occurs from a mutation of the *BIGH3* gene on chromosome 5q31.

◆ Presentation

Patients present with recurrent erosion symptoms of blurred vision, pain, photophobia, tearing, and redness. Examination reveals a superficial gray-white reticular haze more concentrated in the central cornea. Significant scarring can lead to Salzmann nodules and an irregular corneal surface (**Fig. 5.14**).

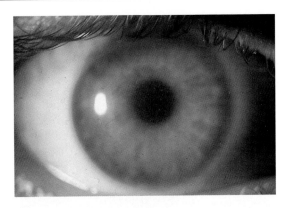

Fig. 5.14 Reis-Bücklers dystrophy.

◆ **Differential Diagnosis**

Meesmann dystrophy, EBMD, granular dystrophy

◆ **Management**

Initial treatment is directed at recurrent corneal erosion treatment as with EBMD. Surgical procedures may include lamellar keratoplasty, penetrating keratoplasty, or phototherapeutic keratectomy. Recurrence is common with penetrating keratoplasty.

Stromal Corneal Dystrophies

Granular Dystrophy

Granular dystrophy is a common bilateral autosomal dominant stromal dystrophy linked to a mutation in the *BIGH3* gene on chromosome 5q31. Stromal deposits consist of hyaline, which can be highlighted with Masson trichrome stain on corneal histopathology. Several forms of this dystrophy exist.

◆ **Presentation**

Symptoms typically occur as a result of recurrent erosions and may include blurred vision, pain, foreign body sensation, photophobia, and tearing. Examination shows bread crumb–like opacities, typically in the central portion of the anterior stroma, with sparing of the limbus (**Fig. 5.15**).

◆ **Differential Diagnosis**

Avellino dystrophy, macular dystrophy

◆ **Management**

Treatment is directed at recurrent erosions. Phototherapeutic keratectomy, lamellar keratoplasty, and penetrating keratoplasty can be used for treatment. Keratoplasty has a good prognosis in cases with poor vision, but recurrence is possible.

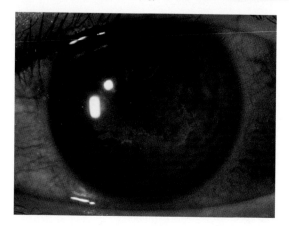

Fig. 5.15   Granular corneal dystrophy.

Lattice Dystrophy

This is a bilateral autosomal dominant stromal dystrophy linked to a mutation in the *BIGH3* gene on chromosome 5q31. Stromal deposits consist of amyloid, which can be highlighted on corneal histopathology with Congo-red stain. Several types of this dystrophy exist, including an autosomal recessive form.

◆ **Presentation**

Patients are asymptomatic unless recurrent erosions develop. Decreased vision can result from deposits. Examination reveals central refractile branching lines within the anterior corneal stroma that are best seen on retroillumination. The limbus is spared (**Fig. 5.16A,B**).

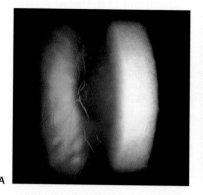
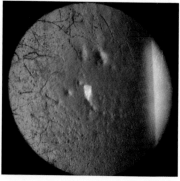

A   B

Fig. 5.16   **(A)** Lattice corneal dystrophy. **(B)** Lattice corneal dystrophy on retroillumination. (Both images courtesy of Mark J. Mannis, MD)

◆ Differential Diagnosis

Enlarged corneal nerves, ghost vessels of interstitial keratitis

◆ Management

No management is required if the patient is asymptomatic. Treat recurrent erosions as described in section on Recurrent Erosions (p. 156). Recurrence is common despite corneal transplantation, but the procedure can be beneficial in some patients with a good long-term prognosis.

Macular Dystrophy

Macular dystrophy is a rare bilateral autosomal recessive corneal dystrophy with mucopolysaccharide deposition in any or all portions of the stroma. Alcian blue stain can detect the deposits on corneal histopathology.

◆ Presentation

There may be recurrent erosion symptoms. Decreased vision can occur early in the course. Examination shows gray-white opacities with poor margins, separated by intervening haze or cloudiness within the stroma. Lesions often coalesce with time and often involve the entire cornea, limbus to limbus (**Fig. 5.17**).

◆ Differential Diagnosis

Atypical lattice or granular dystrophy

◆ Management

Recurrent erosion symptoms can be treated. Penetrating keratoplasty or deep lamellar keratoplasty is often the only surgical option because of the depth of stromal opacities. Larger graft sizes may limit recurrences.

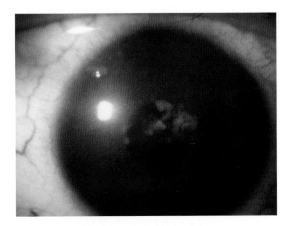

Fig. 5.17 Early macular corneal dystrophy.

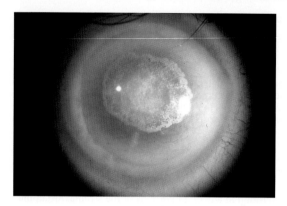

Fig. 5.18 Central crystalline dystrophy of Schnyder. (Courtesy of Mark J. Mannis, MD)

Schnyder Corneal Dystrophy

This condition is a bilateral, slowly progressive autosomal dominant stromal dystrophy, which is often referred to as Schnyder crystalline corneal dystrophy. It can be detected as early as 1 year of age with accumulation of cholesterol and phospholipids within the stroma secondary to abnormal corneal lipid metabolism.

◆ **Presentation**

Decreased vision is a presenting symptom. Examination shows central corneal opacification with sparing of the limbus. The epithelium remains intact with associated corneal arcus development in the second or third decade of life. Subepithelial crystals may be present along with midperipheral corneal opacification in some cases (**Fig. 5.18**).

◆ **Differential Diagnosis**

Other stromal dystrophies, central corneal scars, hyperlipoproteinemia

◆ **Management**

Check the patient's fasting lipid profile because 50% have elevated cholesterol. If vision decline progresses, penetrating keratoplasty is warranted, with a potential for recurrence.

Fleck Dystrophy

Fleck dystrophy is an uncommon nonprogressive autosomal dominant condition that begins early in life. Affected keratocytes contain two abnormal substances: glycosaminoglycan and lipids.

◆ Presentation

Discrete, flat, gray-white, dandruff-like opacities appear throughout the stroma. Symptoms are minimal, and vision is not affected. The condition may be associated with decreased corneal sensation, limbal dermoid, keratoconus, atopy, or pseudoxanthoma elasticum.

◆ Differential Diagnosis

Posterior polymorphous dystrophy, pre–Descemet dystrophy, ichthyosis

◆ Management

No treatment is required.

Central Cloudy Dystrophy of François

This is a bilateral symmetrical stromal dystrophy that is slowly progressive and autosomal dominant. It can be associated with megalocornea.

◆ Presentation

Patients are asymptomatic. Examination shows central corneal opacities with polygonal gray areas separated by intervening clear zones resembling cracks. Haze extends into the anterior corneal stroma unlike with posterior crocodile shagreen (**Fig. 5.19**).

◆ Differential Diagnosis

Posterior crocodile shagreen, other stromal dystrophies

◆ Management

No treatment is necessary because vision is usually not reduced.

Pre–Descemet Dystrophy

This is an acquired condition.

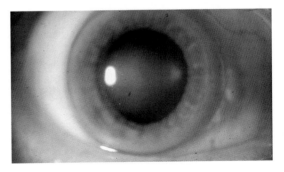

Fig. 5.19 Central cloudy dystrophy of François.

◆ **Presentation**

Patients are generally asymptomatic but visual acuity can be affected. Small linear or punctate gray-white flecks are appreciated in the deep stroma. The condition can be associated with keratoconus, posterior polymorphous dystrophy, and epithelial basement membrane dystrophy.

◆ **Differential Diagnosis**

Fleck dystrophy, posterior polymorphous dystrophy, ichthyosis

◆ **Management**

No treatment is required.

Posterior Amorphous Stromal Dystrophy

This is a rare, bilateral, slowly progressive, autosomal dominant condition presenting in childhood.

◆ **Presentation**

Patients present with diffuse, gray-white lesions in the posterior stroma, usually involving the central area, but may involve up to the limbus. Corneal thinning with flat topography and resulting hyperopia, central corneal thinning, and peripheral iris processes may be seen.

◆ **Management**

Rigid gas permeable contact lenses are used to correct the astigmatism. Visual acuity is rarely affected.

Congenital Hereditary Stromal Dystrophy

This is an autosomal dominant, bilateral, symmetrical, nonprogressive stromal dystrophy seen in the newborn.

◆ **Presentation**

Central corneal clouding is seen in the newborn with sparing of the peripheral stroma. Infants develop amblyopia with nystagmus and squint.

◆ **Differential Diagnosis**

Congenital hereditary endothelial dystrophy, congenital glaucoma, mucopolysaccharidosis, birth trauma, posterior polymorphous corneal dystrophy

◆ **Management**

Penetrating keratoplasty is the treatment of choice.

Posterior Corneal Dystrophies

Corneal Guttae

This is a focal accumulation of collagen on the posterior surface of the Descemet membrane associated with endothelial dysfunction, corneal clouding, and potential visual loss.

◆ Presentation

The lesion appears as a wart or excrescences in relation with the endothelial cells. The lesions, called Hassall–Henle bodies, appear at the periphery of the cornea and are associated with aging. A "beaten metal" appearance, visible during the specular reflection, is associated with melanin deposits.

◆ Differential Diagnosis

Fuchs endothelial dystrophy, Hassall-Henle bodies

◆ Management

Consider specular microscopy. Handling of the cornea must be gentle during intraocular surgeries because this may hasten endothelial compromise.

Fuchs Endothelial Dystrophy

This is a bilateral endothelial dystrophy resulting in progressive damage to the endothelium. It is rarely symptomatic before 50 years of age. Reduction in the number and function of sodium and potassium adenosine triphosphatase pumps in the endothelium occur, creating progressive corneal edema and guttae. The condition is autosomal dominant or sporadic.

◆ Presentation

Symptoms include decreased vision (worse in the morning), foreign body sensation, photophobia, tearing, and pain. Examination results can vary from mild guttae to severe microcystic and stromal edema with bullae formation. The Descemet membrane becomes thickened with an increase in corneal thickness as fluid retention increases within the corneal stroma. Subepithelial fibrosis and scarring may occur in later stages (**Fig. 5.20A,B,C**).

◆ Differential Diagnosis

Hassall-Henle bodies, pseudophakic or aphakic bullous keratopathy, Chandler syndrome, herpes simplex keratitis

◆ Management

Begin with supportive therapy, including artificial tears and in particular sodium chloride drops or ointment. Hair dryers can increase fluid evaporation from the cornea if used carefully. Definitive surgical treatment includes either a penetrating keratoplasty or endothelial keratoplasty (becoming a preferred technique with Fuchs dystrophy). Graft survival prognosis is good.

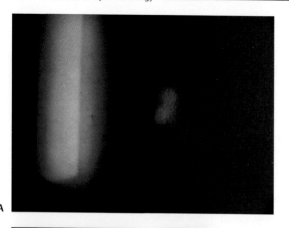

A

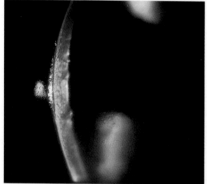

B

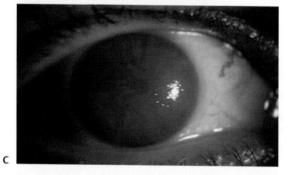

C

Fig. 5.20 **(A)** Guttae seen on retroillumination in Fuchs endothelial dystrophy. **(B)** Microcystic and stromal edema seen in Fuchs endothelial dystrophy. **(C)** Fuchs endothelial dystrophy with subepithelial bullae.

Posterior Polymorphous Dystrophy

This type of dystrophy is a bilateral endothelial dystrophy with gradual progression. It may be autosomal dominant or recessive and has been mapped to chromosome 20q11.

◆ Presentation

Decreased vision and pain may develop, but patients are often asymptomatic. Examination of the posterior cornea reveals grouped vesicles, geographic gray lesions, and/or broad bands with scalloped edges. Associated findings can include corneal edema, haze, corectopia, and iridocorneal adhesions as well as glaucoma. Infants may present with cloudy corneas (**Fig. 5.21A,B**).

◆ Differential Diagnosis

Iridio-corneal endothelial syndrome, congenital hereditary endothelial dystrophy, aphakic or pseudophakic bullous keratopathy, Fuchs dystrophy

◆ Management

Penetrating keratoplasty is required for cases with symptomatic decreased vision. Observe carefully for concurrent open-angle glaucoma.

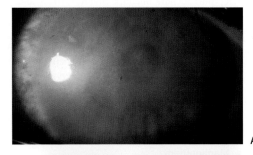

A

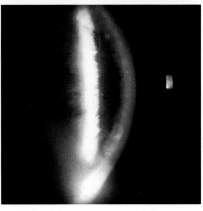

B

Fig. 5.21 **(A)** Edema and haze seen in posterior polymorphous dystrophy. **(B)** Broad bands seen on slit illumination in posterior polymorphous dystrophy.

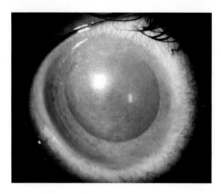

Fig. 5.22 Diffuse epithelial and stromal edema in child with congenital hereditary endothelial dystrophy.

Congenital Hereditary Endothelial Dystrophy

This is a bilateral corneal dystrophy with autosomal dominant and recessive forms. It causes endothelial dysfunction.

◆ **Presentation**

Symptoms include bilateral cloudy corneas and diffuse epithelial and stromal edema with a normal intraocular pressure and thickened Descemet membrane. The recessive form presents with bilateral corneal edema at birth with nystagmus. This condition appears without photophobia and tearing, and there is a lack of dystrophy progression. The dominant form is evident by age 2 with gradual progression of the dystrophy. Pain and tearing are present in the absence of photophobia (**Fig. 5.22**).

◆ **Differential Diagnosis**

Congenital glaucoma, mucopolysaccharidosis, congenital hereditary stromal dystrophy, posterior polymorphous corneal dystrophy, birth trauma

◆ **Management**

Topical sodium chloride drops or ointments are helpful. Penetrating keratoplasty is used in cases with corneal decompensation. There is a concern for amblyopia in infants.

◆ Ectatic Disorders

Keratoconus

Keratoconus is a common bilateral, but often asymmetrical, disorder of corneal thinning in which the central or inferior paracentral cornea undergoes progressive thinning to take on the shape of a cone. It begins in adolescence and progresses slowly with stability in late adulthood. A genetic predisposition is suspected with gene linkages in certain families, but eye rubbing and eye trauma remain a sig-

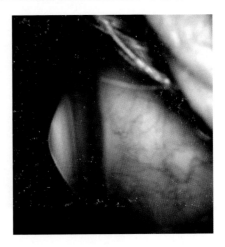

Fig. 5.23 Central corneal thinning and protrusion with keratoconus.

nificant factors. There is a high association with conditions such as atopy, Down syndrome, Marfan syndrome, floppy eyelid syndrome, and Leber congenital hereditary optic neuropathy. Acute hydrops can occur.

◆ Presentation

Vision is decreased as a result of progressive myopic astigmatism from alteration of the shape of the cornea. Keratoconus typically develops in the oblique axis and is associated with irregular astigmatism. Examination shows scissoring of the red reflex and apical corneal thinning. Associated findings may include breaks in the Descemet membrane, apical corneal scarring, stress lines in the stroma (Vogt striae), and iron line formation (Fleischer ring) (**Fig. 5.23**).

◆ Differential Diagnosis

Contact lens scarring, pellucid, keratoglobus

◆ Management

Corneal topography, keratometry, or photokeratoscopy can improve accuracy of diagnosis by demonstrating inferior corneal steepening. Scissoring reflex on retinoscopy is pathognomonic. Treat with spectacle correction of myopic astigmatism or rigid gas permeable or hybrid contact lenses when spectacle correction is poor owing to irregular astigmatism. Intacs corneal implants (Addition Technology, Inc., Sunnyvale, CA) can help in some cases of contact lens intolerance and potentially provide increased corneal stability with or without corneal collagen cross-linking. Penetrating or deep anterior lamellar keratoplasty provides the ultimate cure.

Keratoglobus

Keratoglobus is a rare noninflammatory condition that presents at birth as opposed to other corneal ectatic disorders with midperipheral corneal thinning. Acute hydrops can occur.

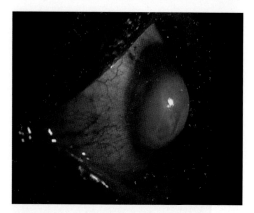

Fig. 5.24   Corneal hydrops in keratoglobus.

◆ **Presentation**

Examination shows a globular shape of both corneas with large corneal diameters. Associated generalized thinning occurs, more concentrated in the midperiphery. The anterior chamber is very deep (**Fig. 5.24**).

◆ **Differential Diagnosis**

Keratoconus

◆ **Management**

A lamellar or penetrating keratoplasty is usually required. Prognosis is guarded because of the necessary large graft diameter.

Pellucid Marginal Degeneration

Pellucid marginal degeneration is a nonhereditary, bilateral, peripheral corneal thinning disorder that most often involves the inferior corneal periphery but may occur in the superior peripheral cornea. It presents in early adulthood, typically between 20 and 40 years of age.

◆ **Presentation**

Patients experience blurred vision as a result of progressive, against the rule astigmatism or oblique astigmatism. Examination demonstrates corneal protrusion above the area of thinning. Stromal scarring can occur within the thinned areas, and rarely perforation may develop (**Fig. 5.25**).

◆ **Differential Diagnosis**

Keratoconus, Terrien marginal degeneration, collagen vascular disease

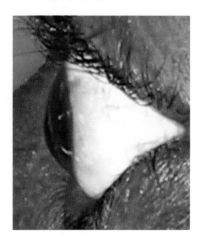

Fig. 5.25 Inferior corneal thinning with pellucid marginal degeneration.

◆ **Management**

Rigid gas permeable lenses are recommended. Spectacle correction is often not helpful. Crescentic lamellar or penetrating keratoplasty can occur in severe cases of vision loss or corneal ectasia.

◆ Corneal Degenerations and Deposits

Arcus Senilis

Arcus senilis is an accumulation of extracellular lipid in the peripheral corneal stroma. It can be associated with hyerlipidemic states.

◆ **Presentation**

Patients are asymptomatic, but the condition can be visible cosmetically as a ring of peripheral opacification that begins in the superior and inferior peripheral corneal stroma with a thin, clear zone between the limbus. It typically presents in a 360-degree ring and can be associated with corresponding carotid artery disease (**Fig. 5.26**).

◆ **Differential Diagnosis**

Hyperlipoproteinemia, pseudogerontoxin, arcus juvenilis

◆ **Management**

No ocular treatment is necessary. Consider obtaining a lipid profile in young adults.

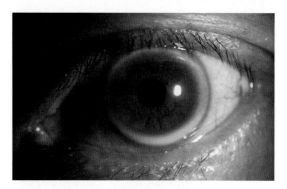

Fig. 5.26 Peripheral lipid deposition with arcus senilis.

Limbal Girdle of Vogt

An elastotic degeneration of collagen develops in the peripheral cornea and may contain particles of calcium.

◆ Presentation

An asymptomatic, peripheral corneal opacity typically begins at 3 and 9 o'clock along the limbus. There may be a clear lucid interval between the opacity and limbus, depending on which type of limbal girdle develops. Chalklike opacification is common (**Fig. 5.27**).

◆ Management

No treatment is needed because visual function is not affected.

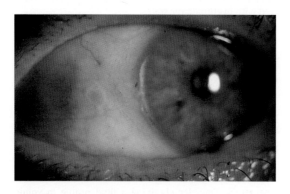

Fig. 5.27 Vogt limbal girdle.

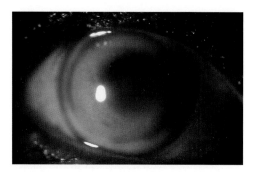

Fig. 5.28   Dense primary lipid keratopathy.

Primary Lipid Keratopathy

A yellow- or cream-colored lipid deposition composed of cholesterol develops in the superficial or deep corneal stroma. Unlike secondary lipid keratopathy where an antecedent corneal inflammatory condition such as herpes simplex, herpes zoster, or trachoma is present, primary cases lack corneal neovascularization and previous infection or inflammation.

◆ Presentation

Patients are asymptomatic unless decreased vision develops from obscuration of the visual axis. Cream or yellow deposits develop in the paracentral or central cornea (**Fig. 5.28**).

◆ Differential Diagnosis

Crocodile shagreen, central cloudy dystrophy of François, Schnyder corneal dystrophy, hyperlipoproteinemia

◆ Management

No treatment is necessary unless the visual axis causes decreased vision. A deep anterior lamellar keratoplasty or penetrating keratoplasty may be needed depending on the depth of lipid deposition in the corneal stroma.

Corneal Keloid

Corneal opacities are composed of irregular patterns of collagenase bundles. They can be associated with oculocerebrorenal (Lowe) syndrome, an autosomal dominant condition in children, in which they are bilateral. Adult cases typically occur after previous corneal perforation or corneal trauma.

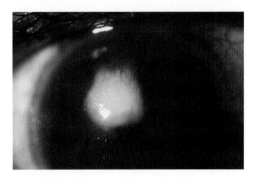

Fig. 5.29 Corneal keloid.

◆ **Presentation**

Patients present with decreased visual acuity and foreign body sensation. A white, elevated, corneal lesion can progressively enlarge and cover the visual axis of the cornea (**Fig. 5.29**).

◆ **Differential Diagnosis**

Scar from infectious corneal ulcer; dermoid

◆ **Management**

If visual acuity is compromised, a lamellar keratectomy or penetrating keratoplasty may be needed for vision rehabilitation. Bilateral cases in children should receive a systemic evaluation for Lowe syndrome with referral to a pediatrician.

Calcific Band Keratopathy

This condition consists of calcific degeneration of the superficial cornea involving the Bowman layer. Systemic causes may include renal disease, hypercalcemic states, gout, sarcoidosis, and elevated phosphorus levels. Conditions of chronic ocular disease such as glaucoma, keratitis, uveitis, and the presence of intraocular silicone oil may also cause this condition. A hereditary form is present. Chronic mercury exposure may be another cause.

◆ **Presentation**

Fine gray-white dustlike opacities develop in the Bowman layer in the peripheral cornea, typically at 3 and 9 o'clock. A lucid interval separates the opacities from the adjacent limbus. The deposits typically coalesce to form a horizontal band of corneal opacification in the interpalpebral zone of the cornea (**Fig. 5.30**).

◆ **Management**

Determine the underlying cause. Any underlying electrolyte or renal disease must be corrected. If pain or foreign body sensation is significant, a lamellar keratectomy with adjunct disodium ethylenediaminetetraacetic acid (EDTA) (1, 1.5, or 2%) can be used to remove calcific deposits. If underlying conditions are not corrected,

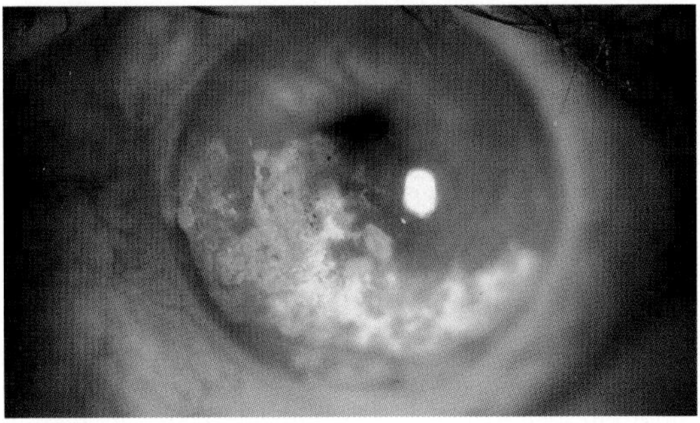

Fig. 5.30 Band keratopathy.

the calcific deposits will recur. Phototherapeutic keratectomy may also be used to remove the deposits.

Salzmann Nodular Degeneration

A noninflammatory corneal degeneration develops either from idiopathic causes or as a sequela of prior chronic keratitis. Some causes may include phlyctenulosis, blepharitis, trachoma, contact lens keratitis, or interstitial keratitis. It may also be associated with recurrent corneal erosions and epithelial basement membrane dystrophy.

◆ Presentation

Patients either may be asymptomatic or may present with foreign body sensation, tearing, and decreased vision. Elevated gray-white or bluish nodules develop representing fibrillar material that has replaced the Bowman layer. The nodules often develop in a circular fashion in the central or paracentral cornea, although they may also be presenting adjacent to the limbus (**Fig. 5.31**).

◆ Differential Diagnosis

Phlyctenulosis, keloid, staphylococcal marginal ulcer, corneal scar from infectious keratitis

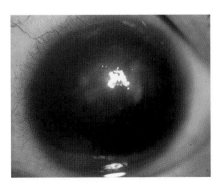

Fig. 5.31 Salzmann's nodular degeneration.

◆ **Management**

Supportive care with artificial tears, gels, or ointment can help. If recurrent erosions are present, a temporary bandage lens or topical osmotic agent such as sodium chloride drops may improve the symptoms. If visual acuity is decreased or significant discomfort develops, a superficial keratectomy can be performed to remove the nodules. Recurrence may develop despite debridement. Penetrating procedures are not commonly needed for this condition.

Spheroidal Degeneration

Spheroidal degeneration is also referred to as corneal elastosis, Labrador keratopathy, climatic droplet keratopathy, and Bietti nodular dystrophy. It is a bilateral condition seen mainly in men, known to have an association with ultraviolet exposure.

◆ **Presentation**

The patient presents with irritation and foreign body sensation. In extreme cases visual impairment may occur. Clinical examination reveals small amber-colored granules in the superficial stroma of the peripheral interpalpebral cornea. Increased opacification, coalescence, and central spread occur in the late presentations.

◆ **Management**

Lamellar keratoplasty and penetrating keratoplasty are options when there is visual impairment.

Polymorphic Amyloid Degeneration

Bilateral corneal opacities containing amyloid develop in late adulthood within the corneal stroma.

◆ **Presentation**

Patients are often asymptomatic with no vision reduction. Gray to white polymorphic and/or filamentous flecks appear in the mid- to deep stroma within the central or paracentral cornea. The deposits appear refractile but are translucent on retroillumination. The intervening stroma is clear (**Fig. 5.32**).

◆ **Differential Diagnosis**

Corneal guttae, corneal farinata, lattice dystrophy

◆ **Management**

Visual acuity is typically not involved so no treatment is necessary.

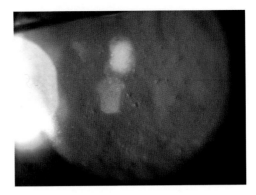

Fig. 5.32 Polymorphic amyloid deposits seen on retroillumination.

Iron Lines

Iron deposition occurs in the epithelium as a result of tear pooling abnormalities from asperity of the corneal surface (**Fig. 5.33**).

◆ Presentation

- *Hudson-Stähli line*: A horizontal line at the junction of the lower third and upper two thirds of the cornea
- *Ferry line*: A line anterior to the edge of the conjunctiva from a filtering bleb
- *Stocker line*: A line anterior to the head of a pterygium
- *Fleischer ring*: A continuous circular or elliptical pattern surrounding the area of corneal steepening in keratoconus
- *Mannis line*: A continuous 360-degree ring just anterior to the sutures of a corneal graft

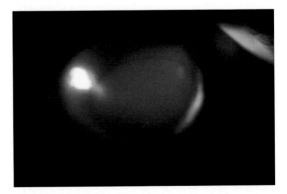

Fig. 5.33 Fleischer ring from keratoconus outlined with cobalt blue light filter.

◆ **Management**

No management is necessary.

Kayser-Fleischer Ring

This is a rare autosomal recessive disorder in which copper deposition occurs throughout the body, including the Descemet membrane. It is also known as hepatolenticular degeneration.

◆ **Presentation**

Corneal findings are asymptomatic, but examination by gonioscopy or slit lamp reveals a Kayser-Fleischer ring (a golden brown to green 360-degree ring pattern at the limbus within the Descemet membrane).

◆ **Management**

Systemic penicillamine causes the ring to disappear gradually. Liver transplantation is often required.

Corneal Verticillata

Lysosomal or lipid deposits occur in the basal epithelial layer of the cornea in association with several systemic medications. This can also occur in Fabry disease.

◆ **Presentation**

Patients are usually asymptomatic but may experience blurred vision.

◆ **Differential Diagnosis**

Fabry disease (**Fig. 5.34A**), amiodarone (**Fig. 5.34B**), chloroquine, hydroxychloroquine, phenothiazines, indomethacin, naproxen, striate melanokeratosis (**Fig. 5.34C**)

◆ **Management**

Observe or perform epithelial debridement if vision is decreased. If the condition is severe, consider discontinuation of systemic medication unless it is essential for treatment of systemic disease.

◆ Peripheral Thinning

Mooren Ulcer

This is an aggressive peripheral ulcerative keratitis with a high risk of corneal melting and perforation not associated with systemic collagen vascular disease. An autoimmune role is thought to play a role in the development of ulceration and stromal melting based on known suppressor T-cell deficiency, increased immunoglobulin A antibody levels, and increased levels of plasma cells, lymphocytes, immunoglobulins, and complement factor in the peripheral cornea and adjacent

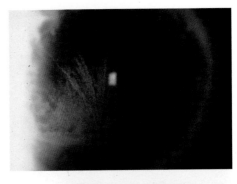

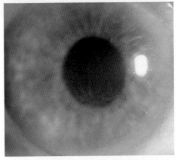

Fig. 5.34 **(A)** Corneal verticillata seen with Fabry disease. **(B)** Corneal verticillata from amiodarone. **(C)** Striate melanokeratosis with melanin deposition in the corneal epithelium.

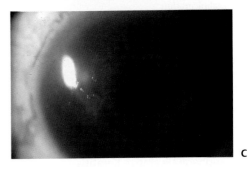

conjunctiva. Risk factors include prior ocular trauma or ocular surgery as well as a subset with prior parasitic infection with helminths.

◆ Presentation

Symptoms include intense pain, redness, tearing, and photophobia. A chronic and progressive corneal ulceration begins in the peripheral cornea with circumferential spread followed by centripetal spread. A leading edge of deepithelialized tissue is present with keratolysis. Significant corneal neovascularization and fibrosis can develop. Patients are often in late adulthood with unilateral presentation. A second form of ulceration occurs in patients with preceding parasitic helminth

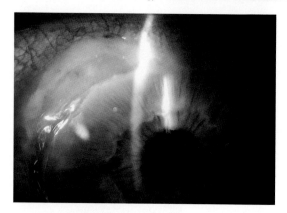

Fig. 5.35   Mooren ulcer.

infection; this form is more common in endemic areas of Africa with high populations of parasitemia. This form is often bilateral and highly associated with corneal perforation. Mooren ulcer can be associated with concurrent hepatitis C infection (**Fig. 5.35**).

◆ Differential Diagnosis

Peripheral ulcerative keratitis, infectious keratitis, rosacea, staphylococcal marginal ulceration

◆ Management

A conjunctival recession can be utilized for initial treatment of ulceration, perhaps by severing connection of the limbal vasculature and associated inflammatory cells from the region of ulceration. Lamellar keratoplasty is often needed in cases with impending or frank perforation. Systemic immunosuppressive agents such as oral corticosteroids, methotrexate, cyclosporine, and cyclophosphamide have shown promise in treatment. Hepatitis C–associated cases have shown improvement with interferon therapy. Despite treatment options, this form of ulceration often has a poor prognosis with a high corneal perforation rate.

Peripheral Ulcerative Keratitis

A peripheral corneal ulceration is associated with epithelial breakdown and keratolysis. The condition can be associated with any connective tissue disorder (collagen vascular disease) but is most commonly seen with rheumatoid arthritis.

◆ Presentation

Presentation includes pain, redness, and decreased vision in the setting of a connective tissue disorder. Peripheral corneal infiltration is present with an associated epithelial defect except in the early stages. Stromal melting may be the first sign of systemic disease and is correlated with exacerbations of systemic disease activity. Symptoms are usually unilateral but may be bilateral in presentation. Associated limbal vaso-occlusion can be seen with the adjacent limbal vessels (**Fig. 5.36A,B**).

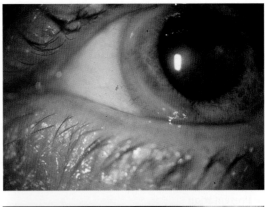

A

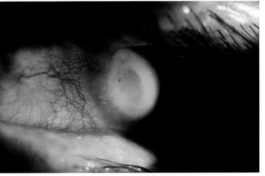

B

Fig. 5.36 **(A)** Peripheral ulcerative keratitis from rheumatoid arthritis. **(B)** Peripheral corneal ulcer associated with systemic lupus erythematosis.

◆ Differential Diagnosis

Infectious keratitis, Mooren ulcer, Terrien marginal degeneration, furrow degeneration, rosacea, exposure keratitis

◆ Management

The goal of therapy is to prevent corneal melting and promote reepithelialization. Surface lubricants such as artificial tears, gels, or ointments should be used every 1 to 2 hours with or without a bland ophthalmic antimicrobial antibiotic such as erythromycin to treat the immune-mediated dry-eye disease. Temporary or permanent punctal cautery can also increase the surface moisture. Systemic collagenase inhibitors (macrolides) may be useful. Control of systemic inflammation is essential with immunosuppression medications such as prednisone, cyclosporine, azathioprine, cylcophosphamide, or methotrexate; this can be administered in concert with a rheumatologist depending on the ophthalmologist's comfort with systemic therapy. Cyanoacrylate glue or therapeutic bandage lenses may be needed in cases of severe stromal thinning. A conjunctival recession of adjacent limbal conjunctiva can promote healing of the adjacent peripheral stromal melting and ulceration, perhaps because of elimination of a source of inflammatory cells and collagenolytic enzymes from severing the connection to the limbal vessels. Lamellar and penetrating keratoplasty may be needed in cases of impending or frank perforation.

Terrien Marginal Degeneration

This is an idiopathic peripheral corneal thinning disorder that can be localized or diffuse. The ocular surface typically shows only mild inflammation in association with the peripheral corneal thinning. The condition is usually bilateral but may be unilateral or asymmetrical in presentation. Electron microscopy reveals the presence of histiocytes in the corneal lamellae, indicating a possible immune-mediated role.

◆ Presentation

Symptoms include foreign body sensation, blurred vision, and only minimal signs of redness or conjunctival injection. Peripheral corneal thinning occurs most often superiorly and progresses in an annular pattern with an overlying intact epithelium. The thinning is accompanied by an anterior lipid border and bridging vessels extending toward the lipid base. The anterior lipid border is often steep, with sloping of the limbal border. Against-the-rule-astigmatism often develops as the thinning progresses. Spontaneous perforation is rare but may occur, especially with ocular trauma (**Fig. 5.37**).

◆ Differential Diagnosis

Peripheral ulcerative keratitis, furrow degeneration, atypical pellucid marginal degeneration, Fuchs superficial marginal keratitis

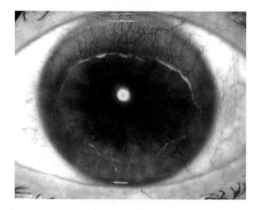

Fig. 5.37 Terrien marginal degeneration.

◆ **Management**

Management often consists of supportive care with lubricant tears, gels, or ointments. Topical cyclosporine may add benefit in some cases. Lamellar corneal patch grafts can be useful in cases of impending perforation. Annular lamellar grafts have also been used in severe cases with 360 degrees of progressive peripheral thinning.

Furrow Degeneration

This may be an optical illusion, though sometimes true thinning does occur.

◆ **Presentation**

The patient is usually asymptomatic. This may occur as an idiopathic condition in the elderly as a lucid area separating the corneal arcus from the limbus. Corneal thinning is evident. The epithelium is intact with no vascularization.

◆ **Differential Diagnosis**

Terrien marginal degeneration

◆ **Management**

No treatment is required.

◆ Aphakic and Pseudophakic Bullous Keratopathy

Refer to the chapter 7 section on corneal edema as a complication of cataract surgery.

◆ Corneal Surgery

Penetrating Keratoplasty

Penetrating keratoplasty consists of a full-thickness replacement of diseased cornea using a donor cornea harvested from a healthy corneoscleral donor rim. Indications for surgery include corneal edema, corneal scarring, corneal dystrophies, keratoconus, corneal ulceration or perforation, infection, and failed corneal transplants, among others. The donor tissue is secured to the peripheral host corneal rim with a variety of suture placement techniques, including interrupted sutures, a continuous running suture, or combined techniques.

Risks of surgery include but are not limited to suture infections and graft rejection. Graft rejection may be epithelial, subepithelial, or endothelial in nature (**Fig. 5.38A,B**).

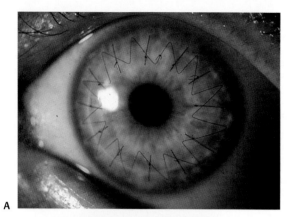

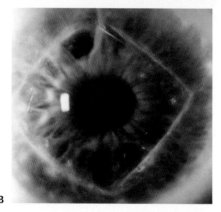

Fig. 5.38 **(A)** Penetrating keratoplasty with combined interrupted and running suture technique. **(B)** Castroviejo square graft.

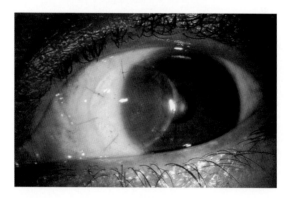

Fig. 5.39 Lamellar keratoplasty for recurrent pterygium.

Lamellar Keratoplasty

This is a partial replacement of the cornea with donor corneal tissue. The procedure can be used in keratoconus, anterior corneal dystrophies, anterior corneal scars, recurrent pterygia, and corneal melts. Lamellar grafts can be performed using an artificial anterior chamber and microkeratome or using a whole globe with handheld partial-thickness donor tissue dissection (**Fig. 5.39**).

Endothelial Keratoplasty

This corneal transplant technique replaces the diseased endothelium with a posterior donor corneal button consisting of endothelium, Descemet membrane, and a thin layer of posterior corneal stroma. It is used for diseases of the endothelium when the epithelium and stroma are essentially normal, such as Fuchs dystrophy, bullous keratopathy, endothelial graft failure, and iridocorneal endothelial syndrome. Tissue can be prepared using an artificial anterior chamber and microkeratome or by handheld dissection. Descemet stripping endothelial keratoplasty (DSEK) has become a popular method of performing this technique with stripping of the Descemet membrane and endothelium, followed by replacement with a thin donor posterior cornea. The partial-thickness donor cornea is held in place with air tamponade (**Fig. 5.40A,B**).

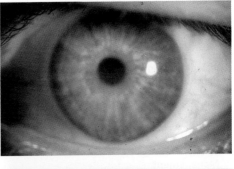

A

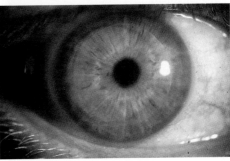

B

Fig. 5.40 **(A)** Endothelial keratoplasty. Preoperative corneal edema from Fuchs dystrophy. **(B)** Endothelial keratoplasty. Postoperative Descemet stripping automated endothelial keratoplasty.

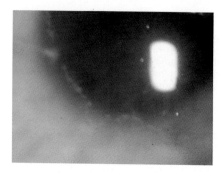

Fig. 5.41 Khodadoust line with endothelial rejection of penetrating keratoplasty.

Graft Rejection

The 5-year failure rate for corneal grafts is ~35% across the United States. Corneal graft rejection is the most common cause of graft failure in the late postoperative period. Diagnosis of corneal graft rejection should be made only in grafts that have remained clear for at least 2 weeks following keratoplasty.

◆ **Presentation**

Patients may complain of a decrease in visual acuity, redness, photophobia, pain, and irritation. Epithelial rejection is marked by an elevated epithelial rejection line that stains with fluorescein or rose bengal or by the presence of subepithelial infiltrates. Stromal rejection is characterized by peripheral full-thickness haze with limbal injection in a previously clear graft. An arc-shaped infiltrate may be noted peripherally at the graft–host junction that progresses centrally. Classic endothelial rejection presents with an endothelial rejection line (Khodadoust line) that usually begins at a vascularized portion of the peripheral graft–host junction and progresses (**Fig. 5.41**). The combination of keratic precipitates, an anterior chamber reaction, circumcorneal injection, and regions of corneal edema should be diagnosed as corneal graft rejection.

◆ **Management**

Rejection may be prevented with steroids, cyclosporine A, and other immunomodulators.

Keratoprosthesis

An artificial device is used to restore vision in conditions of corneal blindness. Commonly used devices include the Boston Dohlman Keratoprosthesis and Alpha-Cor (Addition Technology, Inc., Des Plaines, IL; the Type I device is manufactured and currently available through the Massachusetts Eye and Ear Infirmary at cost: http://www.masstechportal.org/IP1416.aspx). Indications include multiple failed cadaveric allograft surgeries with little hope for success using future cadaveric tissue. This method avoids allograft rejection, but corneal melting, infections, and glaucoma remain a concern with this device. It can also be used for stem cell disease in patients who are poor candidates for immunosuppression (**Fig. 5.42A,B**).

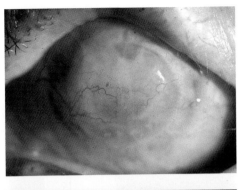

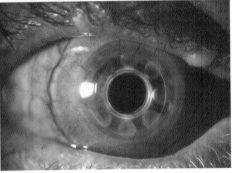

Fig. 5.42 (**A**) Dense corneal opacification prior to Dohlman keratoprosthesis placement. (**B**) Postoperative Dohlman keratoprosthesis with 20/40 uncorrected Snellen visual acuity.

Anterior Staphyloma Managed by Anterior Segment Transplantation

An anterior staphyloma is a challenging entity. Multiple causative factors have been noted in the literature, the common ones being keratitis and congenital malformations, with sporadic reports of disorders such as neurofibromatosis and sarcoidosis .The surgical options for anterior staphyloma and similar diffuse corneal lesions include a conventional keratoplasty, overlay grafts, and partial- or full-thickness sclerokeratoplasty. However, anterior staphyloma is associated with additional problems other than corneal ectasia. The lens is often cataractous with compromised zonules, which has to be taken care of at the time of the surgery. In addition, staphylectomy leads invariably to loss of iris tissue, creating an iatrogenic aniridia. Therefore, an ideal transplant for an anterior staphyloma or a similar diffuse anterior pathology should address these issues. Soosan Jacob has developed a new method of anterior segment transplantation that can be used to treat a malformed anterior segment and transplant a new, bioprosthetic graft simulating the anterior segment (**Figs. 5.43A,B**). This technique is an extension of the glued intraocular lens (IOL) technique invented by Amar Agarwal.

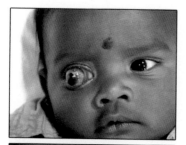

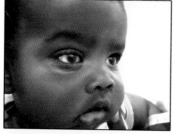

A

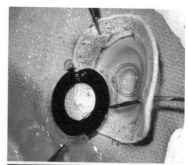

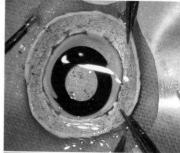

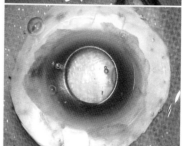

B

Fig. 5.43 (A) Anterior segment transplantation done on a 4-month-old child with anterior staphyloma. (*Top*) Preoperative appearance. (*Bottom*) Postoperative day 1 appearance. **(B)** Biosynthetic graft being prepared for transplantation. One haptic of the aniridia IOL being externalized (top). Biosynthetic graft seen after both haptics have been externalized (center). The bioprosthetic graft prepared for anterior segment transplantation. Note the aniridia intraocular lens haptics externalized at the scleral level below scleral flaps (bottom). The graft has biological components: the cornea and sclera, and synthetic components: the IOL optic, the artificial iris, and the edge of the artificial iris forming the pupil.

◆ **Presentation**

Diffuse corneal involvement and cicatrization of the uveal tissue along with high intraocular pressure results in a large ectatic area of the cornea and limbus.

◆ **Differential Diagnosis**

Peters anomaly, diffuse corneoscleral keratitis

◆ **Management**

The bioprosthetic graft consists of a biological and a prosthetic part. The biological part is fashioned from a cadaveric whole globe (cornea and sclera), and the prosthetic part consists of an aniridia IOL (iris, pupil, and IOL). Two partial-thickness, limbal-based scleral flaps of 3-mm size are created 180 degrees apart on the donor sclera. Two straight sclerotomies are then made with an 18-gauge needle 1.5 mm from the limbus under the existing scleral flaps. A corneo-scleral rim is then cut the entire length of the sclera, including in the scleral flaps. A cyclodialysis is then induced to separate the uveal tissue from the dissected corneoscleral button. The corneoscleral graft is placed concave (i.e., endothelial side up), and the aniridia IOL haptics are externalized through the sclerotomy under the scleral flaps using a 23-gauge forceps. The biosynthetic assembly thus consists of a donor cornea and sclera and an artificial iris and lens (aniridia IOL). In the recipient eye, the staphylomatous cornea is excised. Underlying cataract is managed with lensectomy and vitrectomy. The biosynthetic graft is then placed on the host and sutured. The IOL haptics are then tucked into a scleral pocket created at the edge of the scleral flaps, and the flap is then glued down with tissue glue (Tisseel, Baxter, Deerfield, IL). The conjunctiva is then closed by gluing.

◆ Enlarged Corneal Nerves

◆ Presentation

Prominent corneal nerves may be seen radiating centrally from the corneal periphery.

◆ Differential Diagnosis

Multiple endocrine neoplasia type IIb, icthyosis, Refsum disease, leprosy, keratoconus, Fuchs endothelial dystrophy, osteogenesis imperfecta, ocular pemphigus, neurofibromatosis, phthisis bulbi, posterior polymorphous dystrophy, herpes simplex, herpes zoster, primary amyloidosis

◆ Management

Management is aimed at the underlying condition.

◆ Corneal Neovascularization

The cornea is typically devoid of blood vessels; however, in conditions of infection, inflammation, or ocular surface insult, blood vessels can abnormally extend into the cornea. This is often referred to as corneal neovascularization or pannus. It is mainly seen in inflammatory corneal diseases such as trachoma.

◆ Presentation

Pannus presents as a vascular ingrowth into the cornea from the limbal vasculature. It can be superficial or deep (**Fig. 5.44**).

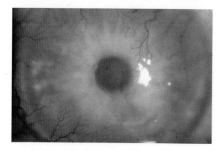

Fig. 5.44 A slit-lamp photograph demonstrating severe corneal neo-vascularization from diffuse stem cell deficiency.

◆ Differential Diagnosis

Trachoma, leprosy, herpes simplex or herpes zoster keratitis, phlyctenular kerato-conjunctivitis, toxic conjunctivitis, acne rosacea, bullous keratopathy, molluscum contagiosum, vernal conjunctivitis, keratoconjunctivitis sicca, contact lens use, inclusion conjunctivitis (micropannus), superior limbic keratoconjunctivitis, contact lens keratitis, Fuchs marginal keratitis, hypoparathyroidism, vitamin B deficiency, and pellagra.

◆ Management

Management is aimed at the underlying condition.

◆ Leukocornea

Leukocornea may arise due to a wide variety of conditions including infection, inflammation, anomalies, hereditary conditions, and trauma.

◆ Presentation

Opacification of the cornea is evident, even without the slit-lamp examination.

◆ Differential Diagnosis

- *Infections*: Bacterial, fungal, herpetic ulcers, stromal scarring, trachoma, *Acanthamoeba*
- *Inflammatory*: aphakic and pseudophakic bullous keratopathy, Steven Johnsons syndrome, graft rejection, ocular cicatricial pemphigoid
- *Congenital*: Anterior chamber cleavage syndromes, sclerocornea, congenital glaucoma, dermoid, amyloidosis
- *Hereditary*: Congenital hereditary corneal dystrophy, Down syndrome, Patau syndrome, inborn errors of metabolism (mucopolysaccharidosis, Lowe syndrome, mucolipoidosis)
- *Trauma*: Descemet tear (birth trauma), thermal injury, chemical burns

◆ Management

Management consists mainly of doing a corneal transplantation in suitable cases. Any underlying cause should also be addressed.

◆ Chemical Burn

See the chapter 1 section on chemical exposure burns.

Intraocular Inflammation

Soosan Jacob, Dhivya Ashok Kumar, Athiya Agarwal, and Amar Agarwal

◆ Acute Anterior Nongranulomatous Uveitis

HLA-B27-Associated Uveitis

Ankylosing Spondylitis

Ankylosing spondylitis (AS) is an arthropathy characterized by back pain and stiffness after inactivity. HLA-B27 is found in up to 90% of patients with AS. The chance that an HLA-B27–positive patient will develop spondyloarthritis or eye disease is 1 in 4. Not all HLA-B27–positive patients develop disease.

Sacroiliac x-ray films should be obtained when indicated by a suggestive history in a patient with ocular disease consistent with HLA-B27 syndrome. Sacroiliac x-ray films show sclerosis and eventual narrowing of the joint space, ligamentous ossification.

◆ Complications

Bony deformity, pulmonary apical fibrosis, aortitis, aortic valvular insufficiency

◆ Uveitis

◆ Management

Topical steroids and cycloplegics. Sacroiliac joint radiograph, HLA-B27 screening rheumatology consultation

Reiter Syndrome

Reiter syndrome is characterized by the following:

- ◆ Nonspecific urethritis
- ◆ Polyarthritis
- ◆ Conjunctival inflammation, often accompanied by iritis

◆ Presentation

This is commonly seen in young adult males (90%), whereas females constitute only 10%. Arthritis is typically asymmetric and in oligoarticular distribution, involving knees, ankles, feet, and wrists. Sacroiliitis is present in as many as 70% of patients.

Keratoderma blennorrhagicum (a scaly, erythematous disorder of the palms and soles) and circinate balanitis (a persistent, scaly, erythematous, circumferential rash of the distal penis) may be found.

Less common findings are plantar fasciitis, Achilles tendinitis, sacroiliitis, nailbed pitting, palate ulcers, and tongue ulcers.

Ocular involvement ranges from conjunctivitis (mucopurulent and papillary) to keratitis (punctate and subepithelial) to anterior, nongranulomatous inflammation.

◆ **Uveitis**

◆ **Management**

Topical steroids and cycloplegics

◆ HLA-B27 screening because it is present in 85 to 95% of patients
◆ Rheumatology consultation

Inflammatory Bowel Disease (IBD)

Ulcerative colitis (diffuse inflammation of the colonic mucosa) and Crohn disease (granulomatous iliocolitis) are both associated with acute iritis.

◆ **Presentation**

Between 5 and 12% of patients with ulcerative colitis, and 2.4% of patients with Crohn disease develop acute anterior uveitis (AAU). Of patients with inflammatory bowel disease, 20% may have sacroiliitis, and of these patients, 60% are HLA-B27 positive. Ocular involvement may occur first and may include anterior uveitis, conjunctivitis, keratitis, episcleritis, scleritis, extraocular muscle palsies, optic neuropathy, retinal vasculitis, neuroretinitis, and orbital inflammation. Systemic symptoms include bloody diarrhea, crampy abdominal pain, skin rash, arthralgia, erythema nodosum, pyoderma gangrenosum, sacroiliitis, renal stones, and hepatobiliary abnormalities.

◆ **Uveitis**

◆ **Management**

Topical steroids and cycloplegics. Treat in conjunction with an internist.

Psoriatic Arthritis

◆ *Ocular involvement*: Nongranulomatous, anterior inflammation, nodular episcleritis, keratitis, keratoconjunctivitis sicca

  Uveitis is not associated with psoriasis without arthritis.

◆ *Systemic*: Erythematous, hyperkeratotic rash, nail pitting, and distal interphalangeal joint arthritis

◆ **Uveitis**

◆ **Management**

Topical steroids, cycloplegics, immunosuppressives. Treat in conjunction with an internist.

Glaucoma-Related Uveitis

Posner-Schlossman Syndrome

◆ **Presentation**

Manifests as unilateral mild acute iritis symptoms that include discomfort, blurred vision, or haloes. Signs include markedly elevated intraocular pressure, corneal edema, fine keriatic precipitates, low-grade, and slightly dilated pupil.

Posner-Schlossman syndrome may be associated with HLA-B54 gene locus.

◆ **Management**

Topical steroids and intraocular pressure–lowering agents

Uveitis-Glaucoma-Hyphema Syndrome

Irritation of the iris root by the warped footplates of poorly made, rigid, anterior chamber intraocular lens implants causes the uveitis-glaucoma-hyphema triad.

◆ **Presentation**

Increased intraocular pressure, anterior chamber inflammation, and hyphema formation in the presence of an intraocular lens

◆ **Management**

Topical steroids, cycloplegics, and intraocular pressure–lowering agents

Phacolytic Uveitis/Glaucoma

This involves an acute increase in intraocular pressure caused by blockage of the trabecular meshwork by lens protein and engorged macrophages.

◆ **Presentation**

Low-grade anterior chamber inflammation, increased intraocular pressure, lack of keratic precipitates, and synechiae. Aqueous tap may reveal swollen macrophages.

◆ **Management**

Intraocular pressure reduction with osmotic agents as well as topical medications. The cataract needs to be removed.

◆ Chronic Nongranulomatous Uveitis

Juvenile Rheumatoid Arthritis–Associated Uveitis

Juvenile rheumatoid arthritis (JRA) is a group of diseases with onset before 16 years of age.

◆ **Presentation**

◆ *Systemic onset*: Usually seen in children under the age of 5 years, of which < 6% present with uveitis; rash, fever, lymphadenopathy, hepatosplenomegaly, pericarditis, anemia, psoriasis; patients presenting with systemic onset account for ~20% of all cases of JRA.
◆ *Polyarticular onset*: Shows involvement of five or more joints in the first 6 weeks of the disease. It constitutes 40% of JRA cases overall but only 7 to 14% of cases of JRA-associated iridocyclitis.
◆ *Panciarticular onset*: This includes the vast majority (80 to 90%) of patients with JRA who have uveitis.
   ◆ *Type 1*: Girls under age 5, positive for antinuclear antibody (ANA). Chronic iridocyclitis occurs in up to 25% of these patients.
   ◆ *Type 2*: Older boys, seronegative spondyloarthropathy (75% are HLA-B27 positive). Uveitis tends to be acute and recurrent rather than chronic as in type 1.
◆ *Ocular involvement*: It usually occurs within 5 to 7 years of onset of arthritis, but the risk remains into adulthood. Ocular inflammation occurs in 2 to 12% of all cases and is usually bilateral. Unilateral cases often progress to bilateral within 12 months. The ocular and joint disease activity are not associated. It may be antinuclear antibody test positive, rheumatoid factor negative.

Children are often asymptomatic with insidious disease onset. There may be mild ocular pain, headache, photophobia, and decreased vision. A white eye with active anterior chamber inflammation, keratic precipitates, posterior synechia, cataract formation, glaucoma, and band shaped keratopathy may even be found on the first examination.

◆ **Management**

Uveitis is treated with topical steroids and cycloplegics. Systemic or periocular steroids are sometimes needed. Ethylenediaminetetraacetic acid (EDTA) chelation is done for band-shaped keratopathy. Rheumatology consultation is often necessary.

Fuchs Heterochromic Iridocyclitis

◆ **Presentation**

Presentation is usually unilateral; symptoms vary from none to mild blurring and discomfort.

◆ **Signs**

◆ Diffuse iris stromal atrophy with variable pigment epithelial layer atrophy
◆ Small white stellate keratic precipitates scattered diffusely over the entire endothelium
◆ Cells present in the anterior chamber as well as the anterior vitreous.
◆ Synechiae almost never form.
◆ Glaucoma and cataracts occur.
◆ Abnormal vessels may bridge the angle on gonioscopy.
◆ Fundus lesions are absent; sometimes toxoplasma scars have been reported.

◆ **Management**

◆ Cataract surgery and intraocular lens implant can be done successfully.
◆ Glaucoma is difficult to control and may need surgery.

◆ Granulomatous Uveitis

Syphilis

◆ Presentation

Syphilitic involvement of the uveal tract can present in two ways:

1. *Congenital syphilitic uveitis*: Here the involvement is bilateral, the periphery of the retina is involved, and occasionally one or two quadrants of the posterior pole can be involved rarely. Thus the vision is not affected. The typical appearance is that of a salt and pepper fundus due to areas of pigment accumulation interspersed with areas of pigment loss. An associated ocular feature is the presence of bilateral interstitial keratitis.

   Secondary retinal pigment degeneration may be seen, which is a condition that is progressive and is associated with constriction of the blood vessels of the retina and the choroids in the form of sclerosis. The optic disk is pale with sharply defined borders. Pigments dispersed are also sharply demarcated with a star shape or bony corpuscle formation. The posterior pole or the periphery can be affected, and the condition is bilateral.

2. *Acquired syphilis*: This has three components: iritis, chorioretinitis, and neuroretinitis. The iritis is characterized by three forms: iritis papulosa, iritis nodosa, and iritis roseata. Chorioretinitis is characterized by vitreous haze, fine punctate gray to yellow exudation areas, pigment accumulation along the optic nerve and blood vessels, and flame-shaped hemorrhages with chorioretinal edema. Neuroretinitis consists of optic nerve head involvement with vascular involvement of the surrounding retinal vessels.

◆ Management

Blood tests in the form of Venereal Disease Research Laboratory test (VDRL) and the fluorescent treponemal antibody–absorption test (FTA-ABS) are done. Uveitis is treated with topical steroids and cycloplegics. The systemic disease should be treated in conjunction with an internist.

Sarcoidosis

Sarcoidosis is a chronic granulomatous uveitis of unknown etiology. It may also affect the lungs, eyes, and skin.

◆ Presentation

◆ *Ocular*: Symptoms of uveal involvement are variable and frequently include mild to moderate blurring of vision. It may involve all structures of the eye. A sizable proportion of patients develop chronic granulomatous iridocyclitis. Typical findings are mutton fat keratic precipitates, Koeppe and Busacca iris nodules, and snowballs in the infectious anterior vitreous. Nummular corneal infiltrates, endothelial opacification, and large iris granulomas also occur. Posterior synechiae can be extensive and may lead to iris bombé and angle closure glaucoma. Peripheral anterior synechia may be extensive, involving 360 degrees in advanced cases. Secondary glaucoma can be severe.

Posterior segment involvement is characterized by nodular granulomas measuring ¼ to 1 disc diameter that occur in both the retina and the choroid. Irregular nodular granulomas along venules have been termed *candlewax drippings* or *taches de bougie*. Linear or patchy retinal periphlebitis presents as sheathing. Cystoid macular edema is common; retinal neovascularization, disk edema, and optic nerve granulomas also occur. Palpebral and bulbar conjunctival nodules also occur.

◆ *Lungs*: Hilar adenopathy.
◆ *Central nervous system (CNS):* Cranial and peripheral neuropathy, aseptic meningitis.
◆ *Cardiovascular system*: Cardiac arrhythmias, pericarditis, arthritis, myositis, erythema nodosa, renal involvement hepatosplenomegaly and bone marrow infiltration.

◆ Management

Serum angiotensin-converting enzyme and lysozyme levels are increased. Chest x-ray shows hilar adenopathy.

◆ Uveitis

Topical, periocular, and systemic steroids, topical cycloplegics. Treat in conjunction with an internist.

Tuberculosis

◆ Presentation

Tuberculous uveitis can present include the following ways:

◆ Acute nongranulomatous infection—immunological or allergic in nature
◆ Nodular granulomatous infiltrates that are fulminating and caseating. Two types of nodules are present as shown in **Table 6.1**.
◆ Relapsing and recurrent iritis
◆ Low-grade chronic inflammation that presents with cataract, glaucoma, or pthisis bulbi
◆ Choroidal lesions appear as raised multiple yellow nodules with blurred margins. Retinal periphlebitis and subretinal vascularizations are seen.
◆ Other ocular features of tuberculosis include phlyctenulosis, episcleritis, nodular scleritis, and optic neuritis.

◆ Management

Antituberculous treatment is started in conjunction with an internist. Steroids should be started only after starting antituberculous treatment.

Table 6.1   Two Types of Nodular Granulomatous Infiltrates

Solitary or conglomerate nodule	Miliary nodules
Otherwise healthy immune responsive patients	Immunocompromised patients, severely debilitated patients
Single large tumorlike nodule yellow to white	Multiple nodules over the iris at the papillary margin and ciliary body with dissemination of bacilli

◆ Intermediate Uveitis/Pars Planitis

◆ Presentation

The disease is typically seen in children. It is also known as chronic cyclitis. Patients have visual symptoms like blurred, distorted vision secondary to macular edema. They also complain of floaters. The active vitreous inflammation shows cells that are small, round, nonpigmented, and numerous. The old vitritis has cells that are irregular, pigmented, and remain in the formed vitreous. At the edges of the ora serrata there is snow banking that is characteristic of deposition of inflammatory cells at this region. Anterior segment inflammation signs such as congestion and tenderness are absent. The symptoms of pain or photophobia are also absent or minimal.

There are several key differentiating features:

◆ Peripheral retinitis
◆ Perivasculitis
◆ Vitritis
◆ Snow banking at the inferior peripheral retina

◆ Differential Diagnosis

Multiple sclerosis, sarcoidosis, tuberculosis, toxocariasis, syphilis, Lyme disease

◆ Management

Steroids are given via topical, subtenons, or oral route. Systemic immunosuppressants and vitrectomy may also be necessary in some cases.

◆ Posterior Uveitis

Toxoplasmosis

Toxoplasmosis is the most common cause of chorioretinitis, congenital in origin. When the mother is affected in the first trimester, there is a 40% risk of transmission to the fetus.

◆ Presentation

Two forms of toxoplasmosis exist: congenital and adult. Both forms are characterized by acute focal chorioretinitis (**Fig. 6.1**).

◆ *Congenital toxoplasmosis*: It is bilateral in 85% of children and 80% have chorioretinitis. When CNS symptoms such as convulsions, hydrocephalus, mental retardation, and intracranial calcifications are absent, congenital lesions are diagnosed when the child presents with esotropia or exotropia or decreased vision.

The clinical characteristics of the congenital form are as follows:
  ◆ Bilateral
  ◆ Multiple chorioretinal lesions, especially in the macular area
  ◆ Punched-out lesion due to full-thickness necrosis
  ◆ Heavily pigmented scar, mistaken to be congenital colobomas

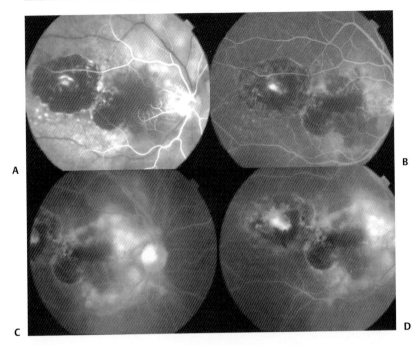

Fig. 6.1 **(A)** Arterial phase fluorescein angiogram (FA) demonstrating active toxoplasma chorioretinitis adjacent to a classic chorioretinal scar. **(B)** Arteriovenous phase FA demonstrating the classic old pigmented lesion with hypofluorescence at the center and hyperfluorescence at the margins of the lesion. **(C)** Late-phase FA showing juxtapapillary multiple hyperfluorescent areas corresponding to new, active lesions. **(D)** Active lesions, areas of hyperfluorescence, are usually seen in the vicinity of old scars, as evidenced here. (Courtesy of J. Fernando Arevalo, Venezuela)

◆ *Adult toxoplasmosis*: There is reactivation of inflammation at the edges of a pre-existing scar; this is called a satellite lesion. Vitritis is severe and the margins of the lesion are yellow and blurred. There is a hypersensitivity reaction to the trophozoites that are released from the cysts.
The following terms have been used to describe the lesion:
  ◆ *Searchlight in fog*: Yellow lesions seen through the vitreous haze
  ◆ *Grapevines*: Of the membranes and cells of vitritis
  ◆ *Wet snow*: Sticky vitreous exudates in vitritis

◆ **Differential Diagnosis**

In children, differentials include congenital colobomas, cytomegalovirus inclusion chorioretinitis, herpes simplex chorioretinitis, toxocariasis, retinoblastoma, and cerebral trauma.
  In adults, differentials include tuberculous chorioretinitis, candidiasis, and histioplasmosis.

◆ Management

Antibiotics in the form of Bactrim DS (double strength), clindamycin, or pyrimethamine with folinic acid are given for 6 weeks in conjunction with an internist. Oral steroids may be indicated when the disease spreads close to the optic nerve or macula.

Presumed Ocular Histoplasmosis

Histoplasma capsulatum causes the characteristic presumed ocular histoplasmosis syndrome (POHS). Immunocompromised patients are affected by the presence of an isolated granuloma or endophthalmitis.

POHS typically affects young people and is responsible for bilateral visual loss. The characteristic features of the syndrome are the appearance of isolated disciform macular lesions and scars that are well circumscribed. These are quiet lesions without the presence of active inflammation and the presence of peripapillary pigment atrophy (**Fig. 6.2**).

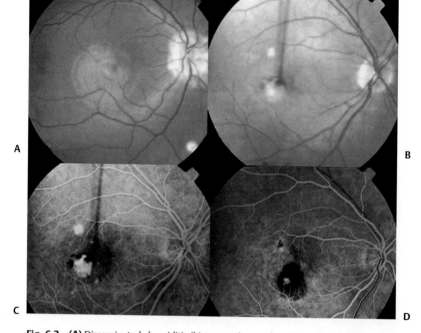

Fig. 6.2   **(A)** Disseminated choroiditis (histo spots), maculopathy, and peripapillary chorioretinal degenerative changes in a patient with the presumed ocular histoplasmosis syndrome. **(B)** Disseminated choroiditis (histo spots), maculopathy, and peripapillary chorioretinal degenerative changes in another patient with the presumed ocular histoplasmosis syndrome. **(C)** Fluorescein angiography of the patient in **Fig. 6.2B**, revealed serosanguinous retinal detachment with faint pigment halo in right macula and choroidal neovascularization. **(D)** Fluorescein angiography of patient in **Fig. 6.2B**, revealed hypofluorescence after photodynamic therapy with verteporfin. (Courtesy of Steve Bloom, MD).

◆ Management

Follow up for development of choroidal neovascular membrane and treat accordingly.

White Dot Syndrome

Multifocal Choroiditis

Multifocal choroiditis is a rare disorder involving idiopathic inflammation of the choroid and retinal pigment epithelium (RPE).

◆ Presentation

Presentation is usually bilateral, with symptoms such as photophobia, blurred vision, eye pain, and decreased visual acuity. The patient may also have metamorphopsia, floaters, scotomas, and photopsia. There may be signs and symptoms of anterior uveitis.

Multiple, small, yellow/gray-white spots may be seen along with cystoid macular edema, choroidal neovascular membrane, and subretinal fibrosis.

◆ Management

Corticosteroids are helpful in resolving the lesions.

Multiple Evanescent White Dot Syndrome

Multiple evanescent white dot syndrome (MEWDS) is an acute but benign, rare, unilateral disease of unknown etiology involving the RPE and choroidal capillaries. It usually affects young females. It can rarely be bilateral (**Fig. 6.3**).

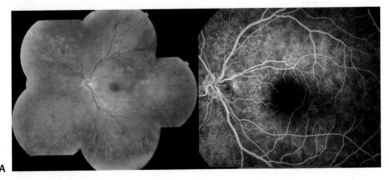

A   B

Fig. 6.3   Multiple evanescent white dot syndromes (MEWDS). **(A)** Fundus examination revealed small and large spots scatted through the fundus in the left eye. **(B)** Fluorescein angiography showed punctate hyperfluorescence. (Courtesy of Antonio Ciardella, MD). (*Continued on page 204*)

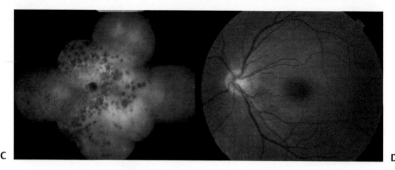

C   D

Fig. 6.3 (*Continued*) Multiple evanescent white dot syndromes (MEWDS). **(C)** Indocyanine green videoangiography demonstrated small and large hypofluorescent spots. A
diagnosis of MEWDS was made. **(D)** One month later the spots in the fundus had disap-
peared, and visual acuity recovered. (Courtesy of Antonio Ciardella, MD).

◆ **Presentation**

Multiple white dots at the level of the RPE and optic nerve head swelling may be
seen. The macula often has a granular appearance. Visual-field defects in the form
of an enlarged blind spot and paracentral and central scotomas may also be seen.
Visual loss, even if significant initially, almost always returns to normal later. The
patient may also have photopsia.

◆ **Management**

Fundus fluorescein angiography shows focal areas of early punctate hyperfluorescence that correspond to the white dots. The changes on indo-cyanine green
angiography maintain longer than fundus photo and FFA. The prognosis for visual
acuity in MEWDS is very good, and it resolves on its own.

Acute Multifocal Posterior Placoid Pigment Epitheliopathy

This condition closely resembles MEWDS. It may be associated with HLA-B7.

◆ **Presentation**

Similar to MEWDS, it can also present with a viral predrome followed by transient
visual loss in young to middle-aged adults. It is usually bilateral. Retinal lesions
consist of multiple yellow-white placoid lesions, which are larger than in MEWDS,
involving the RPE **(Fig. 6.4)**.

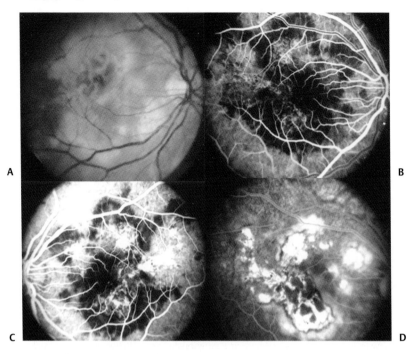

A

B

C

D

Fig. 6.4 **(A)** Early phase fluorescein angiography in acute posterior multifocal placoid pigment epitheliopathy (APMPPE) shows irregular areas of blocked fluorescence characteristic of acute lesions. **(B)** At the arteriovenous phase, acute lesions still block fluorescence and are well demarcated. **(C)** Mid- and **(D)** late-phase angiograms demonstrate progressive, diffuse, even staining of the acute lesions. (Courtesy of J. Fernando Arevalo, Venezuela)

◆ **Management**

FFA shows early blocked fluorescence with late staining. The lesions slowly heal with scarring and leave behind extensive RPE defects that persist.

Serpiginous Choroiditis

This is a recurrent inflammatory disease of the RPE and choroid that is generally bilateral.

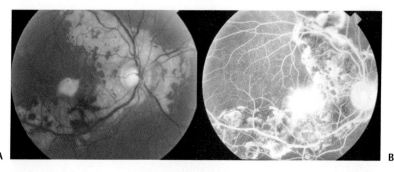

A B

Fig. 6.5 **(A)** Fundus photograph and **(B)** hyperfluorescence on fluorescein angiography of a patient with serpiginous choroiditis demonstrating choroidal neovascularization. (Courtesy of J. Fernando Arevalo, Venezuela)

◆ Presentation

Serpiginous choroiditis is seen most commonly in adults in the fourth to sixth decade of life. Blurred vision is the first symptom. Vitreous varies from clear to mildly cellular. A serpiginous or geographic (maplike) pattern of scars may present in the posterior fundus. Edges of these lesions may be active, with a yellow-gray and edematous appearance. As active lesions become atiophied over weeks to months, new lesions can occur elsewhere or contiguously in a snail-like pattern. Scotomas may be seen. FFA shows early hypofluorescence with late hyperfluorescence of lesions during active disease (**Figs. 6.5** and **6.6**).

◆ Management

Oral steroids along with immunosuppressants

Birdshot Retinochoroidopathy (Vitiliginous Chorioretinitis)

This is a cause of chronic posterior uveitis, with a female predilection. It is also associated with HLA-A29.

◆ Presentation

Multiple small white/yellow spots are seen scattered about the posterior pole in the deep retina and choroid. Vitritis and macular edema with or without epiretinal membrane formation may be seen. Disk edema and optic nerve inflammation with peripapillary atrophy may be seen (**Fig. 6.7**).

◆ Management

Though it generally runs a benign course, it is potentially blinding secondary to macular inflammation and permanent damage. Hence, in cases with significant inflammation or vision-affecting macular edema, aggressive treatment should be given.

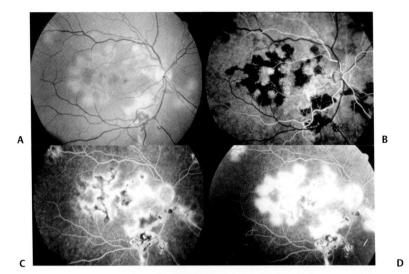

Fig. 6.6 Serpiginous choroiditis. **(A)** Color fundus photo. **(B)** Fluorescein angiography shows early blockage. **(C)** As the angiogram proceeds, the active margins progressively become hyperfluorescent **(D)** and spread toward the center of the lesion as it absorbs dye from the choriocapillaris. (Courtesy of J. Fernando Arevalo, Venezuela)

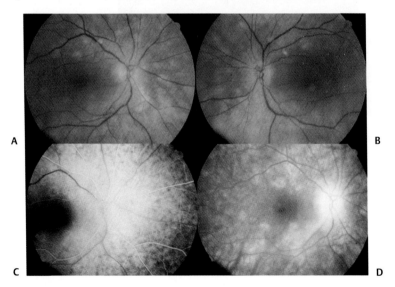

Fig. 6.7 Birdshot retinochoroidopathy. **(A)** Color fundus photo of right and **(B)** left eye. **(C)** Early fluorescein angiography with choroidal infiltration and minimal retinal pigment epithelium atrophy. The spots are hypofluorescent. **(D)** The lesions become mildly hyperfluorescent in the late phases of the study as dye from the choriocapillaris stains the extrachoroidal vascular space. (Courtesy of J. Fernando Arevalo, Venezuela)

Cytomegalovirus (CMV) Retinitis

◆ **Presentation**

Congenital CMV: Most commonly seen at the posterior pole with overlying vitreous haze and pigment clumps. There can be mild chorioretinitis or a severe necrotizing chorioretinitis. The lesions are multiple, and hyperplastic macular scarring can be seen. The vision loss can be secondary to optic nerve abnormality.

Immunosuppressed CMV retinitis: Retinal infarcts manifesting as cotton wool spots, retinal hemorrhages, retinal necrosis, vitreous haze, and retinal vasculitis are seen (**Figs. 6.8** and **6.9**).

◆ **Management**

CMV retinitis is treated with intravenous ganciclovir (5 mg/kg every 12 hours) or intravenous foscarnet (60 mg/kg every 8 hours) or cidofovir. Intravitreal injections may also be given.

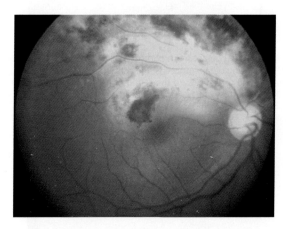

Fig. 6.8   Cytomegalovirus retinitis.

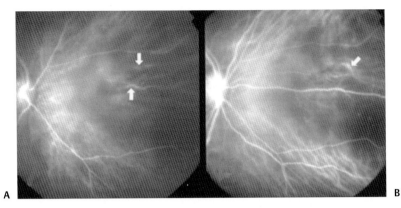

A   B

Fig. 6.9   Cytomegalovirus (CMV) retinitis in an AIDS patient. **(A)** Early indocyanine green angiography (ICG-V) frame shows the onset of fluorescence. Engorged leaking choroidal vessels (white arrows) indicating inflammatory choroidal vasculopathy. **(B)** Maximum fluorescence on ICG-V of leaking choroidal vessels (white arrow). (Courtesy of J. Fernando Arevalo, Venezuela)

Acute Retinal Necrosis Syndrome

◆ Presentation

This syndrome is a form of severe posterior uveitis that is caused by varicella zoster virus and herpes simplex virus types 1 and 2. It is defined by the following very definite clinical characteristics: presence of focal, defined areas of retinal necrosis in the peripheral retina outside the vascular arcades, rapid progression to confluent circumferential necrosis, occlusive vasculopathy, marked vitritis, and iritis.

Other features are optic atrophy, scleritis, and pain.

◆ Management

Systemic antivirals such as acyclovir and valacyclovir are given initially followed by oral steroids. Anticoagulant therapy may be required. Prophylactic laser photocoagulation or pars plana vitrectomy may be required.

◆ Vogt-Koyanagi-Harada Syndrome

◆ Presentation

◆ Headache, nausea
◆ Bilateral vitritis, choroiditis, and multiple oval detachments of the retina that are exudative
◆ Retinal and peripapillary neovascularizations
◆ Mutton fat keratic precipitates
◆ Papillary nodules and shallow anterior chambers
◆ Differential diagnosis: sympathetic ophthalmia, sarcoidosis, acute posterior multifocal placoid pigment epitheliopathy
◆ Associated findings include alopecia, vitiligo, poliosis, and hearing loss (**Figs. 6.10** and **6.11**).

◆ Management

Treat aggressively with cycloplegics; topical, periocular, and systemic steroids; and/or immunosuppressive agents.

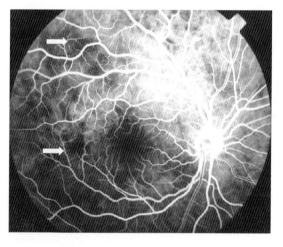

Fig. 6.10   Occlusion (*arrows*) of choroidal vessels in a patient with Vogt-Koyanagi-Harada syndrome. (Courtesy of J. Fernando Arevalo, Venezuela)

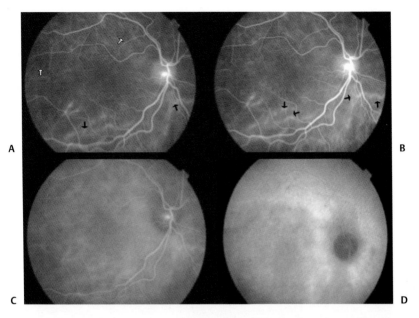

A   B   C   D

Fig. 6.11 Vogt-Koyanagi-Harada syndrome. **(A)** Individual leaking choroidal vessels (*black arrows*) indicating inflammatory choroidal vasculopathy and patchy hypofluorescent areas (*white arrows*) were visible in the early-phase indocyanine green videoangiography (ICG-V) in the acute disease. **(B)** Note marked decrease in the number of large choroidal vessels (*black arrows*) in the early phase ICG-V in the acute disease. **(C)** Evenly sized hypofluorescent spots are observed in the intermediate phase ICG-V at the acute phase of the disease. **(D)** Some of the spots are persisting into the late phase. (Courtesy of Leyla Atmaca, MD)

◆ Behçet Syndrome (Oculo-Oro-Genital Syndrome)

It was first described by Behçet as a syndrome characterized by recurrent oral aphthous ulcers, genital ulcers, and uveitis (**Fig. 6.12**).

◆ Presentation

◆ Major features
- ◆ Recurrent aphthous ulceration of the oral mucous membrane
- ◆ Skin lesions (erythema nodosum–like lesions), subcutaneous thrombophlebitis, folliculitis (acnelike lesions), cutaneous hypersensitivity
- ◆ Eye lesions (iridocyclitis, chorioretinitis, retinouveitis) and a definite history of chorioretinitis or retinouveitis
- ◆ Genital ulcers

◆ **Minor features**
- ◆ Arthritis without deformity and ankylosis
- ◆ Gastrointestinal lesions characterized by ileocecal ulcers
- ◆ Epididymitis
- ◆ Vascular lesions
- ◆ CNS symptoms

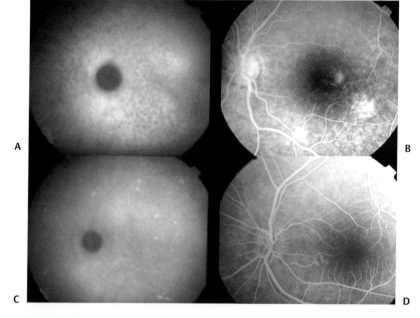

Fig. 6.12   Behçet syndrome. **(A)** Hypofluorescent spots in the late phase of indocyanine green videoangiography (ICG-V). **(B)** These spots cannot be seen on fluorescein angiography. Hyperfluorescence due to pigment epithelial changes can be observed. **(C)** Hyperfluorescent spots in the late phase of ICG-V. **(D)** These spots cannot be seen on fluorescein angiography. (Courtesy of Leyla Atmaca, MD)

Differential Diagnosis

◆ *Complete*: Four major features
◆ *Incomplete*: (1) Three major features, (2) two major and two minor features, or (3) typical ocular symptom and one major or two minor features
◆ *Possible*: (1) Two major features or (2) one major and two minor features

Management

Corticosteroids and other immunosuppressives have been tried. Empirical treatment is given.

◆ Sympathetic Ophthalmia

Presentation

◆ *Characteristic symptoms*: Pain, photophobia, and decreased accommodation
◆ *Characteristic signs*: Inflamed and thickened uveal tissue with edematous iris, disk swelling, nodules, papillitis, and yellow nodules called Dalen-Fuchs nodules
◆ *Characteristic associations*: vitiligo, poliosis, alopecia
◆ *Differential diagnosis*: Vogt Koyanagi Harada, lens-induced uveitis

Treatment

Steroids via all routes and immunosuppressants are indicated.

◆ Endophthalmitis

Traumatic Endophthalmitis

Bacteria or fungi are introduced at the time of injury in traumatic endophthalmitis. It can occur in up to 13% of cases of penetrating globe trauma. The causative organism differs from other endophthalmitis with gram-positive bacteria accounting for 61.0% cases, gram-negative bacteria for 10.2% of cases, fungi in 8.3% cases, and polymicrobial infections in 15.6% cases. The most common gram-positive organisms were coagulase-negative *Staphylococcus* (21.5%) and *Bacillus* species (18.5%), followed by *Streptococcus* species (14.8%) and *Staphylococcus aureus* (8%).

Presentation

Because ocular trauma generally occurs in a nonsterile environment, most injuring objects are contaminated with multiple infectious agents. Patients with a larger area of laceration, delay in surgery, ruptured lens capsule, retained intraocular foreign body, nonmetallic foreign body, and dirty wound are more commonly associated with posttraumatic endophthalmitis. The patient presents with pain, photophobia, and decreased vision occurring a variable period, even years, after penetrating ocular trauma. Signs of intraocular infection are seen.

◆ **Management**

Early repair of the injury is necessary. A retained intraocular foreign body may require a vitrectomy. If the risk of endophthalmitis is greater, consider taking an aqueous and vitreous tap for culture and sensitivity. Intravitreal antibiotics such as vancomycin hydrochloride (1 mg in 0.1 mL) and amikacin (0.4 mg in 0.1 mL) or ceftazidime (2.25 mg in 0.1 mL) may be given at the time of surgery along with intracameral and intensive postoperative antibiotics, which are changed according to culture and sensitivity reports.

Once the infection is controlled, steroids may be added to decrease the inflammation.

Postoperative Endophthalmitis

Any surgical procedure on the eye that disrupts the integrity of the globe, however minor the breach may be, can lead to postoperative endophthalmitis, such as cataract, glaucoma, vitrectomy, and radial keratotomy. Postoperative endophthalmitis represents 70% of infective endophthalmitis. The large majority of cases follow cataract surgery, with an approximate prevalence of 0.082 to 0.1%. It can occur secondary to periocular flora gaining access into the eye during surgery, organisms being carried into the eye as surface fluid refluxes through the wound during surgery, secondary to intraocular lens contamination if it touches the ocular surface, or with the use of contaminated irrigation solutions (**Fig. 6.13**).

◆ **Presentation**

The patient generally presents with pain, redness, decreased vision, lid edema, hazy cornea, and hypopyon. Three forms of presentation may be seen:
◆ *Acute form*: Usually fulminant, occurs 2 to 4 days postop, most commonly due to *S. aureus* or streptococci
◆ *Delayed form*: Moderately severe, occurs 5 to 7 days postop, due to *Staphylococcus epidermidis*, coagulase-negative cocci, rarely fungi
◆ *Chronic form*: Occurs as early as 1 month postop, due to *Propionibacterium acnes*, *Staphylococcus epidermidis*, or fungi

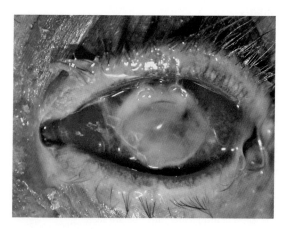

Fig. 6.13   Endophthalmitis—conjunctivitis.

◆ Management

Certain measures, such as 3 days of preoperative prophylactic antibiotics and pre-operative povidone-iodine (5%) scrub, can help reduce the risk of postoperative endophthalmitis (POE). Primary use of preoperative topical fourth-generation fluoroquinolones such as moxifloxacin and gatifloxacin is beneficial and is better for preventing resistance.

The Endophthalmitis Vitrectomy Study was a multicenter randomized trial performed at 24 centers in the United States (1990 to 1994) to determine the role of intravenous antibiotics in the management of POE and the role of initial vitrectomy in management. The study concluded that systemic antibiotics were of no benefit and that initial vitrectomy was only beneficial for patients presenting with a very poor visual acuity.

Cultures should be taken from the aqueous and vitreous. The possibility of isolating an organism from the vitreous is 56 to 70%, whereas from the aqueous it is 36 to 40%. In established endophthalmitis, oral or intravenous antibiotics have poor penetration into the vitreous cavity. Hence intravitreal injections are the treatment of choice. For gram-positive organisms, a single dose of intravitreal vancomycin 1 mg in (0.1 mL) has adequate antibiotic concentrations for over 1 week. Amikacin (0.4 mg in 0.1 mL) and ceftazidime (2.25 mg/0.1 mL) are effective against gram-negative organisms. Thus vancomycin combined with amikacin or ceftazidime appears to be the best combination for the treatment of POE.

◆ *Dose of subconjunctival antibiotics*: Vancomycin (25 mg in 0.5 mL) and ceftazidime (100 mg in 0.5 mL) or amikacin (25 mg in 0.5 mL)
◆ *Dose of topical fortified antibiotics*: Vancomycin (50 mg/mL) and amikacin (20 mg/mL), alternating every 1 to 4 hours
◆ *Dose of corticosteroids*: Topical, sub-conjunctival injection (dexamethasone, 6 mg in 0.2 mL), oral (prednisolone 30 mg by mouth twice a day for 5 to 10 days), or intravitreal

Endogenous Endophthalmitis

Endogenous endophthalmitis is generally of hematogenous origin and usually affects adults with predisposing conditions such as diabetes, urogenital and gastrointestinal tract disorders, endocarditis, and patients on immunosuppressives or having undergone invasive procedures. The etiological organism may be gram-positive or negative bacteria or fungi. In the pediatric age group, neonatal infection has been seen with group B streptococcal or *Candida albicans*.

◆ Presentation

It may present acutely or as a slowly progressive condition. The patient may present with pain and decreased visual acuity. Examination may show a spectrum of clinical signs ranging from minimum signs of inflammation, hypopyon, vitritis, Roth spots, retinal periphlebitis, to panophthalmitis in severe cases. White chorioretinal infiltrates with fluffy white vitreous opacities ("string of pearls" appearance) may be seen in *Candida endophthalmitis*.

◆ Management

Blood cultures, intraocular cultures obtained from both chambers, and cultures from other sites such as an indwelling catheter are taken. Early intravenous antibiotic therapy is crucial. The patient should be worked up systemically to determine the etiology, source, and cause for the endogenous endophthalmitis. The role of intravitreal antibiotics and vitrectomy is controversial unlike in exogenous endophthalmitis. Topical and periocular antibiotic/antifungal agents along with cycloplegics may be used.

◆ Masquerade Syndromes

Masquerade syndromes are disorders that occur with intraocular inflammation and are often misdiagnosed as a chronic idiopathic uveitis. These are malignancies that present with reactions in the anterior and posterior segment of inflammation thus masquerading as cases of uveitis (**Table 6.2**).

Intraocular Lymphoma

Most patients with intraocular lymphoma have immunosuppression. They generally present with blurry vision and floaters, with slit lamp examination often showing mild cells and flare and keratic precipitates. Vitritis may also be seen with subretinal yellow infiltrates and sometimes hemorrhagic retinal vasculitis.

Intraocular Leukemia

Intraocular leukemia may present with hypopyon, vitreous and optic nerve infiltration, and vasculitis.

Retinoblastoma

Retinoblastoma should be ruled out in children less than 3 years of age presenting with uveitis. Pseudohypopyon may be seen along with vitreous seedlings.

Choroidal Melanoma

Approximately 5% of uveal melanomas present with ocular inflammatory reactions. A black hypopyon may be seen (see chapter 11, section on Choroidal Melanoma).

Table 6.2 Masquerading Cases of Uveitis

Retinoblastoma	Juvenile xanthogranulomas	Malignant leukemias and lymphomas
Pseudohypopyon nodules on iris Retinal lesions X-ray shows calcification	Recurrent hyphema yellow, poorly defined tumors.	Anterior chamber Aspirate Iris tissue biopsy Central nervous system lymphoma presents with vitritis and choroidal nodules

Intraocular Foreign Body

A retained intraocular foreign body can cause siderosis, manifesting as a focal low-grade inflammation, cataract formation, or chronic inflammation.

Schwartz-Jampel Syndrome

Rhegmatogenous retinal detachment may be associated with anterior chamber reaction and glaucoma.

Juvenile Xanthogranuloma

Juvenile xanthogranuloma is a rare pediatric disorder affecting the histiocytes of the skin. It may sometimes affect the eye and can present with many differing ocular manifestations such as masquerade uveitis, heterochromia, hyphema, or glaucoma.

Paraneoplastic Syndrome

Tumor-associated retinopathy secondary to cutaneous melanoma or bronchial carcinoma may sometimes occur. Such patients may have bilateral retinopathy and loss of vision.

7 Lens and Cataract

Athiya Agarwal, Soosan Jacob, and Amar Agarwal

◆ Posterior Polar Cataract

The posterior polar cataract has a unique circular whorl-like appearance located in the central axis near the nodal point of the eye with the rest of the lens remaining clear. It is frequently associated with a weakened or deficient posterior capsule. Missing the diagnosis in a posterior polar cataract can be catastrophic and a nightmare.

◆ Presentation

The bull's-eye appearance is pathognomonic of posterior polar cataracts. However, this entity could be camouflaged under a dense nuclear sclerosis or a total white cataract (**Fig. 7.1A**).

◆ Differential Diagnosis

Interdigitation with the posterior capsule is characteristic as opposed to a posterior subcapsular cataract.

◆ Management

A small, continuous curvilinear capsulorhexis is aimed for in the eventuality of the intraocular lens having to be placed in the sulcus. Hydrodissection may cause hydraulic perforation at the weakened area of the capsule; hence only a careful, controlled hydrodelineation is preferred. This epinuclear shell provides additional protection by tamponading any vitreous or capsular breach during phacoemulsi-

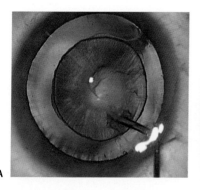 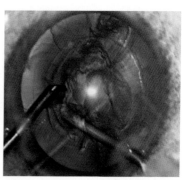

A   B

Fig. 7.1 **(A)** Posterior polar cataract. Note hydrodelineation only done. No hydrodissection has been done. **(B)** Microphakonit is started. Note the 0.7-mm irrigating chopper and 0.7-mm phako tip without the sleeve inside the eye. All instruments are made by MicroSurgical Technology, Redmond, WA. The assistant continuously irrigates the phaco probe area from outside to prevent corneal burns.

fication. A small amount of viscoelastic can be injected just under the rim of the rhexis all around to form a mechanical barrier for fluid from accidentally entering the subcapsular plane while performing hydrodelineation. Because the nucleus after hydrodelineation is very small, it can be removed easily either by carouselling (constantly rotating the nucleus to prolong occlusion and allow more effective breakdown of the cataract) it out with the phaco tip or by using a chop maneuver. Phaco chop is especially helpful in case of associated nuclear sclerosis. If the central plaque was not removed at the time of surgery, it can be tackled by a yittrium aluminum garnet capsulotomy postoperatively.

Sub 1 mm 700-Micrometer Cataract Surgery—Microphakonit

Microphakonit or bimanual phacoemulsification through two 0.7-mm instruments (an irrigating chopper and a phaco tip) can be used effectively to tackle a posterior polar cataract. Hydrodelineation can be done through both ports here. Another advantage of this technique is that one can easily revert to bimanual vitrectomy in case of vitreous loss. The advantage of microphakonit over phaco is that one has a closed chamber throughout surgery because both the incisions are so small (**Fig. 7.1B**).

◆ Subluxated Cataract

Subluxated cataracts pose a risk of nucleus drop during cataract surgery, and hence require special precautions.

◆ Presentation

There can be a zonular dehiscence or weakness present.

◆ Differential Diagnosis

Coloboma of the lens. There can be coloboma with a subluxation (**Fig. 7.2A**).

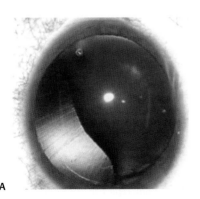
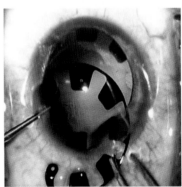

A   B

Fig. 7.2 **(A)** Subluxated colobomatous lens. **(B)** Aniridia rings being implanted. (**[A]** Courtesy of Lincoln L. Freitas)

◆ Management

Cataract surgery in the presence of zonular weakness or a subluxated lens is a great challenge. In the past, surgical intervention in these cases was difficult, leading to complications. The use of an endocapsular flexible polymethyl methacrylate (PMMA) ring has changed the surgical approach to subluxated cataracts. Implantation of a capsular tension ring (CTR) stabilizes a loose lens and allows the surgeon to place the intraocular lens in the most desirable place—the capsular bag. There are numerous other advantages: vitreous herniation to the anterior chamber is reduced, a taut capsule gives countertraction to all traction maneuvers making them easier to perform, capsular support for an "in the bag" implant is obtained, and most importantly, the capsular bag maintains its shape, avoiding capsular fibrosis syndrome and intraocular lens decentration.

Do not use trypan blue in subluxated cataracts because the trypan blue will go into the vitreous cavity through the zonular dehiscence and make the whole vitreous cavity blue. When zonular dehiscence is large in extent or progressive in nature, capsular bag shrinkage resulting in intraocular lens decentration and pseudophakodonesis may occur even after a successful surgery with a capsular ring. Complete luxation of the bag and its contents has also been reported. For such cases, Cionni's modified design with a fixation hook is a good solution. The hook is kept in the area of dialysis and is pulled peripherally using a transscleral fixation suture to counteract capsular bag decentration and tilt. In severe cases, two such rings or the two-hooked model can be used. An alternative in cases of severe decentration is to make a small equatorial capsulorrhexis through which a standard capsular tension ring can be inserted. A scleral suture can then be passed around the exposed capsular tension ring, which is then used to center the lens before capsulorrhexis. Peribulbar anesthesia is suitable for creation of scleral windows and transscleral suturing of the capsular ring or of the intraocular lens if necessary.

CTRs can also be placed to cover sector iris defects or coloboma. These coloboma shields have an integrated 60- to 90-degree sector shield to protect against glare and monocular diplopia. More than one capsular tension ring can be used if more than 90 degrees of defect is present. Multisegmented coloboma rings are available for aniridia as well as for cases with large permanently dilated pupils secondary to any cause. Insertion of two of these rings so that the interspaces of the first ring are covered by the sector shields of the second makes a contiguous artificial iris possible (**Fig. 7.2B**).

◆ Miotic Pupil Cataract

A well-dilated pupil is the gateway to a smooth, easy, and rewarding cataract surgery. But the surgeon may not be lucky enough to sail smoothly through the well-charted path of a dilated pupil each time. Sometimes the door looks narrow and uninviting even for the best. A miotic pupil is a common bugbear that every surgeon faces at some time.

◆ Presentation

A small pupil affects all steps of phacoemulsification, right from capsulorrhexis to intraocular lens insertion. Difficult maneuvering causes iris damage, sphincter tears, zonular dialysis, bleeding, and so on. Poor exposure through a small pupil forces the surgeon to make a smaller rhexis, adding to the difficulty and frequently leading to capsular dehiscence and nucleus drop—the worst nightmare. The prolonged surgical time takes its toll thereafter. Corneal edema, uveitis, secondary glaucoma, cystoid macular edema, distorted pupil—the list is endless.

◆ Differential Diagnosis

Causes of small pupil

◆ Management

Sphincter-Sparing Techniques
Pharmacological mydriasis alone may not be effective in cases with posterior synechiae, pupillary membrane, or scarred pupils. Such pupils need intraoperative procedures such as high-molecular-weight cohesive viscoelastics, synechiolysis, viscomydriasis, and/or pupillary membrane stripping.

Sphincter-Involving Techniques
Minisphincterotomies (less than 1 mm) limited to the sphincter tissue can be made with either Vanass scissors or the vitreoretinal scissors. Dilatation can also be achieved by pupillary stretching using push-pull instruments. Bipronged, tripronged, and quadripronged pupil stretchers are also very effective. Other alternatives are commercially available iris hooks, pupil ring expanders, and the Malyugin ring (**Fig. 7.3A,B**).

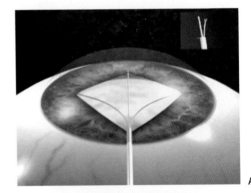

A

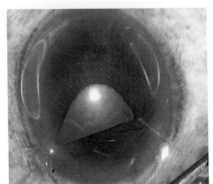

B

Fig. 7.3 (A) Tri-pronged pupil stretchers. **(B)** Iris hooks inserted to enlarge the pupil.

◆ Mature Cataract

One of the biggest bugbears for a phaco surgeon is to perform a rhexis in a mature cataract. Once one performs rhexis in mature and hypermature cataracts, then phaco can be done in these cases and a foldable intraocular lens can be implanted.

◆ Presentation

The solution to mature cataracts is to have a dye that stains the anterior capsule. This dye is trypan blue (**Fig. 7.4A,B**). One can also use indocyanine green.

◆ Differential Diagnosis

Check for various causes of mature cataracts.

◆ Management

The problem when one operates a mature cataract is the creation of the rhexis, which can be solved using a dye. The other problem is surge. One should understand the working of a phaco machine for understanding surge. When an occluded fragment is held by high vacuum and then abruptly aspirated, fluid rushes into the

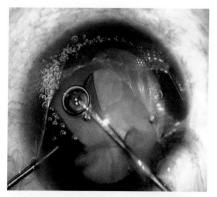

A

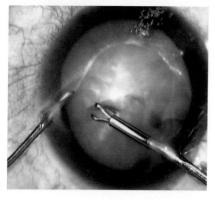

B

Fig. 7.4 **(A)** Rhexis being done in a mature cataract with cystotome. **(B)** Rhexis forceps (MicroSurgical Technology, Redmond, WA) used to perform the rhexis in a mature cataract. Note the trypan blue (Blurhex, Dr. Agarwal Pharma Ltd., Chennai, India) staining the anterior capsule.

phaco tip to equilibrate the built-up vacuum in the aspiration line, causing surge. This leads to shallowing or collapse of the anterior chamber. Different machines employ a variety of methods to combat surge. Another method is the air pump. An automated air pump is used to push air into the infusion bottle, thus increasing the pressure with which the fluid flows into the eye. This increases the steady-state pressure of the eye, making the anterior chamber deep and well maintained during the entire procedure. It makes phakonit and phacoemulsification a relatively safe procedure by reducing surge even at high vacuum levels (**Figs. 7.5, 7.6, 7.7, and 7.8**).

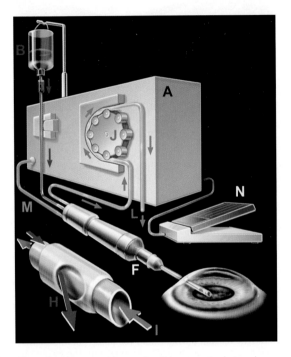

Fig. 7.5   The principles of how the phaco machine works. This conceptual view shows the three main elements of most phaco systems. (1) The irrigation (*red*): Intraocular pressure is maintained and irrigation is provided by the bottle of balanced salt solution (B) connected via tubing to the phaco handpiece (F). It is controlled by the surgeon. Irrigation enters the eye via an infusion port (H) located on the outer sleeve of the bi-tube phaco probe. Height of the bottle above the eye is used to control the inflow pressure. (2) Aspiration (*blue*): (I) enters through the tip of the phaco probe, passes within the inner tube of the probe, travels through the aspiration tubing, and is controlled by the surgeon by way of a variable-speed pump (J). The peristaltic type pump is basically a motorized wheel exerting rotating external pressure on a portion of the flexible aspiration line, which physically forces fluid through the tubing. Varying the speed of the rotating pump controls the rate of aspiration. Aspirated fluid passes to a drain (I). (3) Ultrasonic energy (*green*) is provided to the probe tip via a connection (M) to the unit. All three of these main phaco functions are under control of the surgeon by way of a multicontrol foot pedal (N). (Courtesy of Benjamin F. Boyd, MD, FACS, Editor-in-Chief, "The Art and the Science of Cataract Surgery." *Highlights of Ophthalmology*, English Edition, 2001.)

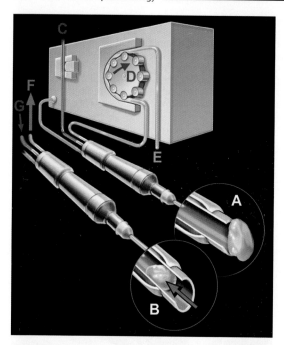

Fig. 7.6 Mechanism of the undesirable surge phenomenon. One problem area of the closed phaco system occurs during abrupt dislodging of an occluding piece of lens material so that it no longer occludes the aspiration port of the phaco tip. A sudden drop in intraocular pressure occurs as the fluid rate into the eye fails to immediately match the sudden fluid rate out of the eye. This is known as the surge phenomenon. (A) A piece of lens material occluding the aspiration port of the phaco tip is held in place by vacuum pressure created by the operating pump (D). (Note there is no drainage (E) from the blocked system.) Infusion from the irrigating bottle (C) has ceased, but it is still providing controlled intraocular pressure due to its elevated position above the eye. With sufficient vacuum pressure from the pump and/or emulsification from the ultrasonic energy, the nuclear piece will abruptly enter the aspiration port and the fluid system will once again open (B). Because the plastic infusion/aspiration lines and the eye walls are flexible in absorbing the sudden inflow–outflow pressure differential, there occurs a moment when the infusion fluid (G, *small arrow*) does not effectively enter the eye fast enough to replace the fluid suddenly moving out of the unblocked system (F, *large arrow*). Outflow rate from the force of the pump is momentarily greater than the replacing infusion rate. This out-of-balance system (out of balance in not providing constant intraocular pressure) in which the eye momentarily absorbs the inflow–outflow rate differential may traumatically collapse the eye for a short period. (Courtesy of Benjamin F. Boyd, MD, FACS, Editor-in-Chief, "The Art and the Science of Cataract Surgery." *Highlights of Ophthalmology*, English Edition, 2001.)

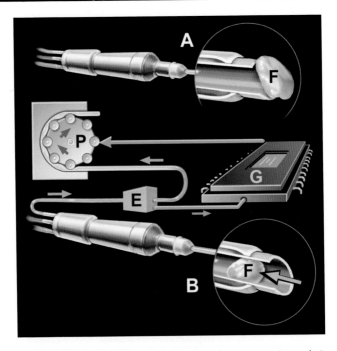

Fig. 7.7   Technical solution to prevent the undesirable surge phenomenon. One technical solution for eliminating the surge phenomenon involves the use of a high-tech microprocessor. When a nuclear piece (F) occludes the aspiration port and then suddenly (B) is aspirated (F, *arrow*) by the vacuum pressure of the pump (P), a sensor (E) located on the aspiration line signals a microprocessor (G) in the unit that an abrupt surge in aspiration flow has begun to take place. Within milliseconds, the microprocessor directs the motor of the pump (P) to slow down. The reduction in aspiration rate resulting from the slowed pump occurs before the eye can collapse from any volume differential encountered between sudden inflow and outflow rates. The potentially dangerous surge phenomenon is avoided. This elimination of the surge phenomenon allows the surgeon to safely use higher vacuum rates (necessary in some situations) with a reduction in the need to use potentially damaging high ultrasonic power settings. Surgery becomes safer and faster. (Courtesy of Benjamin F. Boyd, MD, FACS, Editor-in-Chief, "The Art and the Science of Cataract Surgery." *Highlights of Ophthalmology*, English Edition, 2001.)

Fig. 7.8 Diagrammatic representation of the connection of the air
pump to the infusion bottle.

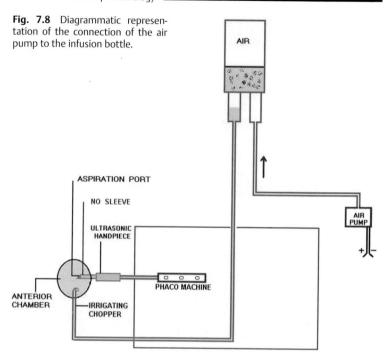

◆ Senile Cataract

One should perform cataract surgery well in senile cataracts (**Fig. 7.9**).

◆ Presentation

The fundamental goal of Phaco is to remove the cataract with minimal disturbance
to the eye using the least number of surgical manipulations. Each maneuver should
be performed with minimal force, and maximal efficiency should be obtained.

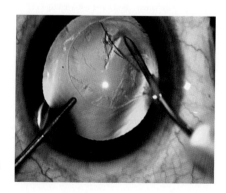

Fig. 7.9 Rhexis being done in a
case of senile cataract.

◆ Differential Diagnosis

Other systemic causes of cataract

◆ Management

After viscoelastic is injected into the eye through a 26-gauge needle, a globe stabilization rod is inserted and a clear corneal incision is made. One can then remove the cataracts using the divide and conquer techniques. We prefer the chopping technique (**Figs. 7.10** and **7.11**). The Phaco probe is inserted through the incision slightly superior to the center of the nucleus, and the phaco tip is embedded in the nucleus with the tip directed obliquely downward toward the vitreous and not horizontally toward the iris. Once the tip is embedded, while in foot position 2, the nucleus is chopped with a straight downward motion at the end of which the chopper moves to the left on reaching the center of the nucleus (i.e., like a laterally reversed L) (**Fig. 7.12**). The nucleus is then rotated 180 degrees and cracked again to get two halves of the nucleus. This is then repeated to further chop the cataract into smaller pieces, which are then brought into the anterior chamber one by one and emulsified. Once the nucleus and cortex are removed the foldable intraocular lens is implanted (**Fig. 7.13**).

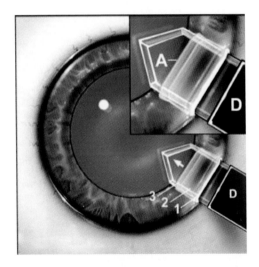

Fig. 7.10   A diamond knife blade (D) enters the first incision (1), the second tunnel incision (2), and is then directed slightly oblique to the iris plane and advanced (*arrow*) into the anterior chamber. This forms the internal aspect of the incision into the chamber (A). This is the third step (3) in the three-step self-sealing incision. (Courtesy of Benjamin F. Boyd, MD, FACS, Editor-in-Chief, "The Art and the Science of Cataract Surgery." *Highlights of Ophthalmology*, English Edition, 2001.)

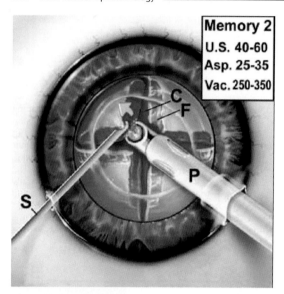

Fig. 7.11 Emulsification of lens fragments: This surgeon's view shows the management of the lens quadrants. The apex of each of the four loose quadrants is lifted with the second instrument (S), the ultrasound phaco tip (P) is embedded into the posterior edge of each, and by means of aspiration the surgeon centralizes each quadrant for emulsification. U.S., ultrasound; Asp., aspiration flow rate; Vac., vacuum; C, capsule; F, fragment. (Courtesy of Benjamin F. Boyd, MD, FACS, Editor-in-Chief, "The Art and the Science of Cataract Surgery." *Highlights of Ophthalmology*, English Edition, 2001.)

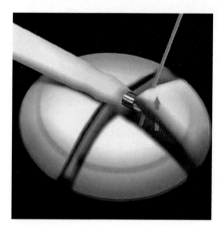

Fig. 7.12 This cross-section view shows the phacoemulsification probe removing the nucleus fragments within the capsular bag. Note the apex of one of the fragments created in the nucleus being lifted with the second instrument (*arrow*) and the ultrasound tip embedded into the posterior edge of each segment ready for emulsification. The epinucleus and cortex will then be removed during the phaco process. If we operate on a softer cataract, the freed fractured pieces are emulsified immediately. (Courtesy of Benjamin F. Boyd, MD, FACS, Editor-in-Chief, "The Art and the Science of Cataract Surgery." *Highlights of Ophthalmology*, English Edition, 2001.)

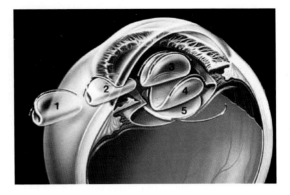

Fig. 7.13 This cross-section view shows the movement of the foldable intraocular lens during insertion. Folding forceps removed for clarity. (1) Folded lens outside the eye. (2) Folded lens passing through small incision. (3) Folded lens placed posteriorly into the capsular bag through anterior capsule opening and then rotated 90 degrees. (4) Lens slowly unfolded in the bag. (5) Final unfolded position of lens within the capsular bag. (Courtesy of Benjamin F. Boyd, MD, FACS, Editor-in-Chief, "The Art and the Science of Cataract Surgery." *Highlights of Ophthalmology*, English Edition, 2001.)

◆ Glued Intraocular Lens

Intraocular lens (IOL) implantation in eyes that lack posterior capsular support has been accomplished in the past by means of an iris-fixated IOL, anterior chamber IOL, and transscleral IOL fixation through the ciliary sulcus or pars plana. Surgical expertise, prolonged surgical time, suture-induced inflammation, suture degradation, and delayed IOL subluxation or dislocation due to broken suture are some of the limitations in sutured scleral fixated IOLs.

It is possible to place a posterior chamber IOL in eyes with a deficient posterior capsule using a glued IOL technique.

◆ Technique

After clamping the superior rectus, an infusion cannula or anterior chamber maintainer is inserted, preferably in the inferonasal quadrant to prevent interference in creating the scleral flaps, which is the next step in the surgery. Two partial-thickness limbal-based scleral flaps ~2.5 × 3.0 mm are then created exactly 180 degrees

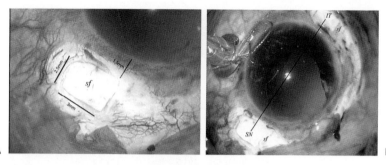

Fig. 7.14 **(A)** Scleral flaps (sf) of 2.5 x 3.0 mm made ~1.5 mm from the limbus. **(B)** Two flaps are made exactly 180 degrees diagonally apart.

diagonally apart (**Fig. 7.14**) up to the limbus. This is followed by vitrectomy via a pars plana or anterior route to remove all vitreous traction. Two straight sclerotomies with a 22-gauge needle are made ~1.5 mm from the limbus under the existing scleral flaps. A corneo-scleral or scleral tunnel incision is then prepared for introducing the IOL in secondary IOL implantation.

While the IOL is being introduced with one hand using a McPherson forceps, an end-gripping 23-gauge MST micro rhexis forceps (MicroSurgical Technology, Redmond, WA) is passed through the inferior sclerotomy with the other hand. The tip of the leading haptic is then grasped with the micro rhexis forceps, pulled through the inferior sclerotomy following the curve of the haptic (**Figs. 7.15** and **7.16**), and externalized under the inferior scleral flap. Similarly, the trailing haptic is also externalized through the superior sclerotomy under the scleral flap. Scleral tunnels are made with a 26-gauge needle at the edge of the scleral flap and the haptics are then tucked into these scleral tunnels for additional stability of the IOL (**Fig. 7.17**). Reconstituted fibrin glue is then injected through the cannula of the double-syringe delivery system under the superior (**Fig. 7.18**) and inferior scleral flaps. Local pressure is given over the flaps for ~10 to 20 seconds for the formation of fibrin polypeptides. In patients who have a luxated IOL, similar lamellar scleral flaps as

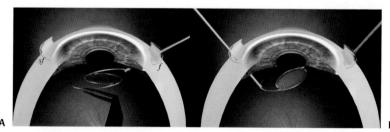

Fig. 7.15 **(A)** The IOL is inserted with a McPherson forceps, and the leading haptic is grasped by an end-gripping 23-gauge micro rhexis forceps (f) passed through a sclerotomy wound. The haptic is then externalised under the scleral flap (sf). **(B)** The trailing haptic is also externalized in a similar manner.

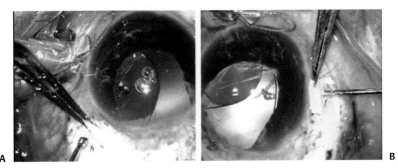

Fig. 7.16 **(A)** One haptic of the IOL is grasped by an end-gripping 23-gauge micro rhexis forceps (f) passed through sclerotomy wound. The haptic (h) is then externalised under the scleral flap (sf). **(B)** The second haptic is also externalized in a similar manner.

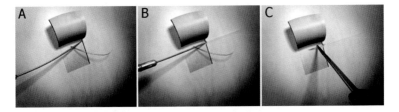

Fig. 7.17 **(A)** The haptics are externalized and a 26-gauge needle is taken to create a scleral tunnel. **(B)** 26-gauge needle is seen making a scleral tunnel near the edge of the flap, parallel to the limbus. **(C)** The haptic is tucked into the tunnel made with the 26-gauge needle. This provides it additional stability.

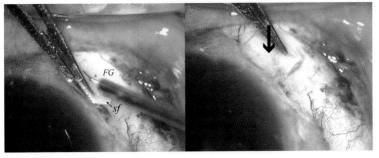

Fig. 7.18 **(A)** Reconstituted fibrinogen and thrombin preparation of fibrin glue (FG) injected beneath the scleral flaps. **(B)** Scleral flaps (*arrow*) sealed well with the scleral bed.

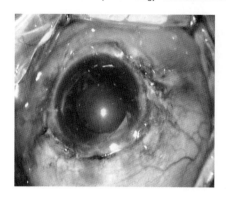

Fig. 7.19 Conjunctiva closed with fibrin glue.

described earlier are made and the luxated IOL haptic is then grasped with the 23-gauge micro rhexis forceps and externalized, tucked into the scleral tunnel made at the edge of the flaps, and then glued under the scleral flaps. The infusion cannula is then removed. Conjunctiva is also closed with the same fibrin glue (**Fig. 7.19**).

This technique is useful in a myriad of clinical situations where scleral-fixated IOLs are indicated, such as a luxated IOL, dislocated IOL, zonulopathy, or secondary IOL implantation. In dislocated posterior chamber polymethyl methacrylate (PMMA) IOL, the same IOL can be repositioned, thereby reducing the need for further manipulation. It can be performed well with a rigid PMMA IOL, IOLs with modified PMMA haptics, or multifocal glued IOLs. One therefore does not need to have special scleral fixated IOLs with eyelets or newer haptic designs. Because

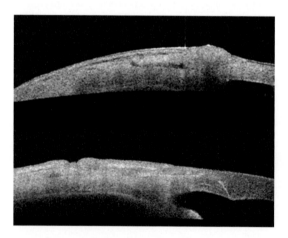

Fig. 7.20 Image of the scleral flap as seen by anterior segment optical coherence tomography on day 1 (above) and well sealed scleral flaps at 6 weeks (below).

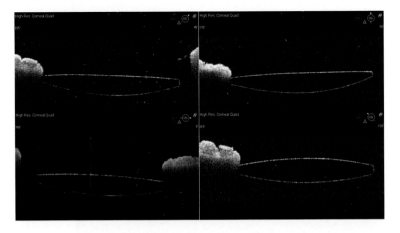

Fig. 7.21 Postoperative anterior segment optical coherence tomography showing 360 degrees well-centered intraocular lens at 6 weeks.

the haptic is being placed in its normal curved configuration without any traction, there is no distortion or change in shape of the IOL optic. Externalization of the greater part of the haptics along its curvature stabilizes the axial positioning of the IOL and thereby prevents any IOL tilt (**Figs. 7.20** and **7.21**).

◆ Temporary Haptic Externalization

One of the most difficult steps of repositioning a dislocated posterior chamber IOL is securing a suture on the haptics. In 1992, Clement Chan first introduced the concept of temporary haptic externalization to enhance the ease of suture placement and changed IOL repositioning from an uncontrolled to a highly controlled setting that allows fixation of the dislocated IOL in the ciliary sulcus on a consistent basis (**Fig. 7.22**).

A three-port pars plana vitrectomy is performed for the removal of the anterior and central vitreous adjacent to the dislocated IOL to prevent any vitreoretinal traction during the process of manipulating the IOL. Two diametrically opposed limbal-based partial-thickness triangular scleral flaps are prepared along the horizontal meridians at 3 and 9 o'clock. Cauterization is done to prevent any bleeding Anterior sclerotomies within the beds under the scleral flaps are made at 1 to 1.5 mm from the limbus. As an alternative to the scleral flaps, the anterior sclerotomies may be made within the scleral grooves at 1.0 to 1.5 mm from the horizontal limbus.

A fiberoptic light pipe is inserted through one of the posterior sclerotomies, while a pair of fine, nonangled positive-action forceps (e.g., Grieshaber 612.8, Alcon Grieshaber, Ltd., Schaffhausen, SZ) is inserted to hold the IOL and bring it anteriorly. A forceps is then passed through the anterior sclerotomy of the oppos-

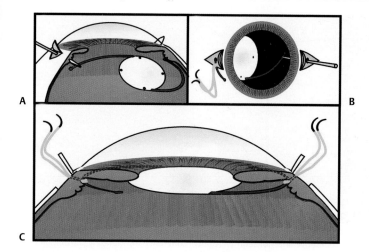

Fig. 7.22 **(A)** A forceps is passed through a sclerotomy made under a scleral flap in the opposite quadrant and one haptic of the dislocated IOL is caught for temporary externalization. **(B)** A double-armed 9–0 or 10–0 polypropylene suture is tied around the externalized haptic to make a secured knot and it is re-introduced into the vitreous cavity. The same process is then repeated for the other haptic. **(C)** The internalized haptics are anchored securely in the ciliary sulcus by taking scleral bites with the external suture needles.

ing quadrant to engage one haptic of the dislocated IOL for the temporary externalization. A double-armed 9–0 (Ethicon TG 160–8 plus, Somerville, NJ) or 10–0 polypropylene suture (Ethicon CS 160–6, Somerville, NJ) is tied around the externalized haptic to make a secured knot. The same process is repeated for the other haptic after the surgeon switches the instruments to the opposite hands. The externalized haptics with the tied sutures are reinternalized through the corresponding anterior sclerotomies with the same forceps. The internalized haptics are anchored securely in the ciliary sulcus by taking scleral bites with the external suture needles on the lips of the anterior sclerotomies. By adjusting the tension of the opposing sutures while tying the polypropylene suture knots by the anterior sclerotomies, the optic is centered behind the pupil, and the haptics are anchored in the ciliary sulcus.

◆ Intraoperative Complications

Posterior Capsular Rupture

If a capsular tear does occur, several steps can help minimize vitreous loss. A closed system should be maintained by injecting viscoelastic before withdrawing the phaco tip. This helps to tamponade the vitreous backward where a capsular dehiscence is present. Cortical removal should then proceed with either low infusion or by a dry technique filling the chamber with viscoelastic material and us-

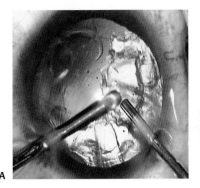 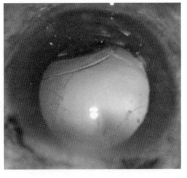

A   B

Fig. 7.23 **(A)** Bimanual vitrectomy being done in a case after posterior capsular rupture and vitreous loss. One should never do a coaxial vitrectomy. **(B)** Case of a dropped intraocular lens and nucleus (see the white reflex) after a posterior capsular rupture.

ing a Simcoe aspirator. If the hyaloid face is broken and vitreous presents through the rupture, a routine two-port mechanized vitrectomy using an Accurus Vitrector (Accurus 800 CS, Alcon Laboratories, Fort Worth, TX) using low-flow and low-vacuum parameters is performed. The tear can then be converted into a round and stable opening. The IOL can then be safely placed into the capsular bag. An uncontrolled tear necessitates implantation into the ciliary sulcus. A 6-mm optic acrylic lens is preferred when implanting in the bag as it unfolds slowly, thus causing less stress on the posterior capsule. The leading edge of the lens should be directed away from the area of a weak capsule. One can develop a dropped IOL and nucleus also (**Fig. 7.23A,B**).

Iridodialysis

One can develop an iridodialysis, which will require suturing (**Fig. 7.24**).

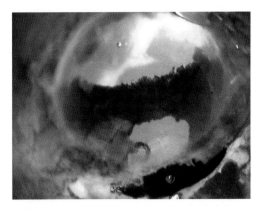

Fig. 7.24 Iridodialysis.

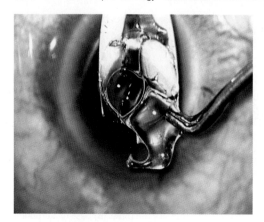

Fig. 7.25 Torn intraocular lens.

Torn Intraocular Lens

An IOL can get torn during implantation. In such a case it should be explanted and replaced (**Fig. 7.25**).

◆ Postoperative Complications

Corneal Edema after Cataract Extraction

Corneal edema after a cataract surgery can be identified immediately after the cataract surgery. It is best appreciated a few hours after the cataract surgery. Most common causes that lead to epithelial or stromal edema after the cataract surgery are mechanical trauma, prolonged intraocular irrigation, inflammation, increased intraocular pressure (IOP), Descemet membrane detachment, intraocular toxins, and a complicated cataract surgery.

◆ Presentation

An associated endothelial abnormality or decompensation has to be ruled out preoperatively. There is an associated increase in the corneal thickness. An increased epithelial thickness with associated hazy cornea, irregular surface, and epithelial defect form the hallmarks of epithelial edema. The thickness returns to normal after a few hours of surgery. Stromal edema is associated with a marked increase in the corneal thickness, corneal haze, and endothelial folds involving mainly the center of the cornea (**Fig. 7.26**). Brown-McLean syndrome, a clinical condition arising after cataract surgery, is characterized by peripheral corneal edema with a clear center.

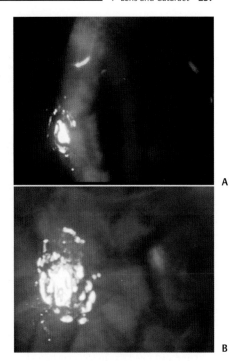

Fig. 7.26 Postoperative striate striate keratitis.

◆ Management

As a rule, if the corneal periphery is clear, the corneal edema reduces in a few hours. Cases with epithelial edema require a medical reduction of IOP if the edema does not resolve in a few hours. A stromal corneal edema persisting for a few days is required to be managed with hypertonic eyedrops and steroids. A vitrectomy is indicated in patients with existing vitreocorneal adherence with associated corneal edema. A Descemet membrane detachment can be handled by injecting air or gas (C_3F_8 or SF_6). Edema existing for more than 3 months usually requires a penetrating keratoplasty.

Hypotony and Wound Leak after Cataract Extraction

Hypotony due to wound leak after cataract surgery is a common complication of the cataract surgery. The leakage can occur from the incision site, the side port, or the bleb in cases with the combined trabeculectomy surgery.

◆ Presentation

Wound leakage can be picked up on slit lamp and by employing a Siedel test. Mild to moderate leaks present with a shallow anterior chamber, leaking wound, irrigation, tearing, contact lens intolerance, infection, and significant hypotony. Severe leaks may be associated with iridocorneal touch with severe corneal edema.

◆ **Management**

Most of the leaks are self-limiting and require observation with patching and use of topical and systemic aqueous suppressants. Temporary reduction of the topical steroids helps in prompter healing by increasing inflammation. In chronic cases use of cyanoacrylate glue, simple wound suturing, and anterior chamber reformation with saline or air followed by wound suturing helps.

Elevated IOP after Cataract Extraction

An IOP fluctuation immediately after cataract surgery is a common but self-limiting problem in most of the cases. Retention of viscoelastic material in the eye during the surgery is one of the most common causes of postoperative inflammation and IOP rise. Other causes of increased IOP after cataract surgery include pupillary block, hyphema, ciliary block, endophthalmitis, retained lens material, iris pigment release, preexisting glaucoma, use of steroids, and peripheral anterior synechiae.

◆ **Presentation**

The patient usually complains of hazy vision and pain. Hazy corneas due to epithelial or stromal edema and associated anterior chamber inflammation are common.

◆ **Management**

Most of the cases are mild and self-limiting and require only monitoring. A rise in IOP noted intraoperatively can be managed by depressing the lower lip of the paracentesis site to evacuate some of the fluid out of the eye. However, a significant and sustained rise in IOP may necessitate timely and specific management of several circumstances. Secondary glaucomas are handled by treating the underlying cause.

Cystoid Macular Edema after Cataract Extraction

Cystoid macular edema (CME) is a painless condition in which cystic swelling or thickening occurs of the central retina (macula) and is usually associated with blurred or distorted vision. When CME develops following cataract surgery and its cause is thought to be directly related to the surgery, it is referred to as Irvine-Gass syndrome. The Müller cells in the retina become overwhelmed with fluid, leading to their lysis. This results in an accumulation of fluid in the outer plexiform and inner nuclear layers of the retina. Usual causes of CME are vascular instability, intraocular inflammation, and mechanical forces (e.g., epiretinal membrane, vitreomacular traction). The incidence of CME is 1% after phacoemulsification and 20% after extra-capsular cataract extraction (ECCE).

◆ **Presentation**

Patients with CME usually present with decreased or blurry vision. Slit-lamp biomicroscopy reveals blunted or irregular foveal light reflex, retinal thickening, and/or intraretinal cysts in the foveal region. Optic disk edema, epiretinal membrane/macular pucker, diabetic retinopathy, and uveitis must be looked for to rule out other causes. On fundus fluorescein angiography a petaloid pattern of leakage in the macula occurs. Optical coherence tomography (OCT) is helpful in establishing a diagnosis and in measuring the therapeutic response (**Fig. 7.27**).

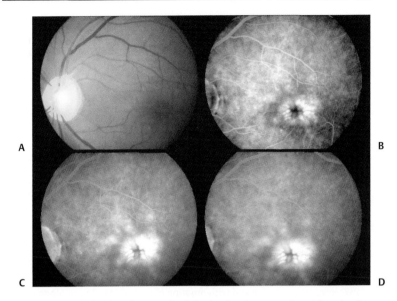

Fig. 7.27 **(A)** Color photograph of the fundus shows an absent foveal reflex with cystoid edema. **(B)** Fundus fluorescein angiography shows a characteristic patelloid pattern of hyperfluorescence in the early venous phase, which increases in intensity in the later phases **(C,D)** of the angiogram.

◆ Differential Diagnosis

Diabetic macular edema, retinitis pigmentosa, juvenile retinoschisis, vitreomacular traction syndrome, epiretinal membrane, Goldmann-Favre syndrome, macular cyst, and foveal schisis in high myopes

◆ Management

Treatment is aimed at the underlying etiology; however, several of the common treatments may help different causes of CME. Medical treatment modalities include corticosteroids (topical, oral, intravitreal, or in the sub-Tenon space), nonsteroidal antiinflammatory drugs, carbonic anhydrase inhibitors, and YAG laser lysis of the vitreous strands.

Surgical therapy includes pars plana vitrectomy to remove vitreous strands tracking to the surgical wound or pupil status after complicated ocular surgery, peeling of the posterior hyaloid face from the surface of the macula in vitreomacular traction syndrome, peeling of the epiretinal membranes, removal of inflammatory mediators from the vitreous cavity, removal of retained nuclear lens fragments, and repositioning of a dislocated or subluxed IOL.

Retinal Detachment, Suprachoroidal Hemorrhage/Effusion after Cataract Extraction

Intraocular surgery is a major risk factor in the development of rhegmatogenous retinal detachment (RRD). Because cataract surgery is the most common intraocular procedure, it is also the most common risk factor for RRD. It has been estimated

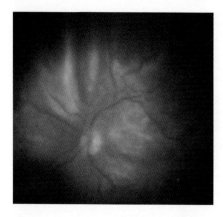

Fig. 7.28 Aphakic retinal detachment.

that 20 to 40% of RRDs occur in eyes that have undergone cataract extraction. Aphakia and pseudophakia, especially after YAG capsulotomy, predispose to posterior vitreous detachment (PVD). Previous studies have shown that the incidence of PVD increased with age and with duration of the aphakia. In pseudophakic patients, peripheral capsular opacification, lenticular remnants, and optical effects induced by the rim of the IOL may impair visualization of the small peripheral retinal breaks by indirect ophthalmoscopy, leading to missed breaks during surgical repair.

◆ Presentation

Because most postoperative retinal detachments are rhegmatogenous in nature, similar symptoms, such as photopsias, floaters, visual-field defects, and central visual loss are experienced by patients. The retinal breaks are often small, difficult to visualize, and located along the posterior border of the vitreous base. RRD is often extensive and commonly involves the macula. The most important postoperative factor is YAG capsulotomy. Anterior chamber IOL and iris clip lenses induce more inflammation, resulting in a higher incidence of proliferative vitreoretinopathy (**Fig. 7.28**).

◆ Differential Diagnosis

IOL dislocation, lattice degeneration, and other types of retinal detachment

◆ Management

B-scan ultrasound is the main investigation. As with all RRDs, the goal is to identify and close all the retinal breaks. Vitrectomy with fluid-air exchange, vitrectomy and scleral buckling, and pneumatic retinopexy are some of the treatment modalities.

Endophthalmitis after Cataract Extraction

Postoperative endophthalmitis is defined as severe inflammation involving both the anterior and posterior segments of the eye after intraocular surgery. Typically, postoperative endophthalmitis is caused by the perioperative introduction of microbial organisms into the eye either from the patient's normal conjunctival and skin flora or from contaminated instruments. Although most cases of postoperative endophthalmitis occur within 6 weeks of surgery, infections seen in high-risk patients or infections caused by slow-growing organisms may occur months or years after the procedure.

◆ Presentation

Patients with acute postoperative endophthalmitis typically present within 6 weeks of intraocular surgery with moderate to severe eye pain and decreased vision. The hallmark findings on ophthalmic examination are posterior and anterior chamber inflammation, hypopyon, conjunctival hyperemia and chemosis, corneal edema, wound abnormalities, and associated eyelid or orbital inflammation. In rare circumstances, patients may develop chronic, infectious endophthalmitis months to years after intraocular surgery (**Fig. 7.29**).

Risk factors for development of postoperative endophthalmitis may include increased operative time, posterior capsule rupture/vitreous loss, retained lens fragments, inadequate sterilization of the operative field, and contamination of surgical instruments. In the endophthalmitis vitrectomy study, the most common organisms isolated were coagulase-negative staphylococci (70%), *Staphylococcus aureus* (9.9%), and streptococci species (9.0%). Infections caused by gram-negative organisms were seen in 6% of cases. In chronic postoperative endophthalmitis, an important causative organism is *Propionibacterium acnes*, a slow-growing, gram-positive bacillus that is associated with a characteristic white, intracapsular plaque that develops weeks to months after cataract surgery.

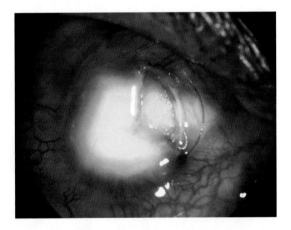

Fig. 7.29 Postoperative endophthalmitis with corneal melt and intraocular lens extrusion.

◆ Differential Diagnosis

Endogenous endophthalmitis, intraocular foreign body, vitreous hemorrhage, glaucoma (lens particle, phacolytic, phacomorphic, and uveitis), and vitreous wick syndrome

◆ Management

Obtain vitreous, aqueous samples and conjunctival cultures for microbiological identification of the offending organism. B-scan is done to confirm the diagnosis. The results of an endophthalmitis vitrectomy study demonstrated no difference in final visual outcomes in patients who underwent initial intraocular antibiotic injection (vitreous tap) or immediate pars plana vitrectomy (vitrectomy) if presenting visual acuity was better than light perception. However, in patients presenting with light perception vision, those who underwent initial VIT were three times more likely to achieve 20/40 vision, twice as likely to maintain 20/100 vision, and had a nearly 50% reduction in the risk of severe visual loss (<5/200), compared with patients who underwent TAP. No long-term difference occurred in media clarity between treatment groups. Intravenous antibiotics had no effect on either treatment outcome.

Vancomycin has been shown effective against greater than 99% of gram-positive endophthalmitis isolates. The aminoglycoside amikacin (0.4 mg in 0.1 mL) is useful for gram-negative coverage. Approximately 90% of gram-negative isolates are susceptible to this agent. Ceftazidime is a reasonable alternative for gram-negative coverage. The use of intravitreal dexamethasone in the treatment of acute postoperative endophthalmitis remains controversial. In chronic postoperative endophthalmitis from *Propionibacterium acnes*, intraocular vancomycin alone has been associated with high rates of persistent inflammation.

The endophthalmitis vitrectomy study recommends rapid intervention with surgery for patients with severe vision loss on presentation.

Intraocular Lens Opacification

It has been more than 50 years since Harold Ridley's first implant, and the cataract-IOL procedure has reached an extraordinarily high level of quality and performance. However, complications such as IOL opacification do occur (**Fig. 7.30A,B**).

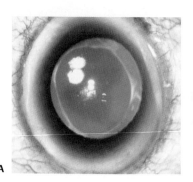
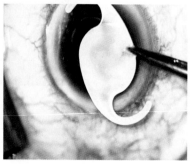

A   B

Fig. 7.30   (**A**) Opacified intraocular lens. (**B**) Opacified intraocular lens explanted.

◆ Presentation

The opacities of the IOL optics may start as scattered white-brown spots within the substance of the IOL optic and remain stable or slowly progressive. Some may gradually increase in intensity and numbers, eventually reaching a point where a visual acuity loss may necessitate removal or exchange of the IOL. In addition to visual loss, the reported symptoms included decrease in contrast sensitivity and various visual disturbances and aberrations, including glare. In the early stages there was usually no effect on Snellen visual acuity, but a gradual decrease of visual acuity was noted in the late stage of the process.

◆ Differential Diagnosis

Cataract

◆ Management

If necessary, one should explant and remove the opacified IOL and replace it with a new one.

8 Glaucoma

Soosan Jacob and Amar Agarwal

◆ Primary Open-Angle Glaucoma

Open-angle glaucoma (OAG) is characterized by a gonioscopically open angle and reduced facility of outflow not due to any obvious disease of the eye. It has a familial tendency.

◆ Presentation

OAG is a bilateral, insidious, slowly progressive, often asymmetric, asymptomatic disease, often not recognized by the patient until late in the disease when vision is lost. Patients have an elevated intraocular pressure (IOP) with open angles all around. The optic nerve shows characteristic changes that include a generalized enlargement of the cup with documented thinning of the neurosensory rim over time progressing from inferior to superior to nasal and then finally to the temporal rim, focal (especially vertical) enlargement of the cup, notching in the rim, acquired pit of the optic nerve, cup:disk (C:D) ratio asymmetry greater than 2, enlarged C:D ratio more than 0.6, nerve fiber layer hemorrhage crossing the rim margin, nerve fiber layer defect, peripapillary atrophy, and bayoneting sign. Initially, the superior and inferior poles of the optic nerve are affected (**Fig. 8.1**).

◆ Differential Diagnosis

Physiological cupping of the optic nerve, secondary OAG, creeping angle-closure glaucoma, ocular hypertension, other causes of optic atrophy, congenital optic nerve defects, and drusen of the optic nerve.

◆ Management

Applanation tonometry, visual fields, anterior-segment optical coherence tomography (OCT), optic nerve-head analysis and retinal nerve fiber layer analysis by posterior segment OCT, scanning laser polarimetry or Heidelberg retinal tomogram, and stereoscopic evaluation of the disk form part of the evaluation of the patient.

Medical management of glaucoma is based on the amount of damage already present, the rate of damage progression, and the risk factors. The only proven method of stopping or slowing optic nerve damage is by reducing IOP. Antiglaucoma medications can be used for this such as topical parasympathomimetics, B-adrenergic blockers, epinephrine derivatives, carbonic anhydrase inhibitors, alpha adrenergic agonist, and prostaglandin analogues. Nonmedical management consists of argon laser trabeculoplasty, selective laser trabeculoplasty, and surgery. Surgical procedures include trabeculectomy, setons, and nonpenetrating procedures such as viscocanalostomy and deep sclerectomy.

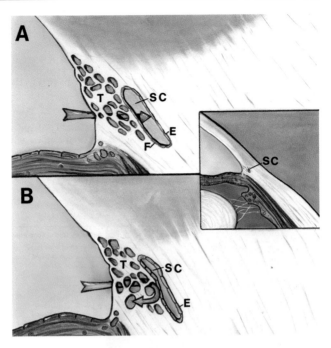

Fig. 8.1   Normal anatomy and fluid dynamics compared with the anatomy and fluid dynamics of a glaucoma patient. (**A**) The normal flow of aqueous humor through the trabecular meshwork (T) to the floor (F) of the Schlemm canal (SC). Active transport of the aqueous humor occurs through the normal endothelium (E) to the lumen of the canal. It is then drained through small openings in the external wall or roof of the Schlemm canal (SC), into scleral collector channels and then into capillaries and veins within the subconjunctival tissues. (**B**) In a diseased eye with open-angle glaucoma, the endothelium (E) of the Schlemm canal is more resistant to aqueous outflow, as is the immediately adjacent trabecular meshwork. This is the site of highest resistance to aqueous flow. Passage of aqueous humor is very slow, resulting in the increased intraocular pressure of glaucoma. (*Inset*) Anatomically, the Schlemm canal (SC) is located slightly behind the limbus. (Courtesy of *Highlights of Ophthalmology*, "Innovations in the Glaucomas: Etiology, Diagnosis and Management," English Edition, 2002. Eds: Benjamin F. Boyd, MD, FACS; Maurice H. Luntz, MD, FACS; Co-Editor: Samuel Boyd, MD.)

◆ Normal-Tension (or Low-Tension) Glaucoma

This is the condition in which optic nerve head loss, loss of nerve fiber layer, and the visual field defects are the same as seen in chronic glaucoma, but there is no rise in IOP. Normal-tension glaucoma (NTG) forms 16% of all the glaucomas.

◆ Presentation

Patients are mostly asymptomatic. Occasionally the patient presents with scotoma. There may be an associated history of episodes of ischemic optic neuropathy, neurological symptoms, migraine, or Raynaud disease.

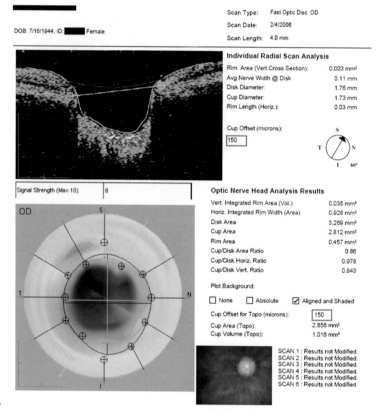

A

Fig. 8.2   (A) Posterior segment optical coherence tomography (OCT) showing optic nerve head analysis in a patient with normal-tension glaucoma and advanced glaucomatous cupping.

IOPs are recorded as normal. The optic disk is typically large in NTG. Cupping is proportionally larger than visual-field loss. A sloping neuroretinal rim edge with shallow cup, higher incidence of optic disk pit associated with it, peripapillary atrophy, optic disk hemorrhages, steeper and deeper visual-field defects close to fixation, a positive family history, myopia, nocturnal hypotension, and a history of carotid artery disease are some of the associated features (**Figs. 8.2A,B**).

◆ Differential Diagnosis

Includes cases with intermittent pressure elevation or diurnal variations in primary open-angle glaucoma (POAG), patients with long-term fluctuations in pressure elevations that have been masked by systemic medications such as β-blockers; other nonglaucomatous optic neuropathy; congenital abnormalities of the optic nerve head

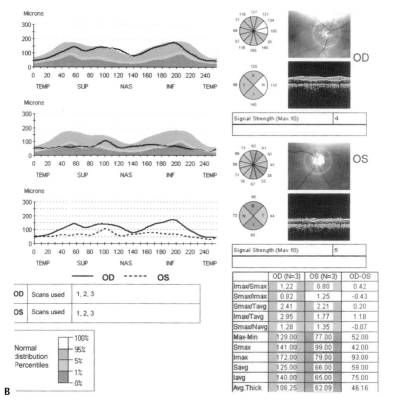

B

Fig. 8.2 (*Continued*) **(B)** Posterior segment OCT showing retinal nerve fiber layer analysis in a patient with bilateral advanced normal-tension glaucoma.

◆ Management

A complete ocular and systemic history is important. History of drug intake, vascular problems, neurological problems, and cardiological problems must be recorded. Careful ocular examination with stereoscopic optic nerve head evaluation, peripheral fundus examination, and gonioscopic and field examination must be done.

A 20 to 25% reduction in the IOP is aimed in early and moderate field changes, and it should be less than 25% in patients with severe field changes. Miotics, α-2 agonist, β-blockers, dorzolamide and latanoprost are good options to reduce IOP. Calcium channel blockers and neuroprotection play a prominent role in the management of NTG. Filtration surgery is an option in advanced field defects.

◆ Secondary Open-Angle Glaucoma

Secondary open-angle glaucoma is OAG that occurs secondary to some other cause.

Pigmentary Dispersion Glaucoma

Pigment dispersion syndrome (PDS) is generally an asymptomatic disorder discovered during routine ophthalmic evaluation. Pigmentary glaucoma is a sequela of PDS. Developmental abnormalities of the iris pigment epithelium are the fundamental defect responsible for the pigment dispersion. The condition is seen in a relatively younger age group and is more common in men than in women. Myopia and a deep anterior chamber are the risk factors for the development of PDS. It is common in persons of European descent.

◆ Presentation

The condition is diagnosed incidentally in most of the cases. Few patients complain of colored halos and smoky vision in the dim light conditions and after vigorous physical exercise. Patients have a raised IOP, defective fields, and optic disk cupping. Other associated findings include Krukenberg spindle, raised central corneal thickness, iris transillumination defect, concave peripheral iris, anisocoria, ring of pigmentation over the peripheral surface of the lens, and a highly pigmented trabecular meshwork (**Fig. 8.3**).

◆ Differential Diagnosis

Pseudoexfoliative glaucoma

◆ Management

Patients with PDS are always considered as glaucoma suspects and IOP spikes, visual fields, cupping, and gonioscopy are checked annually. Myopic patients with PDS have to be checked for peripheral retinal lesions, retinal breaks, and retinal detachment. Miotics, topical β-blockers, and carbonic anhydrase inhibitors form the mainstay of the treatment of pigmentary glaucoma. Patients usually respond well to argon laser trabeculoplasty (ALT). Filtering surgery with antimetabolite is done in advanced and refractory cases.

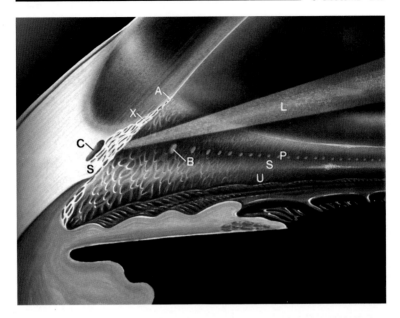

Fig. 8.3 Proper placement of laser application in laser trabeculoplasty. This magnified cross section of the angle area shows a properly placed laser beam (L) being applied to the center of the posterior trabecular meshwork (P) or pigmented band. Notice the laser burns (B) centered on this pigmented band (P). If one were to divide the space between the scleral spur (S) and the Schwalbe line (A) in half (X), the laser burns (B) fall on the center of the posterior half [area between (X) and (S)]. The anterior half of the meshwork [area between (X) and (A)] is left untreated. Posterior to the scleral spur (S) is the uveal meshwork (U). Schlemm canal (C). (Courtesy of *Highlights of Ophthalmology*, "Innovations in the Glaucomas: Etiology, Diagnosis and Management," English Edition, 2002. Eds: Benjamin F. Boyd, MD, FACS; Maurice H. Luntz, MD, FACS; Co-Editor: Samuel Boyd, MD.)

Pseudoexfoliation Syndrome

Pseudoexfoliation syndrome (PEX) is an age-related generalized disorder of extracellular matrix characterized by production and progressive accumulation of fibrillar material in the tissues throughout the anterior segment. PEX is the single most common identifiable cause of OAG, and it is also a risk factor for cataract surgery. Incidence increases with age and is more common in females.

◆ Presentation

Deposition of the grayish white material on the surface of the anterior lens capsule is a common, consistent, and diagnostic finding. The deposition had a classic pattern of three zones (i.e., a relatively homogeneous central disk, a granular layered peripheral zone, and a clear area separating the preceding two).

The PEX material is found deposited on the pupillary border, corneal endothelium, iris furrows, and sometimes even at the extraocular muscles. Other associ-

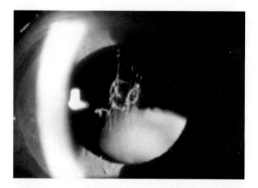

Fig. 8.4 Pseudoexfoliative material seen in a sublux-ated lens. (Courtesy of Lincoln Freitas)

ated features can be peripapillary transillumination defect, insufficient mydriasis, posterior synechiae, Sampaolesi line, less dense but patchy pigmentation of the trabecular meshwork, phacodonesis, and iridodonesis (**Fig. 8.4**).

◆ Differential Diagnosis

True exfoliation, pigmentary glaucoma, other causes for melanin dispersion, primary amyloidosis, senile iridoschisis, POAG.

◆ Management

PEX patients require frequent monitoring of IOP, optic disk, and visual fields. The medical line of management forms the initial line of treatment. ALT is a highly successive treatment for these patients. Filtering surgery is recommended for the advanced cases. Caution should be taken while operating on patients with PEX for cataract surgery, as PEX is associated with an increased incidence of lens subluxation and vitreous loss.

Lens-Induced Glaucoma

Lens-induced glaucomas are either OAGs or angle-closure glaucoma. OAGs include lens protein glaucoma, lens particle glaucoma, and phacoanaphylactic glaucoma. Closed-angle glaucomas include intumescent lens and lens subluxation or dislocation.

Lens Particle Glaucoma
The patient has unilateral pain, defective vision, lacrimation, and photophobia. Increased IOP, cells and flare, white fluffy pieces of lens cortex in the anterior chamber, and open angles are seen. A disruption in the lens capsule by trauma or surgery liberates lens material that obstructs the trabecular meshwork. Inflammation also contributes to the glaucoma. Management consists of reduction of inflammation and IOP followed by removal of the residual lens matter if necessary.

Phacolytic Glaucoma
The patient has unilateral pain, defective vision, lacrimation, and photophobia. Open angles and a hypermature or mature cataract are seen along with increased IOP, iridescent particles, and white material in the anterior chamber and on the lens capsule. Lens protein leaks from an intact cataract and obstructs the trabecular meshwork. Inflammation also contributes to the glaucoma. Aging and cataract formation are the risk factors. Management consists of reduction of inflammation and IOP followed by cataract extraction.

Phacoanaphylactic Glaucoma
Granulomatous inflammation occurs secondary to a hypersensitivity reaction to lens particle released after penetrating trauma or surgery.

Phacomorphic Glaucoma
It is caused by an intumescent lens leading to angle closure glaucoma, secondary to either an enhanced pupillary block mechanism or due to forward displacement of the lens–iris diaphragm.

Ectopia Lentis
Can also cause an angle closure glaucoma. Pupillary block may occur due to the lens being dislocated into the pupil or anterior chamber or the vitreous herniating into the anterior chamber.

Uveitic Glaucoma

Inflammatory cells mechanically obstruct the trabecular meshwork (TBM) and are directly cytotoxic to the TBM. They cause a combination of closed-angle glaucoma secondary to peripheral anterior synechiae (PAS), posterior synechiae, or total synechiae, formation and OAG secondary to increased protein content of the aqueous, aqueous hypersecretion, obstruction by inflammatory cells and debris, trabeculitis, scarring of the TBM, increased episcleral venous pressure, or as a steroid response.

◆ Presentation

It is often unilateral, presenting with pain, photophobia, redness, and decreased vision. On examination, aqueous cells and flare, open angles, irregular pupil, posterior synechiae, PAS, inflammatory precipitates on the posterior corneal surface or trabecular meshwork, ciliary flush, and other signs of uveitis along with signs of glaucomatous damage to the eye may be seen.

◆ Differential Diagnosis

Acute angle-closure glaucoma, neovascular glaucoma, Posner-Schlossman syndrome, Fuchs heterochromic iridocyclitis, steroid response glaucoma

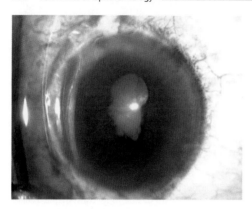

Fig. 8.5 Uveitic evidence seen in an eye with increased intraocular pressure.

◆ Management

Topical steroids and cycloplegics are given for the inflammation, and the glaucoma is managed medically (miotics and prostaglandin analogues are not to be used because they may cause a worsening of the inflammation) and if required surgically with antimetabolites or seton (**Figs. 8.5** and **8.6**).

Elevated Episcleral Venous Pressure

Venous drainage obstruction secondary to retrobulbar tumors, thyroid eye disease, pseudotumor, cavernous sinus thrombosis, jugular vein obstruction, superior vena cava obstruction, and intracranial (Sturge-Weber syndrome, caroticocavernous fistula, dural fistula, venous varix) or orbital arteriovenous fistulas can all lead to increased episcleral venous pressure. It can also increase without any obvious cause.

◆ Presentation

The patient presents with a red eye. The episcleral veins are generally dilated and tortuous with a corkscrew appearance. The angles are open and blood may be seen in the Schlemm canal.

◆ Differential Diagnosis

Conjunctivitis, episcleritis, scleritis, orbital inflammation

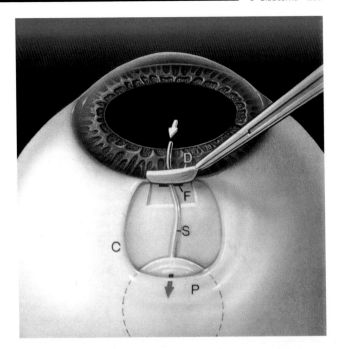

Fig. 8.6 Seton implantation procedure. A fornix-based conjunctival flap (C) is raised and the methylmethacrylate baseplate (P) of the Seton is pushed under the conjunctival flap posteriorly and sutured to the scleral surface. The implant has a biconcave shape with the inferior surface shaped to fit the sclera. A small 3-mm-square half-thickness lamellar scleral flap (D) is raised just as in a trabeculectomy. An incision (F) is made into the anterior chamber under this scleral flap, and the long silicone tube (S) of the Seton is placed into the anterior chamber (the end of the silicone tube can be seen in the anterior chamber near the tip of the *white arrow*). Next, the scleral flap (D) is sutured down around the tube (S) of the Seton. Finally, the conjunctiva is sutured back in place. Aqueous then drains from the anterior chamber (*white arrow*) down through the tube (S) to the baseplate (P) (*black arrow*), where a bleb forms. (Courtesy of *Highlights of Ophthalmology*, "Innovations in the Glaucomas: Etiology, Diagnosis and Management," English Edition, 2002. Eds: Benjamin F. Boyd, MD, FACS; Maurice H. Luntz, MD, FACS; Co-Editor: Samuel Boyd, MD.)

◆ **Management**

Approach to management depends on the cause. Filtering surgery carries the risk of intraoperative choroidal effusion, expulsive hemorrhage, and postoperative flat anterior chamber. Prophylactic sclerotomies in the inferior quadrants should be made prior to starting the filtering surgery. These are left open and covered only with conjunctiva at the end of surgery.

◆ Angle-Closure Glaucoma

Angle-closure glaucoma can be classified as angle-closure glaucoma with pupillary block and angle-closure glaucoma without pupillary block, each of which can be further divided into primary and secondary forms.

Acute Angle-Closure Glaucoma

Any increase in the normal condition of relative pupillary block because of the central iris hugging the anterior lens surface causes the peripheral iris to come in contact with the trabecular meshwork blocking the aqueous outflow, causing an acute rise in pressure.

◆ Presentation

The patient presents with decreased vision, severe pain, redness, blurred vision, colored haloes around lights, nausea, and vomiting. Circumcorneal congestion, corneal microcystic edema, shallow anterior chamber, mild anterior chamber reaction, mid-dilated, vertically oval pupil, and the like are seen. In case of recurrent attacks, posterior synechiae, peripheral anterior synechiae, glaukomflecken (small anterior subcapsular lens opacities), sector or generalized iris atrophy, optic nerve pallor and cupping, permanently increased IOP, and visual-field loss may be seen (**Figs. 8.7** and **8.8**).

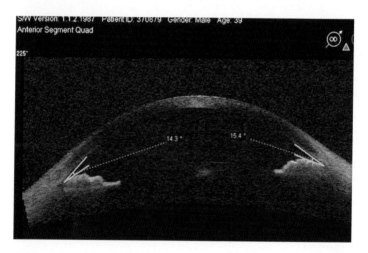

Fig. 8.7 Anterior segment optical coherence tomography in a patient showing narrow angles

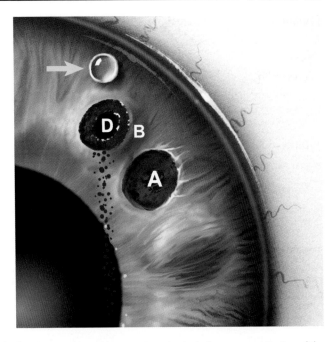

Fig. 8.8 Abraham's argon laser iridectomy two-step technique—surgeon's view of the second burn. The second burn is a penetrating burn aimed at the crest or peak of one of the iris humps (B), which resulted from the first burn. This second burn has now created a hole or iridectomy (D) through the peak of the iris hump (B). The first burn, which was partially penetrating, is shown in (A). Note the iris pigment drifting down while a gas bubble floats superiorly (*arrow*). Use the plano-convex button of the lens only for second coagulation. (Courtesy of *Highlights of Ophthalmology*, "Innovations in the Glaucomas: Etiology, Diagnosis and Management," English Edition, 2002. Eds: Benjamin F. Boyd, MD, FACS; Maurice H. Luntz, MD, FACS; Co-Editor: Samuel Boyd, MD.)

◆ Management

Medical management consists of pilocarpine, topical steroids, antiglaucoma medications, pain killers, and antiemetics. The definitive treatment is laser iridotomy performed with either with an argon or YAG laser. In the case of extensive synechiae with permanently elevated IOP, a trabeculectomy may be required.

Chronic Angle-Closure Glaucoma

Angle synechiae usually begin superiorly and progress in both directions toward the 6 o'clock position.

◆ Presentation

Presentation is similar to primary open-angle glaucoma (POAG). The patient has increased IOP that is asymptomatic until damage has occurred. Diagnosis is by gonioscopy (**Fig. 8.9**).

◆ Differential Diagnosis

Primary or secondary OAG

◆ Management

Medical management and laser iridotomy are used in early cases and trabeculectomy in advanced cases.

Neovascular Glaucoma

Secondary glaucoma is caused by development of new vessels in the angle. Delayed diagnosis and poor management can cause loss of vision. Retinal ischemia or hypoxia and subsequent release of angiogenic factors causes neovascular glaucoma. Elevation of IOP is due to fibrovascular membranes and anterior synechiae blocking the angle.

◆ Presentation

The eye is painful, photophobic, and red. Visual acuity may be as low as counting fingers or no perception of light. IOP may be as high as 60 mm Hg. Conjunctival congestion and steamy cornea are associated findings (**Fig. 8.10**).

A tiny early tuft of new vessels is visible first at the margin of the pupillary border. The vessels later enlarge to form knuckles. The patient's eye is examined under high

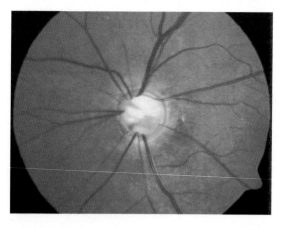

Fig. 8.9   Cupping of the disk.

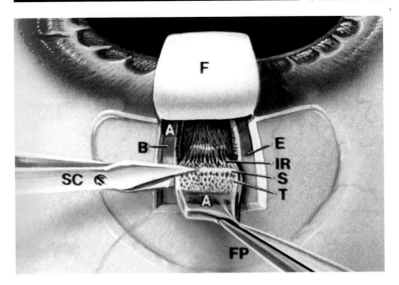

Fig. 8.10 Trabeculectomy with a fornix-based flap—removing the trabecular window— surgeon's view. This is a surgeon's view of the final incision to remove the trabecular window. It also reveals the surgeon's view of the structures most important to proper trabeculectomy. The trabeculectomy flap, which is being excised, has been hinged backward exposing its deep surface to the surgeon's view. The Vannas scissors (SC), make the final cut just in front of the scleral spur (S), on the trabecular tissue, which is here being reflected back with forceps (FP). The scleral spur is localized externally (E) by the junction of the white sclera and gray band (B). A, clear cornea; F, scleral flap; IR, iris root; T, trabeculum. (Courtesy of *Highlights of Ophthalmology*, "Innovations in the Glaucomas: Etiology, Diagnosis and Management," English Edition, 2002. Eds: Benjamin F. Boyd, MD, FACS; Maurice H. Luntz, MD, FACS; Co-Editor: Samuel Boyd, MD.)

magnification. A slight pressure with the gonioscope or dilation of the pupil may obscure the finding. The new vessels then appear on the surface of the iris to reach the iris collarette. Later new vessels extend from the root of the iris to the ciliary body and the scleral spur to arborize the trabecular meshwork. Fibrovascular membranes associated with neovascularization start contracting to tent the iris toward the angle. Anterior synechiae and iridocorneal adhesions are common findings.

◆ **Differential Diagnosis**

Uveitic glaucoma, acute angle-closure glaucoma

◆ **Management**

A thorough history and ophthalmic and retinal examinations are mandatory. Control of IOP and inflammation is the first line of management. Hyperosmotic agents and mydriatic agents play an important role. Panretinal photocoagulation or peripheral cryopexy must be performed at the earliest opportunity. Trabeculectomy with a shunt procedure and application of antimetabolites is preferred. If the IOP is very high and the patient experiences pain with no useful vision, cyclodestructive procedures can be considered.

◆ Iridocorneal Endothelial Syndrome

This is a unilateral condition, seen mainly in women aged 30 to 50 years.

◆ Presentation

The patient usually presents with diminished vision and pain. There is movement of the corneal endothelium onto the iris. Loss of cells from the cornea would lead to corneal swelling, distortion of the iris, melt holes, stretch holes, and a variable degree of distortion of the pupil. The endothelium becomes several layers thick and spreads over the trabecular meshwork, causing glaucoma.

The slit-lamp examination reveals a "fine hammered silver" appearance of the corneal endothelium. Specular microscopy demonstrates pleomorphism in size and shape within certain cells and a loss of clear hexagonal margins. Based on the involvement of the cornea, the disorder is called total, disseminated, or subtotal. Based on the structure involvement the disorder is classified as follows:

◆ Chandler syndrome, which mainly involves the cornea
◆ Cogan-Reese syndrome, which mainly involves the angle, with a pigmented and pedunculated nodule present over the iris
◆ Progressive iris atrophy

◆ Differential Diagnosis

Chandler syndrome, Cogan-Reese syndrome, anterior chamber cleavage syndrome, previous ocular trauma, posterior polymorphous dystrophy

◆ Management

Corneal edema is managed by lowering the IOP, use of hypertonic saline and soft bandage contact lenses, and, finally, penetrating keratoplasty. Glaucoma is best approached with medical management (aqueous suppressants), and, finally, with trabeculectomy in the late stages. Immunotoxins have been found to be effective.

◆ Malignant Glaucoma

Malignant glaucoma may be seen in the postsurgical period on discontinuation of cycloplegics or on addition of miotics. There is posterior misdirection of the aqueous, into the vitreous where it accumulates and displaces the vitreous forward, pushing the ciliary processes, crystalline lens, intraocular implant, or anterior vitreous face forward, causing secondary angle closure.

◆ Presentation

The patient presents with pain, redness, photophobia, and defective vision along with high IOP; a flat or very shallow anterior chamber in the presence of a patent; peripheral iridectomy and in the absence of a choroidal detachment.

◆ Differential Diagnosis

Pupillary block glaucoma, wound leak, choroidal detachment, and suprachoroidal hemorrhage

◆ Management

If there is no iridectomy or if it is not patent, a PI is performed to rule out pupillary block glaucoma. Medical management consists of topical atropine and phenylephrine as well as antiglaucoma medications to control the IOP. All miotics are stopped. Hyperosmotics are given to shrink the vitreous. Surgical management is often required. In aphakic/pseudophakic eyes, the YAG laser may be used to perform an anterior hyaloidotomy and posterior capsulotomy. If the patient is phakic, a vitrectomy may be required to remove the trapped aqueous. A PI should be performed in the contralateral eye. All miotics should be avoided in the patient.

9 Medical Retina

Mandeep Lamba, Soosan Jacob, and Amar Agarwal

◆ Hypertensive Retinopathy

A generalized response to systemic hypertension is vasoconstriction. This causes retinal vasculopathy in both the acute and the chronic stages of systemic hypertension.

◆ Presentation

Most patients are asymptomatic. However, symptoms can range from blurring of vision to profound loss of vision. Ophthalmoscopic examination reveals signs of arteriosclerosis, changed light reflex, copper wiring, sheathing of the vessels, pipestem sheathing, vascular attenuation, arteriovenous nicking, Gunn sign, Salus sign, extravascular retinal lesions (microaneurysms, retinal hemorrhages, macular edema, retinal lipid deposits, and macular star), inner retinal ischemic spots, focal intraretinal periarteriolar transudate, and associated disk edema in malignant hypertension. At arteriovenous crossings, retinal arteries and veins share a common adventitial lining. Obscuration of the retinal veins at these crossings (AV nicking) is considered a hallmark of hypertensive retinopathy. Retinal pigment epithelium (RPE) infarctions become hyperpigmented with time, forming Elschnig

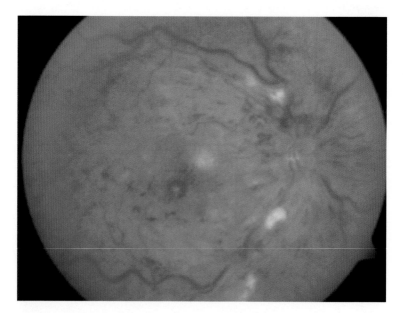

Fig. 9.1 Hypertensive retinopathy. Hypertensive retinopathy grade 4.

spots (peripheral hyperpigmented spots that may be surrounded by a small halo of hypopigmentation). Siegrist streaks are linear hyperpigmented areas directly over choroidal vessels that may have a similar pathophysiology as Elschnig spots. In extreme cases patients can present as hypertensive choroidopathy, serous retinal detachment, and hypertensive optic neuropathy (hemorrhages at the optic disk margin, blurring of disk margins, congestion of retinal veins, macular exudates, and florid disk edema) (**Fig. 9.1**).

◆ Differential Diagnosis

Diabetic retinopathy, collagen vascular diseases, anemia, radiation retinopathy, branch retinal vein occlusion (BRVO), central retinal vein occlusion (CRVO), ischemic optic neuropathy, other causes of neuroretinitis, papilledema, and cherry-red spot

◆ Management

The patient is referred for a cardiological workup. Pharmacotherapy and lifestyle changes are required to prevent further end organ damage.

◆ Diabetic Retinopathy

Retinal vasculopathy affects 25% of the total diabetic population. Diabetes can affect eyes in various ways, most commonly corneal abnormalities, glaucoma, iris neovascularization, cataracts, and neuropathies. However, diabetic retinopathy is the most common and potentially the most blinding of these complications. Native Americans and African Americans are at increased risk of developing diabetic retinopathy (**Fig. 9.2A,B,C,D**).

◆ Presentation

◆ *Nonproliferative diabetic retinopathy (NPDR)*: Most commonly the condition is detected incidentally. However, symptoms can range from mild blurring vision to distortion to visual acuity loss. Common clinical features include the presence of microaneurysms, dot/blot hemorrhages, flame-shaped hemorrhages, retinal edema, hard exudates, cotton wool spots, venous loops/beadings, intraretinal microangiopathies. On the basis of clinical picture, Early Treatment Diabetic Retinopathy Study (ETDRS) has classified NPDR into mild, moderate, and severe types.
◆ *Proliferative Diabetic Retinopathy (PDR)*: This is classified as early and high-risk PDR. Untreated PDR has a 70% chance of leading to total blindness. Symptoms can vary from mild blurring of vision to severe vision loss. Common clinical features include neovascularization of disk (NVD), neovascularization elsewhere (NVE), preretinal and vitreous hemorrhage, fibrovascular tissue proliferation, and traction or combined retinal detachments.
◆ *Maculopathy*: This is the leading cause of vision loss in patients with diabetic retinopathy. It is due to functional damage and necrosis of retinal capillaries. Edema can also be caused by traction in the case of PDR. The definition of clinically significant macular edema (CSME) is given by ETDRS (**Fig. 9.2E,F,G,H**).

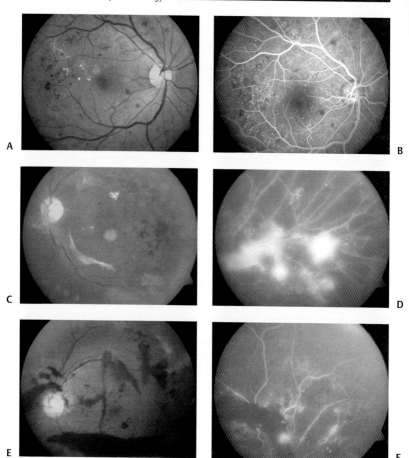

Fig. 9.2 (A) Severe nonproliferative diabetic retinopathy (NPDR) with diffuse diabetic maculopathy. **(B)** Moderate NPDR. **(C)** Proliferative diabetic retinopathy (PDR) with clinically significant macular edema. **(D)** PDR–FFA. **(E)** PDR with preretinal hemorrhage–color fundus photo. **(F)** PDR with preretinal hemorrhage–FFA.

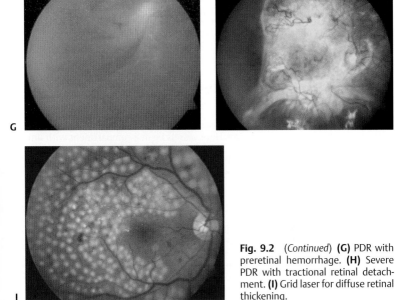

Fig. 9.2 (*Continued*) **(G)** PDR with preretinal hemorrhage. **(H)** Severe PDR with tractional retinal detachment. **(I)** Grid laser for diffuse retinal thickening.

◆ Differential Diagnosis

◆ *NPDR*: CRVO, BRVO, ocular ischemic syndrome, hypertensive retinopathy, radiation retinopathy, sickle cell disease
◆ *PDR*: Neovascularization due to vein occlusion, sickle cell retinopathy, drug abuse, sarcoidosis, Valsalva retinopathy
◆ *Maculopathy*: Cystoid macular edema (CME), central serous retinopathy (CSR), neuroretinitis, parafoveal telangiectasia, macroaneurysm

◆ Management

◆ Fasting glucose level and the hemoglobin A1c (HbA1c) levels are important indicators to monitor control of diabetes mellitus. HbA1c must be maintained between 6 and 7%. Fundus fluorescein angiography is done to diagnose stage and for follow-up of cases of diabetic retinopathy. B-scan is used in diagnosis and follow-up of cases with vitreous hemorrhage.
◆ Laser photocoagulation forms the mainstay of treatment. Focal and grid lasers are done to treat macular edema depending on the number and localization of the leaks. Panretinal photocoagulation is done in PDR. When both the lasers need to be combined, grid laser is done 2 to 3 weeks prior to the PRP (**Fig. 9.2I**).
◆ Intravitreal triamcinolone acetonide and bevacizumab have been tried for treating macular edema. Intravitreal injections of bovine hyaluronidase are used in treatment of vitreous hemorrhages.
◆ Vitrectomy is necessary in cases with longstanding vitreous hemorrhage, traction, or combined retinal detachment.

◆ Follow-up depends on the stage of the diabetic retinopathy (diabetic retino-pathy). Mild NPDR is followed up once in 1 year, moderate NPDR in 6 to 8 months, severe NPDR in 3 to 4 months, CSME in 2 to 3 months, early PDR in 2 to 3 months, and high-risk PDR every 1 to 2 months.

◆ Central Retinal Vein Occlusion

The etiology is thrombus formation posterior to the lamina cribrosa of the optic nerve in the predisposed population. Here vessels lie in a compartment with lim-ited space for displacement. Retinal vein occlusion can be a central or a branch vein occlusion. The pathogenesis of thrombosis can be analyzed by the classic Virchow triad: stasis of blood flow, hypercoagulation, and vessel wall abnormalities. (**Fig. 9.3A,B,C,D**).

◆ Presentation

A detailed history is taken to rule out possible causes. The presenting patient can be asymptomatic or with decreased vision, photophobia, painful blind eye, and redness. Visual loss can be sudden or gradual, over a period of days to weeks. Visual loss ranges from mild to severe. Patients can present with transient obscurations of vision initially, later progressing to constant visual loss. Best-corrected vision is a very good prognostic indicator. Conjunctival congestion, corneal edema, relative afferent pupillary defect (RAPD), iris and angle neovascularization, and periph-eral anterior synechiae are important associated findings. Fundus examination reveals superficial, dot and blot, and/or deep retinal hemorrhages possible in all four quadrants. Whole fundus gives a "blood and thunder" appearance. Veins may be dilated and tortuous. Other associated findings can be optic disk edema, cotton-wool spots, NVD, NVE, optociliary shunt vessels, macular edema with or without exudates, cystoid macular edema, lamellar or full-thickness macular hole, optic atrophy, and pigmentary changes in the macula (**Fig. 9.3E,F**).

◆ Differential Diagnosis

Diabetic retinopathy, acute hypertensive retinopathy, ocular ischemic syndrome, papilledema, papillitis, radiation retinopathy, acute retinitis

◆ Management

Medical examination and laboratory tests are done to find the systemic causes leading to the episode. Ocular hypertension and glaucoma must be ruled out. Dop-pler color imaging, optical coherence tomography (OCT), FFA, and electroretino-gram (ERG) confirm the status of the disease and the likely prognosis. Aspirin, an-tiinflammatory agents, systemic anticoagulants, fibrinolytic agents, and systemic corticosteroids are used as the medical line of treatment.

Intravitreal injection of triamcinolone is the therapy of choice in patients with severe macular involvement. Chorioretinal venous anastomosis, radial optic neu-rotomy, and vitrectomy to remove the posterior hyaloid phase are the surgical ap-proaches used so far. Central vein obstruction study (CVOS) advocated a frequent follow-up in the early months of the episode to look for the iris neovascularization. Neovascularization, macular pucker, macular edema, cellophane maculopathy, and optic atrophy are the complications to be noted in every visit.

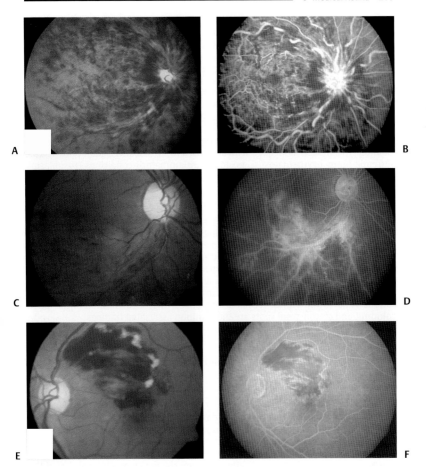

Fig. 9.3 **(A)** Central retinal vein occlusion (CRVO)—color fundus photo. **(B)** CRVO—fundus fluorescein angiography (FFA) late phase. **(C)** Branch retinal vein occlusion (BRVO) involving the macula—color fundus photo. **(D)** BRVO involving macula—FFA. **(E)** Macular retinal vein occlusion—color fundus photo. **(F)** Macular retinal vein occlusion—FFA.

◆ Branch Retinal Artery Occlusion

Of all the acute retinal arterial occlusions, 40% are branch retinal artery occlusions (BRAOs). Pathophysiologically, BRAO resembles central retinal artery occlusion (CRAO), but it involves only a sector of the retina. Ischemia of the inner layers of the retina leads to cellular injury and necrosis. It is most common in the seventh decade of life. Cholesterol emboli, called Hollenhorst plaques, are the emboli most commonly associated with BRAO. Platelet fibrin emboli appear as whitish gray plugs and increases in number with repeated episodes. Calcific emboli appear as large white plaques and usually involve the large arterioles around the disk. Other uncommon sources of emboli are also found, such as leukoemboli (vasculitis, Purtscher retinopathy, septic endocarditis), fat emboli following long-bone fractures, amniotic fluid emboli (complication of pregnancy), tumors (atrial myxoma, mitral valve papillary fibroelastoma), talc emboli (long-term intravenous drug abusers), corticosteroid emboli (complication of intralesional or retrobulbar steroid injection), air emboli following trauma or surgery, synthetic materials used in cardiac and vascular procedures (e.g., synthetic particles from artificial cardiac valves).

Certain nonembolic causes are also responsible for the arterial occlusions, for example, thrombosis associated with atherosclerosis, vasculitis (giant cell arteritis, systemic lupus erythematosus), posterior inflammatory conditions (toxoplasma retinochoroiditis, Behçet syndrome).

◆ Presentation

The patient usually presents with acute, unilateral, painless, partial loss of vision. Many times it can be an incidental finding. A history of associated risk factors like smoking, hypertension, hypercholesterolemia, diabetes, coronary artery disease, or history of stroke or transient ischemic attack and amaurosis fugax may be present. There may be a partial field loss respecting the horizontal meridian.

Fundus examination reveals a grayish white retina along the distribution of the affected vessel. An embolus can be seen in the vessel involved, usually at the bifurcations. A narrowed branch retinal artery, boxcarring, segmentation of the blood columns, and cotton-wool spots are the common associated findings.

◆ Differential Diagnosis

CRAO, cilioretinal artery occlusion, retinitis, retinal contusion, neoplasia, and myelinated nerve fiber layer

◆ Management

The condition is broadly investigated and treated along the same lines as CRAO. All the treatment modalities used in the case of CRAO have been tried but with very little success. Proper systemic investigations are done frequently to diagnose and eliminate the etiological factors. FFA and electroretinography (ERG) play a role in diagnosis of the condition, localization of nonperfusion areas, and viability of the involved retina. Anticoagulants, thrombolysis, and carotid endarterectomy form the treatment options, depending on the results of various investigations.

◆ Central Retinal Artery Occlusion/Ophthalmic Artery Occlusion

Vision loss due to CRAO is attributed to ischemia of the inner retinal layers and pyknosis of the ganglion cell layer. Subsequent ischemic necrosis of the retina causes opacification. Fourteen percent of the population has a cilioretinal artery that is a component of choroidal circulation and supplies the macula with all the components of the maculopapillary bundle. Men in their early sixties are most commonly involved (**Fig. 9.4A,B,C,D**).

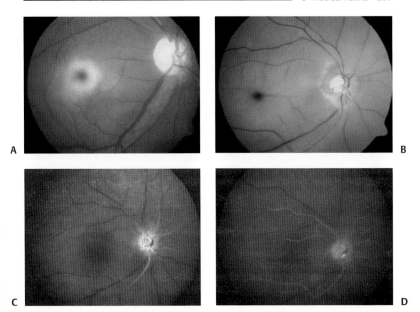

Fig. 9.4 **(A)** Central retinal artery occlusion (CRAO) showing cherry-red spot. **(B)** CRAO—color fundus photo. **(C)** CRAO fundus fluorescein angiography showing poor filling even after 6 minutes. **(D)** CRAO FFA showing poor filling even after 10 minutes.

◆ **Presentation**

CRAO presents as unilateral, acute, persistent, painless loss of vision. It can be bilateral in 2% of the population. Amaurosis fugax and other symptoms of temporal arteritis are other associated findings. A history of drug intake and embolic phenomena are commonly present. Visual acuity may vary from hand movements to a few meters. The presence of a cilioretinal artery portends a better prognosis because the central vision in these patients is well preserved. Afferent pupillary defects, pale disk with splinter hemorrhages, cherry-red spot, ground-glass appearance of the retina, boxcar segmentation of the arteries and veins, and embolus in ~20% of patients are common findings. A cardiac examination can reveal the presence of a bruit or murmurs. A history of temporal tenderness, jaw claudication, muscle weakness, raised erythrocyte sedimentation rate (ESR), and fever may be associated.

◆ **Differential Diagnosis**

Anterior ischemic optic neuropathy, inadvertent intraocular injection of gentamicin, blunt trauma, and other causes of cherry red spot like Tay-Sachs disease, other sphingolipidoses, quinine toxicity, macular hemorrhage, hypertension, Hurler syndrome, macular hole, steroid injections

◆ Management

Laboratory studies such as complete blood count, ESR, fibrinogen, antiphospholipid antibodies, prothrombin time/activated partial thromboplastin time (PT/aPTT), serum protein electrophoresis, fasting blood sugar, lipid profile, and blood cultures are helpful in the etiological diagnosis. Imaging techniques such as carotid ultrasound, which is supposedly more specific than carotid Doppler; magnetic resonance imaging; and FFA help in diagnosing the site of occlusion and the prognosis. FFA shows a generalized delay in the dye flow in all the phases of angiogram. Electrocardiography and echocardiography are indicated to rule out cardiac causes. ERG shows a diminished B-wave response.

- *CRAO with duration of onset less than 24 hours*: Treat as an emergency.
- *Ocular massage*: Apply direct pressure over the eye digitally or with a fundus contact lens. The embolus can lodge down, giving a better perfusion to the retina.
- *Anterior chamber paracentesis*: Intraocular pressure (IOP) is checked before the procedure. Topical anesthesia and a topical antibiotic are given to the patient. After withdrawing 0.1 to 0.2 mL of aqueous from the anterior chamber the IOP is rechecked. The procedure is repeated until the patient's IOP is not less than 10 mm Hg.
- *Acetamide*: 500 mg intravenous
- *Topical drugs*: To lower IOP
- *Carbogen therapy (5% CO_2 with 95% O_2)*: Carbon dioxide dilates the retinal arterioles. Oxygen increases the viability of the ischemic tissues. It is given for 10 minutes every 2 hours for 48 hours.
- *Hyperbaric oxygen*: Most useful if started within 2 hours of the episode; 100% oxygen at 2 atmospheric absolute provides an arterial PO_2 of 1000 to 1200 mm Hg resulting in a threefold increase in the oxygen supply to the ischemic tissues. Studies show a two-line improvement in 40% of the patients subjected to hyperbaric oxygen.
- *Intraarterial fibrinolysis*: Tissue plasminogen activator is preferred.

Approximately 20% of patients present with new vessels of iris within a period of 4 to 5 weeks. To prevent this complication the patient has to be reviewed every 2 weeks after the episode. If any evidence of development of new vessels elsewhere or new vessels at the disk is noted, PRP is done to prevent neovascular glaucoma.

◆ Ocular Ischemic Syndromes

This chronic vascular insufficiency occurs secondary to atherosclerotic disease of the internal or common carotid artery. Giant cell arteritis leads to a state of hypoxia to the ocular structures, which causes neovascularization and other symptoms (**Fig. 9.5**).

◆ Presentation

Patients present largely in their fifties and sixties with transient obscuration of vision (amaurosis fugax) or with gradual or abrupt loss of vision and ocular pain. Anterior segment examination shows signs of congestion, anterior uveitis, iris new vessels, and cataract. Posterior segment examination shows narrowing of the retinal arteries, dilated retinal veins, dot and blot hemorrhage, cotton-wool spots, and optic nerve or retinal new vessels.

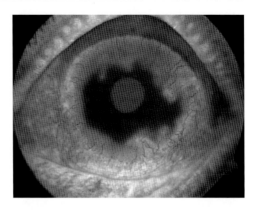

Fig. 9.5 Anterior segment neovascularization in ocular ischemic syndrome seen on anterior segment fluorescein angiography.

◆ **Differential Diagnosis**

CRVO, diabetic retinopathy, panuveitis, and vasculitis

◆ **Management**

Cardiac workup, ESR, and C-reactive protein (CRP) to exclude giant cell arteritis, FFA, and ophthalmodynamometry

◆ Macroaneurysm

Macroaneurysm is an acquired saccular dilatation of the large arterioles of the retina due to weakening of the arteriolar wall seen commonly in women aged 60 to 70 years. Hypertension, arteriosclerosis, and serum lipid abnormalities are the common causes. Other causes are radiation retinopathy, venous occlusive disease, sickle cell, and diabetes.

◆ **Presentation**

Patients present with an asymptomatic, sudden, painless decrease in vision due to vitreous hemorrhage, retinal hemorrhage, or lipid exudates into the macula. The fundus shows aneurysmal dilation of retinal arterioles, circinate exudates, hemorrhage, macular edema, and serous retinal detachment.

◆ **Differential Diagnosis**

Age-related macular degeneration (ARMD), parafoveal telangiectasis, diabetic maculopathy, retinal capillary hemangioma, BRVO

◆ Management

Evaluate cardiovascular disease, control hypertension, lower serum lipids. Fundus fluorescein angiographic evaluation must be done. Spontaneous resolution following thrombosis is the natural course. Lipid exudates and hemorrhage threatening the fovea may be treated with argon laser or yellow-dye laser applied around the aneurysm. Complications include hemorrhage and occlusion of the arteriole.

◆ Vitreous Hemorrhage

Vitreous hemorrhage (VH) is the extravasation of blood from the retinal vessels or new vessels into the vitreous cavity. Causes include diabetic retinopathy, posterior vitreous detachment (PVD) with or without a retinal break, hypertension, retinal vein occlusion, exudative age-related macular degeneration (ARMD), proliferative sickle cell retinopathy, trauma, intraocular tumor, and Eales disease.

◆ Presentation

Patients experience a sudden painless loss of vision, floaters, and cobwebs. Dense VH may reduce the visual acuity to the perception of light. On examination, there is no fundus view with absent red reflex. Chronic vitreous hemorrhage has a chicken-fat appearance owing to organized blood.

◆ Differential Diagnosis

Other causes of sudden loss of visual acuity

◆ Management

Ultrasonography is done when the view of the fundus is obstructed by VH. History and physical examination are important, as well as examination of the other eye. If systemically feasible, anticoagulants and other antiplatelet agents may need to be stopped. Treatment includes limiting physical activity, bilateral patching, and sleeping in an upright position. Partial clearance of the VH with some return of vision may occur over a few months. Pars plana vitrectomy may be required if spontaneous clearing doesn't occur.

◆ Angioid Streaks

Angioid streaks represent dehiscences in the Bruch membrane and appear as dark red bands of irregular contour that radiate from the optic nerve head. Angioid streaks are associated with *Pseudoxanthoma elasticum* (Grönblad-Strandberg syndrome), osteitis deformans (Paget disease), sickle cell anemia, hypertensive cardiovascular disorders, and Ehlers-Danlos syndrome (**Fig. 9.6A,B**).

◆ Presentation

The patient is asymptomatic. Studies report that choroid neovascularization membrane (CNV) occurs in 42 to 86% of patients during follow-up, with most eyes

Fig. 9.6 **(A)** Angioid streaks—color fundus photo. **(B)** Angioid streaks—fundus fluorescein angiography.

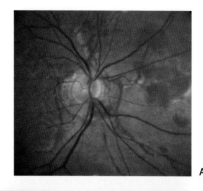

A

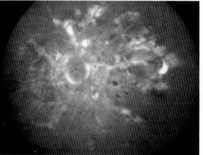

B

progressing to legal blindness. *Pseudoxanthoma elasticum* is associated with peau d'orange and mottled background fundus appearance. Focal midperipheral fine exudates and optic nerve head drusen are also associated. Loose skinfolds and plaquelike lesions can be seen in the neck (chicken skin appearance), and on the flexor aspects of the joints.

◆ **Differential Diagnosis**

Myopic lacquer cracks, choroidal rupture

◆ **Management**

FFA is very helpful in delineating angioid streaks. Fluorescein angiography (FA) reveals early hyperfluorescence due to transmission defects through atrophic RPE present next to the streak. Late-phase FFA shows leakage at the margin of angioid streaks from adjacent choriocapillaries and deep choroidal vessels. Any evidence of choroidal neovascular membrane is also picked on FFA. Indocyanine green angiography is superior to fundus fluorscein in diagnosing the details of a choroidal neovascular membrane. Laser photocoagulation for juxtafoveal and parafoveal lesions and photodynamic theory (with intravitreal triamcinolone acetonide) for subfoveal CNVM have been recommended.

Skin biopsy and cardiological workup for suspected *Pseudoxanthoma elasticum*, serum alkaline phosphatase, and calcium levels for suspected Paget disease and hemoglobin electrophoresis for suspected sickle cell anemia are recommended.

◆ Degenerative Myopia

Progressive myopia of more than –6D or eyes with an axial length greater than 26 mm have structural alterations of the globe resulting in axial lengthening, especially in the posterior pole, leading to stretching of the retina, thinning of the sclera, choroidal degeneration, and potential loss of vision.

◆ Presentation

Decreased best-corrected visual acuity and progressive change in power are seen, usually beyond the fifth decade. Posterior segment findings include vitreous liquefaction, myopic crescent, tilted disk, posterior staphyloma, RPE abnormalities, patchy choroidal atrophy, Fuchs spot (dark area caused by CNV), lattice degeneration in the periphery, and lacquer cracks. Risk for rhegmatogenous retinal detachment is increased, especially with concurrent lattice degeneration (**Fig. 9.7**).

Ocular associations include cataract, primary open-angle glaucoma, pigmentary glaucoma, and retinopathy of prematurity. Systemic associations include Marfan syndrome, Ehlers-Danlos syndrome, and Stickler syndrome.

◆ Differential Diagnosis

Ocular histoplasmosis, gyrate atrophy, congenital staphyloma, age-related choroidal atrophy, ARMD, and angioid streaks

◆ Management

No treatment will regress the progression of staphyloma. Annual to biannual careful examination of the fundus is recommended. Symptomatic retinal breaks should be treated with laser photocoagulation, cryotherapy, or scleral-buckling surgery.

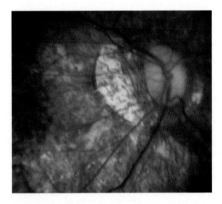

Fig. 9.7   High myopia with chorioretinal degeneration and parapapillary atrophy.

◆ Central Serous Chorioretinopathy

Central serous chorioretinopathy (CSCR) is a localized serous detachment of the neurosensory retina overlying an area of leakage from the choriocapillaris through the RPE. Leaks may be single or double or may be multiple in diffuse RPE dysfunction. Recurrence of 40 to 50% is noted, with 5% of patients developing a choroidal neovascularization or progressive RPE atrophy. It is common in Hispanics and Asian men between 20 and 55 years of age. Type A personalities, patients on exogenous steroids, Cushing syndrome, systemic hypertension, systemic lupus erythematosus, pregnancy, gastroesophageal reflux disease, use of sildenafil citrate, and use of psychopharmacological medications are some precipitating factors for CSCR (**Fig. 9.8A,B**).

◆ Presentation

The patient commonly presents with symptoms of vision loss, micropsia, metamorphopsia, and positive scotoma. Visual acuity ranges from 20/20 to 20/80. The patient usually has a small hyperopic correction with abnormal photo stress test, loss of color saturation, and loss of contrast sensitivity. Clinically CSCR can be associated with pigment epithelial detachments, RPE mottling and atrophy, subretinal fibrin, subretinal lipid, or lipofuscinoid flecks.

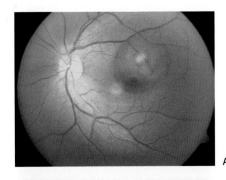

A

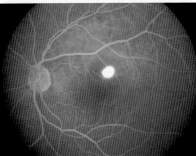

Fig. 9.8 **(A)** Central serous retinopathy—color fundus photo. **(B)** Central serous retinopathy—fundus fluorescein angiography.

B

◆ Differential Diagnosis

Macular hole, different causes of CNV, ARMD, choroidal tumors and metastasis, CME, and retinal detachment

◆ Management

The Amsler grid shows distorted lines or closely crowded lines. FFA demonstrates the site of the leak in a typical smokestack pattern. OCT shows a hyporeflective fluid accumulation between the neurosensory retina and the RPE layer. A deposition of lipofuscin may be associated with CSCR, confusing it with vitelliform dystrophy. OCT confirms the diagnosis by demonstrating the lipofuscin deposited below RPE. ICG angiography may help in some cases. ERG shows a deficit in both eyes in a patient with unilateral CSCR pointing toward a systemic pathology.

Prognosis is generally good, with 85% of the patients gaining back 20/20 vision in 6 to 8 weeks. Laser photocoagulation of the leaking area shortens the disease course. It is done only when the leak is noted 300 μm from the center of the fovea and when the disease process threatens to be chronic. Laser is an option in cases where there is a persistent fluid level for more than 4 months, recurrence in an eye with visual deficit in the other eye, presence of visual deficits in the opposite eye from previous episodes of CSCR, and occupational need requiring prompt recovery of vision.

Plasminogen activator inhibitor 1 has been found to have association with CSCR. Carvalho-Recchia et al and Haimovici et al have derived a significant relationship between patients on exogenous steroids and CSCR. ICG angiography repeatedly demonstrates both multifocal choroidal hyperpermeability and hypofluorescent areas suggestive of focal choroidal vascular compromise in a patient with CSCR. Recently PDT has been used to treat such areas of hyperpermeability in a case with CSCR.

◆ Cystoid Macular Edema

CME is the accumulation of fluid (edema) in the intracellular spaces of outer plexiform and inner nuclear layers of the retina, causing Müller cell degeneration with intracellular vacuolation. CME with a postcataract surgery cause is called Irvine-Gass syndrome. It is the most common type. Other causes can be uveitis, diabetic maculopathy, AMD, retinal vein occlusion, retinitis pigmentosa (RP), vitreomacular traction syndrome, topical epinephrine, CNV, retinal vasculitis, retinal telangiectasias, intraocular tumors, nicotinic acid, and juvenile retinoschisis.

There are many hypotheses to describe the mechanism leading to CME; however, the most acceptable is the one involving intraocular inflammation, which occurs when CME complicates uveitis or traction/distortion of the iris. Inflammatory mediators generated from the arachidonic acid metabolism, such as the prostaglandins and leukotrienes, have been implicated in the pathogenesis (**Fig. 9.9A,B**).

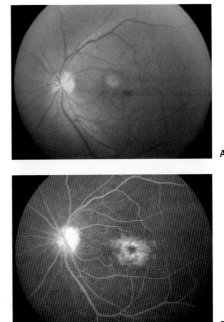

Fig. 9.9 (A) Postoperative cystoid macular edema—color fundus photo. **(B)** Postoperative cystoid macular edema—fundus fluoresein angiography.

◆ **Presentation**

Patient presents with gradual loss of vision or metamorphopsia and a history of a certain precipitating factor. Biomicroscopy reveals characteristic cystic intercellular spaces in the macular region with diminished foveal light reflex and associated foveal thickening. Evidence of intraocular inflammation like ciliary flush, vitreous cells, nerve fiber layer edema, or papilloedema may be present.

In Irvine-Gass syndrome, signs of complicated cataract surgery may be present, such as vitreous traction, vitreous loss, polymerase chain reaction, exchange of intraocular lens (IOL), secondary IOL, old age, post–penetrating keratoplasty, post–YAG capsulotomy, topical epinephrine, or latanoprost.

◆ **Differential Diagnosis**

Retinal telangiectasias, juvenile retinoschisis, phototoxic injury, Berlin edema, CNV, and foveal cysts

◆ **Management**

FFA shows an early and midphase leak from the choriocapillaries surrounding fovea. In the late phase a typical petaloid or spoke-wheel pattern of pooling of dye is evident. An associated condition can also be picked up in FFA. OCT reveals the cystic spaces present in the layers of retina. It can also be used as a monitoring device because it can maintain a serial foveal thickness record of a patient.

Spontaneous resolution occurs in 75% of postcataract patients within a span of 6 weeks. Corticosteroids help by inhibiting the enzyme phospholipase and thus controlling the inflammation in postuveitic causes. It can be administered by all routes, such as topical, oral, posterior subtenon, and intravitreal. Nonsteroidal antiinflammatory drugs (NSAIDs) inhibit the enzyme cyclooxygenase and can also be used in the prevention of CME. NSAIDs, especially ketorolac and flurbiprofen, can be administered topically for 3 to 4 months. Carbonic anhydrase inhibitors such as acetamide are helpful in controlling CME in patients of RP. Prolonged CME due to BRVO responds well to laser photocoagulation.

The role of pars plana vitrectomy is indicated in CME related to uveitis. It is helpful in removing vitreous strands, inflammatory mediators, retained lens fragments, and malpositioned IOLs as well as for greater penetration of topical and oral corticosteroids and suppressing the antigen-specific immune response. Therapies such as antimetabolites, cyclodiathermy, cryotherapy, and photocoagulation have been tried with limited success. The advent of new modes of steroid delivery such as posterior subtenon depot and intravitreal injection of steroids are better options available. Various studies (e.g., Italian diclofenac study group) have reported the superiority of ketorolac over other topical agents in treating CME.

◆ Age-Related Macular Degeneration

Exudative Age-Related Macular Degeneration

In 1995, the International ARM Epidemiologic Study Group redefined age-related macular degeneration (ARMD). Patients with minimal to moderate nonexudative age-related changes at the macula were classified as age-related maculopathy (ARM). Advanced atrophy or the presence of CNV membranes was classified as ARMD. The condition is seen more commonly in women than in men and is diagnosed in individuals over the age of 50. The use of tobacco, obesity, and genetic factors are believed to be strongly associated with the condition (**Fig. 9.10A,B,C,D**).

◆ Presentation

The patient usually presents with a gradual, painless loss of vision associated with delayed dark adaptation, severe metamorphopsia, and field loss. Vision loss is more rapid in exudative ARMD. A sudden loss of vision can be associated with subretinal hemorrhage or pigment epithelium detachment. The Amsler grid and frequent slit-lamp biomicroscopy are the best ways to monitor the condition (**Fig. 9.10E,F,G,H**).

◆ Differential Diagnosis

Nonexudative ARMD, angioid streaks, choroidal rupture, and other causes leading to CNV membrane

◆ Management

◆ FFA is an important tool in diagnosis and classification (subfoveal, juxtafoveal, and extrafoveal) of CNV. ICG angiography provides a more specific diagnosis by pinpointing the feeder vessel in the choroidal vasculature. OCT is used as a tool to follow up after photodynamic therapy (PDT).

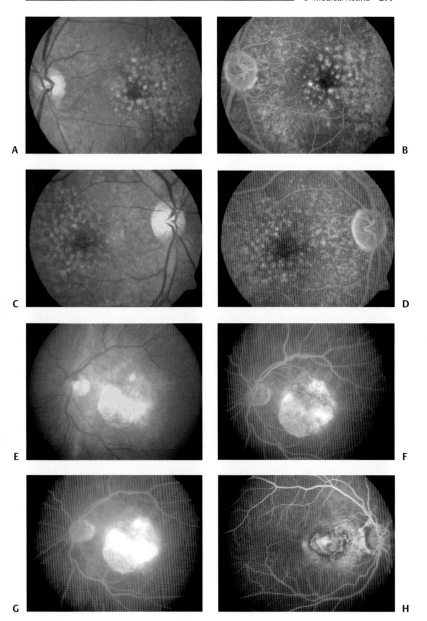

Fig. 9.10 **(A)** Dry age-related macular degeneration (ARMD)—color fundus photo. **(B)** Dry ARMD—FFA late phase. **(C)** Dry ARMD, same patient, other eye—color fundus photo. **(D)** Dry ARMD, same patient, other eye—FFA late phase. **(E)** Wet ARMD—CNVM—color fundus photo. **(F)** Wet ARMD—CNVM—midphase FFA. **(G)** Wet ARMD—CNVM—late phase FFA. **(H)** Wet ARMD, same patient, other eye—venous phase FFA.

◆ Thermal laser photocoagulation and feeder vessel photocoagulation can be used to treat all kinds of CNV membranes.

◆ Transpupillary thermotherapy forms a treatment modality for occult CNV membranes.

◆ PDT using photosensitizers (verteporfin, rostaporfin, motexafin lutetium, talaporfin sodium, ATX-S10) is widely used to treat classic CNV. Target-receptor PDT and combination PDT have also been tried.

◆ Antiangiogenic agents such as vascular endothelial growth factor (VEGF) inhibitors (pegaptanib sodium, ranibizumab, bevacizumab, VEGF trap) form the latest adjuvant in the treatment of CNV membranes.

◆ Steroids like triamcinolone acetonide, anecortave acetate, and implantable corticosteroids have also been tried.

◆ Small interfering RNA therapy, pigment epithelium–derived factor inducer, and microstructure modulation are some of the treatment modalities under trial.

◆ Submacular surgeries, macular translocation, and RPE transplantation are the surgical options at various stages of development.

◆ Stargardt Disease and Fundus Flavimaculatus

Atrophic macular dystrophy with flecks (i.e., Stargardt disease) is the most common type of juvenile macular degeneration. Fundus flavimaculatus (FF) is a variant of Stargardt disease with a significant difference in clinical presentation and prognosis. Almost all cases are determined as autosomal recessive in the pedigree chart. Rarely, cases have been identified as autosomal dominant. The gene locus lies on ABC4R on *1p21–22*. FF is also an autosomal recessive disease.

◆ Presentation

There is considerable confusion related to the terms *Stargardt disease* and *fundus flavimaculatus*. FF was first described as a flecked fundus with yellow-white irregular lesions that extended to the equator. Stargardt disease occurred as flecks in the posterior pole early in life with a progressive macular dystrophy. It is now believed that these two conditions are two different allelic manifestations of the same disease.

The symptoms are mainly bilateral, presenting in the age group from 6 to 20 years. There is associated color vision defect and photophobia. Disappearance of the foveal reflex forms the first sign on ophthalmoscopy. Later, a granular mottling of the macula appears. An oval "snail-slime" or "beaten bronze" appearance of the fovea is the hallmark of Stargardt disease. The flecks may extend to the midperiphery and may give a salt-and-pepper appearance in the region. The disk and vessels are generally normal. FF is usually diagnosed incidentally. The patient can experience a reduced central visual acuity and metamorphopsia in longstanding cases. FF is a bilateral disorder with ill-defined yellowish white flecks ("fishtail-like") extending from the posterior pole to the midperiphery. The fundus has a vermilion tinge in most cases (**Fig. 9.11A,B**).

Fig. 9.11 (A) Stargardt disease fundus flavimaculatus—color fundus photo. **(B)** Stargardt disease fundus flavimaculatus—fundus fluorescein angiography showing early hyperfluorescence.

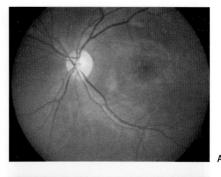

A

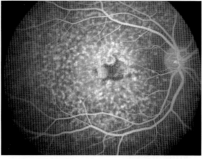

B

◆ **Differential Diagnosis**

Fundus albipunctatus, retinitis puncta albescens, familial drusen, pattern dystrophy, RP inversus, ARMD, histospots

◆ **Management**

FFA shows the most characteristic feature called silent choroid. The evidence of flecks over the contrasting dark choroid with a normal macula is a trademark angiographic appearance of FF. ERG shows a variable photopic response and normal scotopic response. Electro-olfactogram (EOG) is subnormal. Deuteran and tritan defects are present. Prognosis is poor; however, visual acuity usually stabilizes at 6/60.

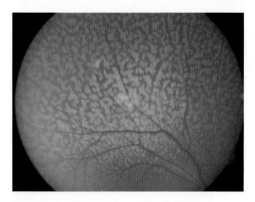

Fig. 9.12 Flecked retina.

◆ Fundus Albipunctatus

Fundus albipunctatus is congenital stationary night blindness with autosomal recessive pattern.

◆ Presentation

Patients may be asymptomatic or have night blindness, usually starting in infancy. Numerous white-yellow dotlike lesions occur in the midperipheral fundus at the level of the RPE (**Fig. 9.12**).

◆ Differential Diagnosis

Retinitis punctate albescence (progressive, behaves like RP), birdshot chorioretinitis, Stargardt disease, familial drusen, Bietti crystalline retinopathy, pattern dystrophy, RP inversus, macular degeneration, pseudoexfoliation, crystalline retinopathy, histospots

◆ Management

ERG shows a prolonged time for dark adaptation to produce normal amplitude due to the delay in regeneration of rhodopsin. Vision and fields remain normal.

◆ Best Disease: Vitelliform Macular Dystrophy

Best disease is an autosomal dominant (variable penetrance) degenerative maculopathy wherein a mutation in the bestrophin gene leads to lipofuscin accumulation in RPE cells.

◆ **Presentation**

Patients may be asymptomatic in childhood and progress to a decrease in vision later in life. Fundus examination shows a large, yellow, yolklike (vitelliform), bilateral, symmetrical macular lesion (pseudohypopyon). Vision may be better than the fundus appearance. The yellow "yolk" eventually breaks down, leaving a mottled geographical atrophy and scarring (scrambled egg appearance). Vision deteriorates in this stage. Choroidal new vessels may be present.

◆ **Differential Diagnosis**

The late scar stage is difficult to distinguish from macular dystrophy or degeneration.

◆ **Management**

The EOG is diminished, whereas the ERG is normal. There is no known treatment. Cases should be followed with an Amsler grid for early detection of CNV.

◆ Pattern Dystrophy

This is an autosomal dominant dystrophy of the RPE due to mutation in the periherin gene, which presents in midlife.

◆ **Presentation**

Visual acuity may be normal or mildly decreased (~20/30), with normal color vision and mild metamorphopsia. Other presenting symptoms include symmetric bilateral hyperpigmentation of the RPE in the macula, butterfly dystrophy, and adult-onset foveomacular vitelliform dystrophy.

◆ **Differential Diagnosis**

Drug-induced degenerations, angioid streaks, rubella retinopathy, myotonic dystrophy

◆ **Management**

The prognosis is good. EOG is subnormal. Fluorescein angiography shows a blocking pattern of the RPE hyperpigmentation. CNV and geographical macular atrophy are the complications. No treatment is known.

◆ Cone Dystrophies

Goodman et al classified various cone dystrophies into seven cone dysfunction syndromes. Sporadic cases are most common among the various patterns of inheritance seen in cone dystrophies. Autosomal dominant is the most commonly established pattern and carries a very grave prognosis. The condition may also present as autosomal recessive and be X-linked.

◆ **Presentation**

The symptoms are exactly the reverse of RP and appear generally in the third decade. The patient most commonly presents with loss of vision and photophobia. The patient sees better in evening hours and prefers to wear dark glasses. Color vision is a problem beginning in the early stages of the condition. Nystagmus can be seen in the advanced stage. The early stage of the disease is marked by a normal fundus or a granular appearance of the macula. Late stages classically resemble a bull's-eye maculopathy. Few signs may be congruent with RP, that is, the presence of bony spicules in the midperiphery, vascular attenuation, and temporal disk pallor. A tapetal-like sheen is noted around the parafoveal region in a colored photograph. Advanced disease is characterized by the typical presence of RPE atrophy, which later develops into a geographical atrophy.

◆ **Differential Diagnosis**

Drug-induced retinopathy, angioid streaks, rubella retinopathy, and myotonic retinopathy

◆ **Management**

FFA findings depend on the stage of the disease and its severity. A transmission defect involving fovea is another presentation similar to bull's-eye maculopathy. Fundus findings may also mimic those of Stargardt disease or FF in the advanced stages of the disease. Photopic response is subnormal or almost unrecordable. Severe deuteron–tritan defects are noted. EOG and dark adaptation are not reliable. Prognosis depends on the extent of rod involvement and mode of inheritance. No treatment is known.

◆ Idiopathic Parafoveal Telangiectasia

In idiopathic parafoveal telangiectasia there is clinically apparent retinal telangiectasia and ectasia of the capillary bed, confined to the juxtafoveal region of one or both eyes. This may result in visual loss from capillary incompetence and exudation. Histopathologic evidence shows this is not a true telangiectasia but rather consists of structural abnormalities similar to diabetic microangiopathy, with deposits of excess basement membrane within the retinal capillaries (**Fig. 9.13A,B**).

◆ **Presentation**

Onset is usually in the fifth to sixth decade. Patients present with mild blurring of central visual acuity.

◆ *Group I*: Unilateral, congenital parafoveal telangiectasia with vascular abnormalities localized to the temporal half of the macula, leading to circinate exudates
◆ *Group II*: Bilateral acquired idiopathic telangiectasia
◆ *Group III*: Bilateral idiopathic parafoveal telangiectasia with retinal capillary obliteration On FFA, leakage is seen from the telangiectatic vessels.

Fig. 9.13 **(A)** Parafoveal telangiectasia leakage—color fundus photo. **(B)** Parafoveal telangiectasia—fundus fluorescein angiography donut-shaped leakage.

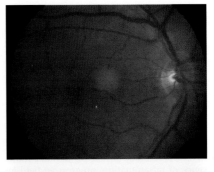

A

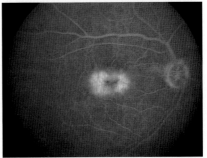

B

◆ **Differential Diagnosis**

Diabetic macular edema, macular edema from other causes, CNV

◆ **Management**

Generally, only observation is required. Laser photocoagulation and intravitreal bevacizumab/ranibizumab have been tried.

◆ Sickle Cell Retinopathy

This hereditary, genetically determined, hemolytic anemia occurs almost exclusively in blacks. HbSS (i.e., sickle cell disease) occurs exclusively in males.

◆ **Presentation**

Ophthalmic manifestations include intravascular occlusions on the surface of the optic disk; retinal artery occlusions; chronic macular changes (sickling maculopathy); choroidal vascular occlusions; nonproliferative sickle retinopathy including venous tortuosity, salmon-patch hemorrhage, schisis cavity, and the black sunburst and proliferative sickle retinopathy with peripheral arteriolar occlusions; arteriolar-venular anastomosis; neovascular proliferation; vitreous hemorrhage; and retinal detachment.

◆ Management

Diathermy, cryotherapy, xenon arc photocoagulation, and argon laser photocoagulation can be tried to treat the proliferative sickle retinopathy. Vitrectomy is indicated in conditions such as nonresolving vitreous hemorrhage and traction or combined retinal detachments.

◆ Retinitis Pigmentosa

RP is a hereditary diffuse pigmentary retinal dystrophy characterized by the absence of inflammation, progressive field losses, and abnormal ERG. RP involves photoreceptors, mainly the rods. Sporadic cases are by far the most common (**Fig. 9.14A,B**).

◆ Presentation

Presentation is always bilateral. Patients present mainly with nyctalopia and a gradual and progressive loss of visual fields. Loss of central vision and metamorphopsia are an indication of associated macular involvement. A few patients also experience episodic light flashes. The classical triad to diagnose RP is arteriolar attenuation, bony spicule–like pigmentation, and waxy pallor of the optic disk.

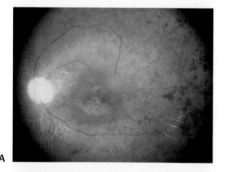

A

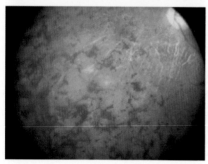

B

Fig. 9.14 **(A)** Retinitis pigmentosa with maculopathy. **(B)** Retinitis pigmentosa—peripheral fundus shows bone spicule pigment hyperplasia.

RP can present atypically as sector RP, pericentral RP, and RP with exudative vasculopathy. RP is associated with posterior subcapsular cataract, open-angle glaucoma, myopia, keratoconus, posterior vitreous detachment, and optic nerve head drusen. Systemic associations of RP are as Bassen-Kornzweig syndrome, Refsum disease, Usher syndrome, Kearns-Sayre syndrome, and Bardet-Biedl syndrome.

◆ Differential Diagnosis

Choroidal dystrophies, vitamin A deficiency, congenital stationary night blindness, phenothiazine toxicity, syphilis, congenital rubella, exudative retinal detachment, myotonic dystrophy.

◆ Management

FFA indicates the associated choroidal sclerosis and indicates the prognosis. A defective dark adaptation, EOG, and scotopic response on ERG are seen. Color vision is normal and perimetry shows circumferential progressive field loss. General ophthalmic care (i.e., refractive status of patient) should be given. Associations such as cataract, glaucoma macular edema, and epiretinal membranes should be managed on respective lines. Psychological counseling, genetic counseling, low vision aid, and vitamin and nutritional supplementation play important roles. Recently, retinal chip device, stem cells, and gene therapy have been tried.

◆ Choroideremia

Choroideremia is a group of X-linked recessive disorders in which there is a mutation in the long arm of chromosome X (*Xq-21.2*; CHM). This focus involves mutation of the CHM gene, which encodes for a protein geranylgeranyl transferase *Rab* escort.

◆ Presentation

The features of the disease are night blindness, constriction of visual field, and ring scotoma, with severe visual loss occurring at later stages of life. The fundus shows patches of choroidal and retinal pigmentary atrophy. The involvement is at the level of choriocapillaries with involvement of large and intermediate choroidal vessels in the late stages when there is a clear visibility of sclera. A subnormal EOG and severely abnormal photopic ERG are characteristic findings.

◆ Differential Diagnosis

RP, gyrate atrophy, albinism

◆ Management

The choroidal phase of the FFA is characterized by clear visualization of the filling of medium- and large-caliber choroidal vessels. This picture presents due to complete absence of the RPE and an associated absence of choriocapillaries under it. There is no known treatment. Genetic counseling helps.

◆ Gyrate Atrophy

This is an autosomal recessive disorder with involvement of chromosome 10 and involves the mutation of gene coding for the enzyme ornithine ketoacid aminotransferase, which is required for ornithine degradation. There are elevated levels of ornithine in the body fluids (i.e., plasma, urine, cerebrospinal fluid, and aqueous humor).

◆ Presentation

The main clinical findings are night blindness associated with axial myopia and astigmatism. Fundus examination shows lobular chorioretinal degeneration in the region behind the equator with vitreous degeneration. These later progress to geographic atrophy with foveal involvement. In advanced stage of the disease, the lesions convalesce to form wider defects and extend in both anterior and posterior directions. Flat ERG in the later stages with subnormal EOG is seen.

◆ Differential Diagnosis

Paving-stone degeneration, choroideremia, high myope

◆ Management

FFA in early stage of the disease is characterized by sharply demarcated multiple, circular window defects, separated by strips of normal retina involving the mid-periphery. The late phase is characterized by fading fluorescence of the choroidal vessels and mild staining of the normal retina forming the margin of the lesions. Treatment involves reduction of ornithine in the diet with vitamin B_6 in high doses. First symptoms are seen in the first or second decade. Visual acuity becomes very poor by the sixth decade of life with involvement of the macula.

◆ Radiation Retinopathy

Irradiation to the head in a total dose exceeding 3000 rads may lead to radiation retinopathy. It may follow plaque therapy, brachytherapy, or external-beam irradiation. Patients with preexisting compromised vasculature such as those with diabetes, hypertension, or collagen vascular disease may develop it at even low doses of radiation.

◆ Presentation

Patients may be asymptomatic or have visual loss delayed 6 months to a year after therapy. Discrete foci of occluded capillaries; irregular dilatation of neighboring microvasculature and vascular sheathing are seen at the posterior fundus along with cotton-wool spots, microaneurysms, neovascularization, exudates, and macular edema. Disk edema may also be seen.

◆ Differential Diagnosis

Diabetic retinopathy, hypertensive retinopathy, Eales disease, Coats disease, sickle cell retinopathy

◆ Management

Macular edema and neovascularization may be treated with laser photocoagulation. Systemic steroids are given for papillopathy.

◆ Solar Retinopathy

Foveomacular retinitis, eclipse retinopathy, solar retinitis, following direct/indirect viewing of the solar eclipse. Secondary to RPE damage caused by shorter wavelengths of ultraviolet-A light.

◆ Presentation

Symptoms appear after 1 to 4 hours of sungazing and include unilateral or bilateral decrease in visual acuity, metamorphopsia, central/paracentral scotoma, and after-image. Yellow-white foveolar lesions that are replaced with a red foveolar depression are seen surrounded by a pigmented halo. Vision improves in 3 to 6 months (usually to > 20/40), but metamorphopsia and scotoma may remain.

◆ Differential Diagnosis

Blunt ocular trauma, RP

◆ Management

There is no treatment. The patient is followed up.

10 Surgical Retina

Clement K. Chan and Dariusz G. Tarasewicz

◆ **Developmental Anomalies and Degenerations**

Cystoid Degeneration

Reticular Cystoid Degeneration

Reticular cystoid degeneration is a type of peripheral retinal cystoid degeneration that highly correlates with age. It occurs in approximately 18% of adult patients and can be bilateral more than 40% of the time. It is not as common as typical cystoid degeneration. It can be radially oriented and often follows the course of retinal vessels. Frequently, it is found posterior to typical cystoid degeneration.

◆ **Presentation**

It is asymptomatic. A stippled appearance to the inner retinal surface is common. Reticular cystoid degeneration is typically found in the inferior temporal quadrant.

◆ **Differential Diagnosis**

Other peripheral retinal degenerations

◆ **Management**

Thorough ophthalmoscopic examination is required. Management consists of observation only.

Typical Cystoid Degeneration

Typical cystoid degeneration is the most common peripheral retinal degeneration. Spaces form in the outer plexiform and inner nuclear layer and coalesce to form tunnels. Where tunnels have not formed, retinal "pillars" remain. These findings occur as early as age 1. It is found in almost all eyes examined. Typical cystoid degeneration is more common in the superior and temporal quadrants.

◆ **Presentation**

No symptoms are notable. The inner retinal surface acquires a stippled appearance. Pillars cause depressions on the surface, whereas domelike areas represent cystoid spaces. The degeneration always begins at the ora serrata and spreads posteriorly.

◆ **Differential Diagnosis**

Other peripheral retinal degenerations

◆ **Management**

Thorough ophthalmoscopic examination is required. Management consists of observation only.

Meridional Folds, Complexes, and Other Peripheral Lesions

A meridional fold is a redundancy of the peripheral retina at the border of the ora serrata. It is most commonly found in the supranasal quadrant and is bilateral for 55% of the cases. Its length can be variable. It has been estimated that 26% of the population has meridional folds.

When a meridional fold is contiguous with a dentate process, it is called a meridional complex. A meridional complex can extend to the pars plana (**Fig. 10.1A**).

An enclosed oral bay (EOB) is a small island of nonpigmented ciliary body epithelium that has become isolated and surrounded by neurosensory retina. Clinically, it may resemble a retinal break (**Fig. 10.1B**).

◆ **Presentation**

Both the meridional folds and the EOB are incidental findings in normal eyes and are usually not associated with any symptoms. The location of meridional folds may aid their diagnosis. They are always close to the ora serrata. They are almost never associated with retinal breaks.

◆ **Differential Diagnosis**

A retinal break is a differential diagnosis for EOB. Scleral indentation shows gradually sloping edges unlike the sharp and abrupt change in retinal breaks. Also the color in the oral bay corresponds to the adjacent pars plana.

◆ **Management**

Careful ophthalmoscopy will differentiate EOB from true retinal breaks. The color within the EOB is the same as the pars plana. A meridional fold is frequently located in the same meridian as an EOB. Unlike retinal breaks, these lesions do not progress rapidly over time. There is no role for prophylactic treatment.

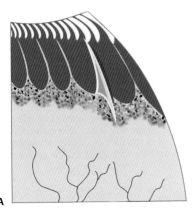 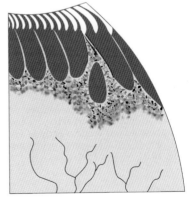

A   B

Fig. 10.1 **(A)** Meridional fold complex. **(B)** Enclosed oral bay.

Pars Plana Cyst

Pars plana cysts are convex, cystoid lesions found anterior to the ora serrata. They are often adjacent to oral bays and can be multiple. The exact etiology is unknown, but they are probably the result of a degenerative process. Microscopically they represent a separation of the nonpigmented from the pigmented epithelial cell layers of the pars plana.

◆ Presentation

Pars plana cysts are asymptomatic. An autopsy series found their presence in 16 to 18% of cases. They are more frequently found on the temporal side. There is no association with other eye diseases.

◆ Differential diagnosis

None

◆ Management

Thorough ophthalmoscopic examination reveals the cyst. No treatment is indicated.

Pars Plana Pearls

Pars plana pearls are striking, glistening white lesions found in the far anterior retinal periphery. They are always beneath a dentate process and represent drusen-like deposits on the inner surface of the Bruch membrane.

◆ Presentation

Pars plana pearls serve as good landmarks in the far peripheral retina. They are always located beneath a dentate process. They are drusen-like structures on the Bruch membrane.

◆ Differential Diagnosis

Other peripheral retinal degenerations

◆ Management

Pars plana pearls have been found in 20% of autopsy subjects and appear in all age groups. There are no known associations with other eye pathologies. Thorough ophthalmoscopic examination is required. No treatment is indicated.

Pavingstone Degeneration

Also commonly termed *cobblestone degeneration*, these are discrete foci of outer retinal atrophy that start at the ora and progress posteriorly. It has been estimated that these lesions occur as early as age 8. Histologically they are characterized by loss of rods, retinal pigment epithelium (RPE), and the underlying choriocapillaris (**Fig. 10.2**).

Fig. 10.2 Pavingstone degeneration.

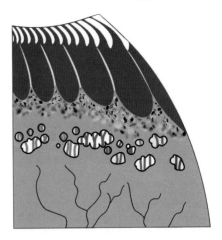

◆ Presentation

In addition to the outer retinal atrophy, these lesions show prominent choroidal
vessels and are easy to see on indirect ophthalmoscopy. They can have a yellowish hue, and pigmented borders are common. These lesions tend to cluster on the
inferior retina.

◆ Differential Diagnosis

Other peripheral retinal degenerations

◆ Management

Thorough ophthalmoscopic examination is required. These lesions are not associated with any symptoms or risk for retinal detachment (RD). Management consists
of observation only; no treatment is indicated.

Senile Tapetochoroidal Degeneration

Tapetochoroidal degeneration represents a pronounced degree of depigmentation
in the peripheral retina. It is caused by a loss of pigment granules in the RPE, usually more pronounced with advancing age.

◆ Presentation

Examination reveals a circumferential band running from the ora serrata to the
equator.

◆ Differential Diagnosis

Other peripheral retinal degenerations

◆ Management

Tapetochoroidal degeneration is found in 20% of patients older than 40 and is bilateral in all cases. Thorough ophthalmoscopic examination is required.

◆ Lattice Degeneration, Retinal Tufts, and Retinoschisis

Lattice Degeneration

Lattice degeneration is a peripheral retinal pathology that carries a moderate risk for a retinal detachment. It has been estimated that lattice degeneration is found in only 6 to 8% of the general population. It is bilateral in up to 48% of nonselected patients. Multiple studies have shown, however, that 20 to 30% of patients with a retinal detachment have lattice degeneration. Lattice degeneration has been associated with multiple names, including snail-track degeneration and retinal and vitreous base excavations, among others. There is a high correlation between lattice degeneration and myopia. No definitive hereditary pattern has been established.

◆ Presentation

A hallmark feature of lattice is its variability in presentation. Classically it is described as a patch of retinal thinning with abnormal overlying vitreous. Vitreous liquefaction over a lattice lesion is common, and vitreoretinal adhesion on its borders is taut and strong. White lines frequently crisscross the retinal surface of lattice degeneration. Peripheral pigmentary changes and white flecks are often found on the posterior surface of the lesion. The white lines correspond to sclerotic vessels, and the flecks are consistent with glial cells.

Progressive thinning of the retinal surface of lattice degeneration leads to formation of atrophic holes. These holes are not associated with vitreous traction. Although mild subretinal fluid may accumulate, asymptomatic atrophic retinal holes associated with lattice degeneration rarely lead to RD.

Lesions of lattice degeneration are usually found between the 11 and 1 o'clock and 5 and 7 o'clock meridians for unknown reasons. The dimensions of lattice patches are highly variable, even within the same eye. Lattice lesions are typically asymptomatic.

◆ Differential Diagnosis

Other peripheral retinal degenerations

◆ Management

Myopia is a well established risk factor for lattice degeneration. Lattice degeneration has been linked to pigment dispersion syndrome, although the reliability of the associated studies has been questioned because of their small sample sizes. Myopia is shared by both conditions, and common etiological factors may contribute to the development of both conditions.

Lattice degeneration is best revealed through careful indirect ophthalmoscopy or peripheral retinal biomicroscopy with scleral depression. Significant debate exists on the treatment of lattice degeneration. The presence of lattice degeneration increases the risk of retinal detachment from 0.01 to 0.5%.

Multiple authors have pointed to the futility of prophylactic treatment of asymptomatic lattice degeneration. Even if atrophic holes are found in a patch of lattice, they rarely result in RD. A retrospective study showed that for eyes with RD, prophylactic treatment of lattice degeneration in the fellow eyes was associated with a risk reduction of RD from 5.9 to 1.8%. Previous studies showed no benefit with prophylactic treatment for eyes with greater than –6 diopters of myopia and myopic eyes with more than 6 clock hours of lattice degeneration.

Close monitoring of asymptomatic lattice lesions is the routine. Prophylactic treatment is reserved for the following situations: symptomatic lattice lesions, signs of prominent vitreoretinal traction, personal or family history of RD.

Retinal Tufts

Cystic Retinal Tufts

These are discrete nodules of glial proliferation that entrap overlying vitreous. Thus the bond between tuft and vitreous is particularly strong. It is considered a congenital variant. Approximately 5% of the population has tufts. Tufts have been found as early as infancy and do not show a particular age predilection.

◆ Presentation

Cystic tufts can be located in all four quadrants. The average diameter is from 0.1 to 1.0 mm. On clinical exam they are usually white and oval in appearance. They are elevated on the retinal surface but not translucent like a retinal break. Because of the tight adhesion between a retinal tuft and the overlying vitreous, a retinal flap tear or an operculated break may develop at the site of the tuft during a posterior vitreous detachment (PVD). Associated symptoms include floaters, flashing lights, "curtain effects," and loss of vision.

◆ Differential Diagnosis

Other peripheral retinal degenerations

◆ Management

Careful indirect ophthalmoscopy or peripheral retinal biomicroscopy with scleral depression. Approximately 10% of RDs are originated from cystic retinal tufts. However, because cystic retinal tufts are found in only 5% of the general population, the overall risk of a retinal detachment from a tuft is calculated to be only 0.28%. Owing to this low incidence, routine prophylactic treatment of asymptomatic tufts is not recommended. If a retinal tear is associated with a tuft, laser or cryotherapy is indicated.

Noncystic Retinal Tufts

These tufts are very thin aggregates of retinal tissue found in clusters at the vitreous base. They are less than 0.1 mm in diameter and consist of processes of Müller cells.

◆ Presentation

Noncystic tufts are found as early as the first decade of life. They are found in 33% of adults and usually on the nasal peripheral retina. There are no symptoms.

◆ Differential Diagnosis

Other peripheral retinal degenerations

◆ Management

Management consists of observation only, with careful indirect ophthalmoscopy or peripheral retinal biomicroscopy with scleral depression.

Zonular Traction Retinal Tuft

Zonular traction tufts (ZTTs) are distinguishable from cystic and noncystic tufts by their greater size, closer location to the ora serrata, and predilection for causing small, full-thickness retinal holes in the far retinal periphery. ZTTs are caused by abnormal zonular connections to the peripheral retina. The result is a taut tuft of tissue pulled anteriorly toward the ciliary body.

◆ Presentation

ZTTs can be further subdivided into juxtabasal or intrabasal tufts. Only intrabasal ZTTs have clinical significance. Retinal tears occur in 4% of all ZTTs. They are the cause for 6% of retinal tears in autopsy eyes. Associated tears are almost always intrabasal (within the vitreous base) lesions. Even when RD occurs, it is localized and nonprogressive. Symptoms occur only if complicated by retinal tears or RD.

◆ Differential Diagnosis

Other peripheral retinal degenerations

◆ Management

ZTTs occur three times more commonly in men and have a prevalence of 15% in autopsy cases. They are also bilateral in 15% of cases and more common in the nasal retina. They are best revealed through careful indirect ophthalmoscopy or peripheral retinal biomicroscopy with scleral depression. Laser or cryotherapy is indicated if there is evidence of a full-thickness retinal break. Prophylactic treatment of ZTTs is not recommended because associated retinal breaks and detachments are usually nonprogressive.

Senile Retinoschisis

Senile retinoschisis is a degenerative process in which the retina splits into two distinct layers at the level of the outer plexiform layer, in contrast to juvenile retinoschisis, in which the retina splits at the nerve fiber layer. Dysfunction of Müller cells likely contributes to the formation of senile retinoschisis. The retinal schisis cavity that forms over time may resemble a retinal detachment. Two forms of schisis have been described: typical degenerative and reticular degenerative.

◆ Presentation

In typical degenerative retinoschisis there are oval areas of retinal splitting and fusiform elevation of the inner retinal layer. The inner layer consists of internal limiting membrane, inner plexiform layer, and retinal vessels. It can have a textured appearance, and white dots can be seen on its surface. The outer layer consists of portions of outer plexiform, outer nuclear, and photoreceptor components. It appears empty and can have a beaten-metal appearance. Retinal breaks are not characteristic for typical degenerative retinoschisis. Posterior extension toward the macula is uncommon.

Reticular degenerative retinoschisis has more extensive retinal involvement. The inner retina can become extremely thin, bullous, and dome-shaped. It consists of only internal limiting membrane, remnants of nerve fiber layer, and residual vessels that appear suspended in mid-air due to the thin retinal appearance. There is complete loss of radial pillars. Typical cystoid degeneration is commonly seen anterior to areas of reticular degenerative retinoschisis. Retinoschisis can be exacerbated by a posterior vitreous detachment. The schisis cavity may enlarge and sometimes progress toward the macula. However, the macula is frequently spared, and the rate of progression is usually very slow.

Outer retinal breaks are more common than inner retinal breaks in reticular degenerative retinoschisis. The appearance of demarcation lines indicates the detachment of the outer retina of a retinoschisis and its eventual conversion to a full-thickness RD. The rate of such a conversion is very slow. The nonprogressive type of detachment occurs much more frequently than the progressive type. However, the formation of inner retinal holes along with the preexisting outer retinal holes may lead to a rapid progression of a full-thickness RD that requires prompt treatment.

Symptoms occur in case of retinal breaks, retinal detachment, or posterior extension toward the macula.

◆ Differential Diagnosis

Other peripheral retinal degenerations

◆ Management

For autopsy eyes, typical degenerative retinoschisis is seen in 1% of the adult population and is bilateral in 33% of cases. Reticular degenerative retinoschisis is seen in 1.6% of adults, and bilateral only 16% of the time. Both lesions are commonly seen in the inferotemporal quadrant.

Management consists of careful indirect ophthalmoscopy or peripheral retinal biomicroscopy with scleral depression.

Routine prophylactic treatment of most retinoschisis is not necessary owing to their usual lack of progression. Their indiscriminate treatment may cause new retinal breaks, retinal detachment, and even proliferative vitreoretinopathy. With signs of progression, treatment may include laser, cryotherapy, scleral buckling, and vitrectomy, depending on the location and extent of the pathology.

◆ Posterior Vitreous Detachment

◆ Presentation

Floaters ("cobwebs," "bugs," "tadpoles," or comma-shaped objects that change position with eye movement), blurred vision, flashes of light, which are more common in dim illumination and are temporally located, are the main complaints of the patient. One or more discrete light gray to black vitreous opacities, often in the shape of a ring (Weiss ring) are suspended over the optic disk. The opacities float within the vitreous as the eye moves from side to side.

◆ Differential Diagnosis

Vitritis, migraine, vitreous hemorrhage, RD

◆ Management

Complete ocular examination, particularly a dilated retinal examination, by using indirect ophthalmoscopy and scleral depression to rule out a retinal break and detachment is mandatory. There is no simple treatment for vitreous floaters. Using the Neo-dymium-YAG laser to break up vitreous floaters is a controversial practice and may be associated with the risk of creating retinal breaks and RD. A vitrectomy is reserved only for very dense vitreous floaters.

◆ Retinal Tears and Retinal Detachment

The posterior fundus structures involved with the development and management of a retinal detachment include the neurosensory retina, choroid, RPE, pars plana, and sclera. A rhegmatogenous RD is the most common type of RD. It is caused by one or more retinal breaks. Most retinal breaks are located between the equator and the ora serrata (28%) or near the equator of the globe (45%). Choroidal vortex veins are the most visible landmarks adjacent to the equator. Peripheral retinal lesions (see Chapter 9), including 12% of small retinal breaks, are frequently located close to the ora serrata, the scalloped junction between the neurosensory retina and the pars plana at the vitreous base.

The distance between the equator and the ora measures between 5 and 6 mm, and it is slightly greater in the temporal than in the nasal retina. The pars plana consists of an inner nonpigmented and an outer pigmented layer that spans ~6 mm from the posterior limbus to the ora serrata radially at the anterior fundus. It represents a surgical "safe" zone, through which needles and surgical instruments may be passed without causing ocular damages. Rare pars plana breaks include focal tears and dialyses associated with certain conditions (e.g., congenital development, trauma, aphakia, and atopic dermatitis). Only 15% of retinal breaks develop posterior to the equator, including macular holes (1%), which may induce a retinal detachment in highly myopic eyes.

Interactions between centrifugal and centripetal forces across the neurosensory retina determine the status of retinal attachment versus detachment. Centrifugal forces that induce retinal detachment include (1) vitreous fluid entry into the subretinal space through retinal breaks and (2) vitreoretinal tractional forces. Centripetal forces that promote retinal attachment include (1) outward hydrostatic vitreous fluid pressure on the retinal surface, (2) mucopolysaccharide adhesives and interdigitating cellular processes between the retinal photoreceptors and the RPE, (3) choroidal oncotic pressure, and (4) metabolic pump of the RPE. An imbalance in favor of centrifugal forces that leads to a retinal detachment is most frequently caused by the onset of retinal break(s).

◆ Presentation

The annual incidence of rhegmatogenous RD is close to 1 per 15,000 people, and the prevalence is 0.3% of the general population. The prevalence is increased for "high-risk" groups: 2% for aphakic patients, 2% for patients with asymptomatic lattice degeneration, 5% for highly myopic patients, and 10% for patients with vitreous loss during cataract extraction.

Most retinal breaks and rhegmatogenous RDs develop spontaneously. The aging process generates vitreous syneresis. The ensuing fibrillar degeneration of the vitreous predisposes an acute PVD and associated retinal breaks/RD. Therefore, the most common age group for RD is between 40 and 70 years. Approximately 40

Fig. 10.3 Types of retinal break. **(A)** flap tear; **(B)** atrophic retinal hole; **(C)** operculated break; **(D)** retinal dialysis.

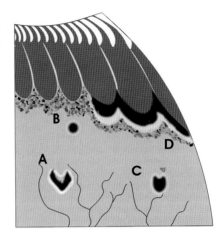

to 50% of RDs are associated with myopia, 30 to 40% are associated with aphakia or pseudophakia, and 10 to 20% are associated with direct ocular trauma. Close to 60% of RDs occur in males, possibly because there are more male than female myopic patients. About 15% of RDs eventually develop in the fellow eyes as well. Bilateral RDs are more common in aphakic eyes (25 to 30%).

Genetic predisposition to RD includes Jewish race and familial tendency (i.e., Jensen disease). The black population has a low incidence of RD.

Visual-field loss and scotomas are common features for all categories of retinal detachment. Macular involvement leads to central vision loss. The location of the retinal detachment is in the opposing quadrant(s) to the visual-field defect owing to the generally contralateral topographical correspondence between the retina and the visual field. Anterior vitreous pigment granules detected on slit-lamp biomicroscopy constitute a reliable hallmark sign (positive Shafer sign) for the presence of retinal break(s). Vitreous hemorrhage is frequently but not always associated with retinal breaks/RD.

There are several types of retinal breaks (**Fig. 10.3**):

◆ *Flap tears*: These are also known as horseshoe tears due to their U-shaped morphology. Anterior vitreoretinal traction on the retinal flaps connected to the anterior margins of the tears makes the flaps point anteriorly toward the vitreous base. Symptomatic flap tears are high risk. Subretinal fluid tends to accumulate around the breaks, and hence, breaks should be treated promptly. A giant tear spans 3 or more clock hours and usually has a scrolled flap that may roll over on itself. It requires a vitrectomy as management.

◆ *Atrophic retinal holes*: These lesions are due to progressive retinal thinning without associated vitreoretinal traction. They are often within patches of lattice degeneration. Most atrophic holes have a low risk and do not require prophylactic treatment, particularly when located inferiorly.

◆ *Operculated breaks*: Persistent vitreoretinal traction may lead to a complete separation of a free-floating vitreous operculum from the underlying break. It tends to locate more posterior than flap tears. It is intermediate in risk (between flap tears and atrophic holes) for an RD. Superior temporal operculated retinal tears are more vulnerable than inferior nasal operculated tears for vision loss. Treatment or observation is on a case-by-case basis.

◆ *Dialysis*: This is a circumferential retinal tear by the ora serrata. Unlike other breaks, vitreoretinal traction is on the posterior margin of the dialysis. It occurs more commonly in the young. Retinal dialysis may be congenital (mostly in the inferior temporal quadrant) or traumatic (usually in the superior nasal quadrant). Retinal dialysis carries moderate to high risk for RD and may require treatment, including laser, cryotherapy, or scleral buckling/vitrectomy.

◆ *Acute*: For acute retinal breaks leading to rhegmatogenous RD induced by PVD, cardinal symptoms include flashing lights, floaters, cobwebs, and a curtain effect. The mechanical disturbance of the retina by vitreoretinal traction is responsible for these photopic phenomena.

◆ **Differential Diagnosis**

Retinal detachments (**Fig. 10.4**) are divided into three types: rhegmatogenous, exudative, and tractional (**Table 10.1**).

◆ *Rhegmatogenous RD*: These are the most common. They involve retinal breaks.

◆ *Exudative RD*: These are caused by excessive accumulation of subretinal serous fluid that may shift with changes in body position. Examples of conditions associated with an exudative RD include central serous chorioretinopathy, various choroidal tumors, and diverse posterior inflammatory diseases.

◆ *Tractional RD*: These are caused by vitreoretinal traction (e.g., proliferative diabetic retinopathy). Whereas a surgical intervention is usually indicated for a rhegmatogenous RD, it is often not required for an exudative RD. A tractional RD involving the macula requires surgery.

A retinoschisis may mimic a retinal detachment. Distinctive features of retinoschisis include a thin and dome-shaped elevated inner layer, absence of demarca-

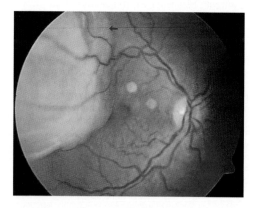

Fig. 10.4 View of a tumor associated with a retinal detachment. The detached retina is denoted with *blue arrow*.

Table 10.1   Differences between Types of Retinal Detachment

Feature	Rhegma-togenous	Exudative	Tractional
1. Retinal break	Yes	No	No primary break; secondary break can occur
2. Shifting fluid	No	Yes	No
3. Choroidal mass	No	May be present	No
4. Intraocular pressure	Low	Varies	Normal
5. Transillumination	Normal	Blocked trans-illumination If pigmented choroidal lesion is present	Normal
6. Retinal mobility	Undulating folds	Smoothly elevated, no folds	Taut retina
7. Extent of RD	Extends to ora quickly	Gravity dependent	Does not extend to ora
8. Pigment in vitreous	Mostly present	No	Present in trauma cases
9. Subretinal fluid	Clear	Turbid	Clear

RD, retinal detachment.

tion lines, and clusters of outer oval retinal holes (**Fig. 10.5**). It is often bilaterally symmetrical and frequently localizes to the inferotemporal quadrant. If diagnosis is uncertain, a laser spot test can be performed. A mild retinal laser uptake on the outer retinal layer confirms the identity of retinoschisis. Most retinoschisis lesions do not progress and require no therapy. Development of both inner- and outer-layer holes may convert a retinoschisis into a rhegmatogenous RD, which requires prompt treatment. A rare progression of a retinoschisis close to the macula also requires barrier laser therapy, scleral buckling, or vitrectomy.

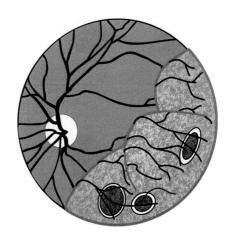

Fig. 10.5   Retinoschisis.

◆ Management

The effective treatment of a rhegmatogenous RD requires the identification and localization of all retinal breaks (**Fig. 10.6**). Indirect ophthalmoscopy with scleral indentation is an indispensable tool for accomplishing this goal. Ancillary techniques for revealing retinal breaks include biomicroscopy and ultrasonography. Historical details of the RD may provide clues of the responsible breaks. For instance, an inferior visual-field defect points to a superior tear and RD. Rapid progression of the

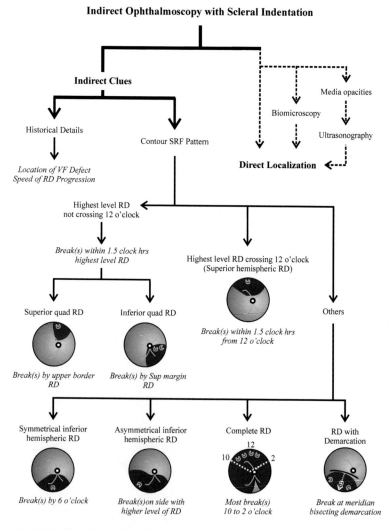

Fig. 10.6 Algorithm for localizing retinal break(s) associated with a retinal detachment. RD, retinal detachment; SRF, subretinal fluid; VF, visual field.

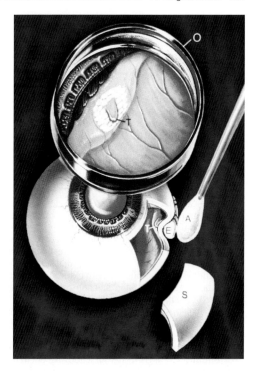

Fig. 10.7 Final view of buckle with proper retinal indentation and positioning of the tear. This internal/external conceptual illustration shows a cross section and the corresponding surgeon's view of the final configuration of a circumferentially placed sponge exoplant (E). The cross section shows a portion of the globe without sclera (S) to enhance clarity for the reader. The surgeon's view is through the indirect ophthalmoscope (O). Note the indented configuration in both views. The retina is reattached and the tear (T) is flat. Also note that the tear is properly positioned on the anterior slope of the buckle, as indicated by the cotton-tipped applicator (A). (Courtesy of *Highlights of Ophthalmology*, "Retinal and Vitreoretinal Surgery: Mastering the Latest Techniques" English Edition, 2002. Editor-in-Chief: Benjamin F. Boyd, MD., FACS; Co-Editor: Samuel Boyd, MD.)

RD suggests a large break, a posterior break, or a superior break. Previous reports also point out the importance of the pattern of subretinal fluid distribution in relation to the locations of the primary retinal breaks.

The closure of all retinal breaks by induction of firm chorioretinal adhesions between the breaks and underlying RPE is the key to successful management of a rhegmatogenous RD. Adhesive modalities include diathermy, cryotherapy, and photocoagulation (**Fig. 10.7**).

Diathermy
Electrical current generates heat at the tip of the diathermy probe, used for localizing retinal breaks. Diathermy lesions on partial-thickness sclera induce strong chorioretinal adhesions as well. Full-thickness treatment is avoided due to scleral necrosis.

Cryotherapy

Low-temperature freezing at the tip of the cryoprobe allows retinal treatment through full-thickness sclera without scleral damage. Direct monitoring with indirect ophthalmoscopy for a whitish ice-ball surrounding the retinal break is the best method.

Photocoagulation

Precise chorioretinal uptakes with laser photocoagulation can be applied only on attached retina or areas of minimal subretinal fluid, limiting its utility in RD repair. Transscleral application of a diode laser shows promising results. Supplemental photocoagulation on the buckle enhances resorption of residual subretinal fluid adjacent to retinal breaks during or after scleral buckling. Intraocular injection of gas before or after supplemental laser for tamponade of the superior retinal breaks on the buckle may further facilitate the resolution of the residual subretinal fluid.

Scleral Buckling

The three cardinal steps for successful scleral buckling include (1) accurate localization of all retinal breaks, (2) induction of chorioretinal adhesions, and (3) support of retinal breaks on the buckle.

Localization of breaks is attained with external scleral marks by diathermy or similar devices under guidance of indirect ophthalmoscopy. Chorioretinal adhesions are achieved with cryotherapy, diathermy, or photocoagulation. Support of retinal breaks is accomplished with external scleral indentation with donor tissues or synthetic materials. Solid silicone rubber or sponges are the most commonly employed buckling elements. They are anchored in place with scleral sutures or scleral belt loops, placing the breaks on the anterior crest of the buckle. Scleral buckling techniques are broadly divided into episcleral versus intrascleral, encircling versus segmental, and drainage versus nondrainage. Episcleral techniques have largely supplanted intrascleral methods in modern scleral buckling. **Table 10.2** outlines the algorithms for choosing encircling versus segmental buckling procedures. Subretinal fluid drainage is performed through a choroidotomy under a radial scleral cut-down with a tapered suture needle, diathermy needle, 27- or 30-gauge needle, or endolaser probe.

Indications for drainage include (1) bullous RD with highly elevated tears, (2) pseudophakic or highly myopic eyes with multiple peripheral breaks, (3) chronic RD with viscous subretinal fluid and cellular elements, (4) eyes with poor choroidal or RPE function, and (5) severe glaucoma or fresh cataract wound not tolerant of ocular hypertension. Recurrent RD due to drainage complications occurs in 12% of cases. Long-term successes of drainage and nondrainage buckling procedures are equivalent.

Table 10.2   Choice of Buckling Procedures

Segmental	versus	Encircling
Few peripheral breaks		Many peripheral breaks
Single break		Extensive breaks
Mobile retina		Rigid retina with folds
Clear vitreous		Cloudy vitreous, vitreous strands and membranes
Healthy sclera		Thin and weak sclera
Good visualization		Suboptimal visualization

Alternative Techniques

Alternative techniques include pneumatic retinopexy, temporary orbital balloon, and primary vitrectomy. Pneumatic retinopexy involves cryotherapy or laser to induce chorioretinal adhesions and injection of a small gas bubble to treat limited superior retinal breaks (within 1 to 2 clock hours apart) of a simple RD. A temporary orbital balloon allows treatment of simple RDs with limited superior or inferior breaks without need of permanent buckling. Vitrectomy achieves direct internal flattening of complex breaks and RDs while avoiding external buckling elements.

Intraoperative and postoperative factors contribute to surgical failure. Intraoperative causes include (1) inadequate localization, chorioretinal adhesion, or support of breaks; (2) marked subretinal or choroidal hemorrhage; (3) inadequate relief of vitreoretinal/chorioretinal traction; (4) complications of subretinal fluid drainage (incarceration, perforation, hemorrhage); (5) inadvertent retinal, choroidal, scleral perforations; and (6) severe choroidal detachment. Postoperative causes include (1) marked exudative retinal and choroidal detachment, (2) anterior segment ischemia, (3) proliferative vitreoretinopathy, (4) extrusion or intrusion of buckling elements, and (5) infections (episcleral, endophthalmitis).

Numerous advances in vitreoretinal surgical techniques promise more precise and quicker surgical treatments for RD on an outpatient basis (**Figs. 10.8, 10.9,**

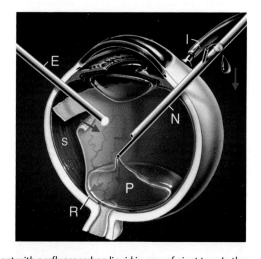

Fig. 10.8   Retinal reattachment with perfluorocarbon liquid in case of giant tear. In the case of retinal detachment with a giant retinal tear, perfluorocarbon liquid (P) is injected into the vitreous cavity via a Chang cannula (N). Because the liquid has a specific gravity greater than water, it gravitates (*blue arrow*) to the posterior pole. This forces the subretinal fluid (S, *red arrows*) out through the giant retinal tear and out of the eye via the Chang cannula. The retina (R) is being forced to reattach (*green arrow*) in this manner. E, endoilluminator; I, infusion cannula. (Courtesy of *Highlights of Ophthalmology*, "Retinal and Vitreoretinal Surgery: Mastering the Latest Techniques" English Edition, 2002. Editor-in-Chief: Benjamin F. Boyd, MD, FACS; Co-Editor: Samuel Boyd, MD.)

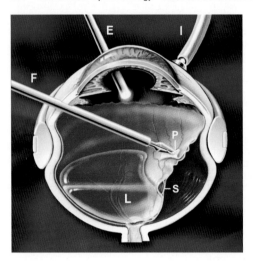

Fig. 10.9   For surgical treatment of proliferative vitreo-retinopathy, perfluorocarbon liquid (L) may be injected. This will reveal any persistent retinal traction related to epiretinal membranes (P) that must be removed. A vitreoretinal pic or Grieshaber mini-diamond forceps (F) is used to remove such a membrane (P). Note the subretinal membrane (S), endoilluminator (E), and infusion terminal (I). (Courtesy of *Highlights of Ophthalmology*, "Retinal and Vitreoretinal Surgery: Mastering the Latest Techniques" English Edition, 2002. Editor-in-Chief: Benjamin F. Boyd, MD, FACS; Co-Editor: Samuel Boyd, MD.)

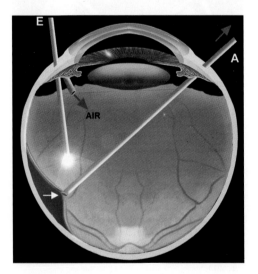

Fig. 10.10   Air-fluid exchange and internal drainage of subretinal fluid (*white arrow*) with an extrusion needle (A) is performed to flatten the retina. E, endoilluminator. (Courtesy of *Highlights of Ophthalmology*, "Retinal and Vitreoretinal Surgery: Mastering the Latest Techniques" English Edition, 2002. Editor-in-Chief: Benjamin F. Boyd, MD, FACS; Co-Editor: Samuel Boyd, MD.)

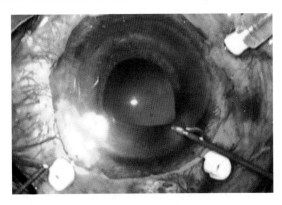

Fig. 10.11   Combined microphakonit (700 μm cataract surgery) and 25-gauge transconjunctival sutureless vitrectomy.

10.10). Pneumatic retinopexy and vitrectomy have become increasingly popular techniques for repairing RD. Recent advances in 25-gauge vitrectomy technology may allow its application on certain simple RDs (**Fig. 10.11**).

◆ Scleral Buckle Procedure

Scleral buckling procedure is a time-honored surgical technique first popularized by Custodis for repairing an RD. Successful scleral buckling requires the fulfillment of several important criteria, including (1) the accurate assessment and localization of all retinal breaks and vitreoretinal traction, (2) appropriate application of retinopexy for all associated retinal breaks, (3) precise placement of scleral buckling elements to support the underlying retinal breaks and relief of vitreoretinal traction, and (4) proper drainage of subretinal fluid. Drainage of subretinal fluid is not always necessary, and some surgeons prefer the nondrainage scleral buckle procedure.

◆ Accurate Localization of Retinal Breaks

The contour of an RD is frequently determined by the locations of its associated retinal breaks. **Figure 10.12** depicts the rules for predicting the location(s) of the retinal break(s) responsible for the RD based on its contour. Lincoff has pointed out that for RDs with an asymmetrical contour not crossing the 12 o'clock meridian, the responsible break is found within 1.5 hours from its highest level. In case the RD crosses the 12:00 meridian, the primary break(s) can be detected within 1½ hours from 12:00. Schepens and Hilton have also indicated a series of rules regarding finding the responsible retinal breaks: (1) the primary break is close to the upper margin of the RD for a superior quadrantic detachment, (2) the primary break is close to 12:00 for a superior symmetrical hemispheric RD, (3) the primary break

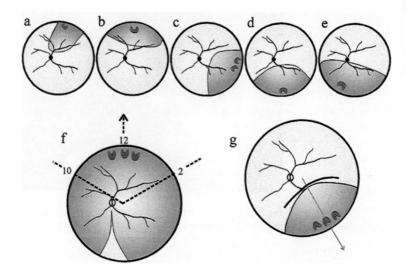

Fig. 10.12   The distribution of the subretinal fluid associated with a retinal detachment (RD) points to the likely location of the retinal break(s): (a) superior RD: break is near the superior edge; (b) superior symmetrical hemispheric RD: break is close to 12:00; (c) inferior quadrantic RD: break is near superior edge; (d) inferior hemispheric detachment: break is by 6:00; (e) asymmetrical inferior RD: break is close to side with higher level; (f) superior RD crossing 12:00: break is within 1½ clock hours from 12:00; (g) RD with a demarcation line: break is along meridian bisecting the demarcation. (Adapted from Agarwal et al. *Textbook of Ophthalmology* (4 Vols.). New Delhi, India: Jaypee Brothers.)

is close to the upper margin or along the meridian bisecting the region of the RD for an inferior quadrantic RD, (4) the primary break is close to 6 o'clock for a symmetrical inferior hemispheric RD, (5) the break is close to the upper margin for an asymmetrical inferior hemispheric RD, (6) the responsible break is usually found within 12:00 to 2:00 meridians in cases of a complete RD, (7) the retinal break is along the meridian bisecting the demarcating zone for an RD with a demarcation line. Deviations from these rules can be expected in case of chorioretinal scarring and traction or reoperations.

◆ **Color-Coded Diagram**

A color-coded chart with specific symbols representing various retinal lesions and treatment modalities allows detailed documentation of the pathology of the RD and its management in an organized manner. **Figure 10.13** demonstrates such a chart frequently used along with scleral buckling techniques.

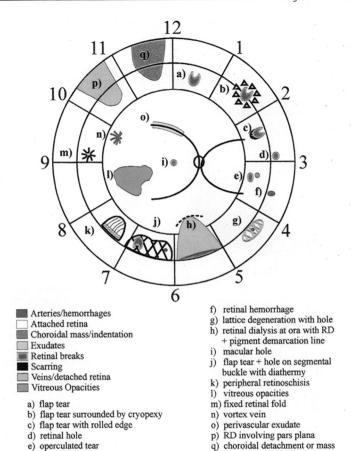

Arteries/hemorrhages
Attached retina
Choroidal mass/indentation
Exudates
Retinal breaks
Scarring
Veins/detached retina
Vitreous Opacities

a) flap tear
b) flap tear surrounded by cryopexy
c) flap tear with rolled edge
d) retinal hole
e) operculated tear

f) retinal hemorrhage
g) lattice degeneration with hole
h) retinal dialysis at ora with RD
   + pigment demarcation line
i) macular hole
j) flap tear + hole on segmental
   buckle with diathermy
k) peripheral retinoschisis
l) vitreous opacities
m) fixed retinal fold
n) vortex vein
o) perivascular exudate
p) RD involving pars plana
q) choroidal detachment or mass

Fig. 10.13 A color-coded fundus chart with specific symbols allows the documentation of the relevant retinal lesions associated with a retinal detachment, and the detailed steps of the associated scleral buckling procedure. (Adapted from Agarwal et al. *Textbook of Ophthalmology* (4 Vols.). New Delhi, India: Jaypee Brothers.)

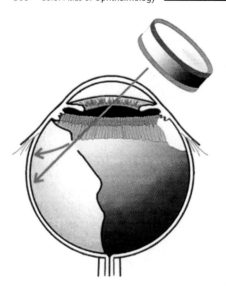

Fig. 10.14 The parallax associated with a bullous retinal detachment tends to cause the mistaken localization of the retinal break to be more posterior than it should be. A compensatory anterior adjustment during the localization is necessary.

◆ Parallax Associated with Viewing

Parallax is a frequently encountered phenomenon when viewing an RD with bullous subretinal fluid, whereby the associated retinal break appears more posterior than its actual location. Thus a compensatory anterior shifting is needed to accurately localize the retinal break (**Fig. 10.14**).

◆ Shafting during Localization

Figure 10.15 shows the phenomenon of shafting that mistakes the location of the compressing diathermy shaft on the globe for the tip of the probe. To avoid this error, the tip of the diathermy probe is placed on the external location of the retinal break first and then arched forward to prevent extensive contact of the shaft of the probe with the globe during localization of the retinal break.

◆ Exoplant Material

Soft and hard silicone exoplants have withstood the test of time to be durable and safe buckling material for supporting retinal breaks in the repair of an RD. **Figure 10.16** showed details of soft silicone sponges and hard silicone rubber. Commonly used silicone sponges include 3, 5, and 7.5 mm diameter sponges. Sponges may also be trimmed to a precise dimension to customize them for specific cases. There are numerous styles of hard silicone rubber with variable diameters. More common styles of solid silicone implants include 20, 40, 41, 42, 220, 240, 276, 277, and 287 bands or tires. A silicone tire has a groove along its long axis to accommodate a silicone band. The groove may be centrally located as in 20, 210, and 277 tires. An off-centered groove (e.g., 276 tire), allows a more posterior buckling effect. The majority of silicone rubbers are designed for circumferential placement, whereas most silicone sponges are designed for radial placement. However, circumferential

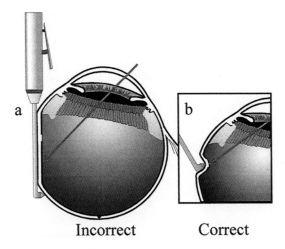

Incorrect   Correct

Fig. 10.15 **(A)** Mistaking the shaft for the tip of the diathermy probe may result in too posterior a placement of the localizing diathermy mark. **(B)** This error may be avoided with an anterior arching of the distal end of the probe, and indenting with only the tip of the probe.

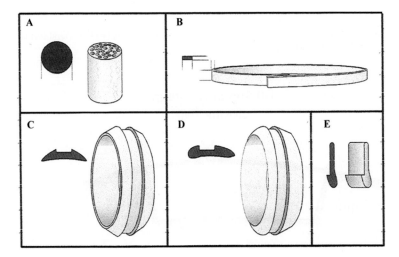

Fig. 10.16 Solid silicone is well tolerated by the eye and is the most commonly used material for an implant or explant during scleral buckling in the modem era. **(A)** It is available in **(A)** the form of soft sponges, or **(B)** solid rubber. A rubber silicone tire has a groove along its long axis to accommodate an encircling band. **(C)** The groove may be centrally located as in a 277 tire, or **(D)** off-centered as in a 276 tire associated with a more posterior buckling effect. **(E)** A meridional silicone wedge allows the radial support of a retinal break.

sponges and radial silicone rubbers (e.g., silicone wedges) are available but used less frequently. A silicone sponge with a hollow interior to accommodate insertion of a circumferential band allows a higher buckling effect corresponding to the location of its placement (e.g., 507T).

◆ Proper Suturing Technique

Spatulated needles are used for anchoring sutures on the sclera. To avoid inadvertent scleral perforation, the angle of the needle must be relatively parallel to the plane of the sclera (**Fig. 10.17**).

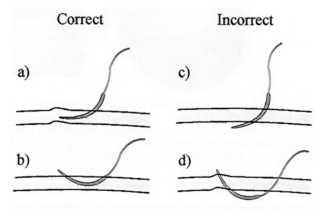

Fig. 10.17 The angle of the spatulated needle must be parallel to the scleral surface to avoid scleral perforation.

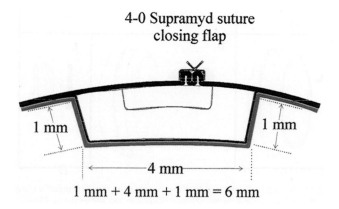

Fig. 10.18 A distance of 6 mm is required between the two circumferentially placed sutures to anchor a solid silicone rubber implant of 4 mm width and 1 mm thickness (1 mm + 4 mm + 1 mm = 6 mm).

◆ Calculating the Distance of Suture Placement for Silicone Exoplant

In general, the cross-sectional circumferential dimension of the silicone exoplant is calculated to estimate the distance of suture placement, as shown by the following examples:

◆ Circumferential implantation of solid silicone rubber with a 4-mm width and 1 mm thickness requires a suture distance of 6 mm (1 mm + 4 mm + 1 mm = 6 mm) (**Fig. 10.18**).
◆ The size of a tear needs to be within 4 mm to fit on the anterior slope of a circumferential buckle created by a 5-mm sponge (π x D/4 = 3.1416 × 5/4 = 3.927) (**Fig. 10.19**).
◆ The anchoring of the mattress suture corresponding to the meridian(s) of the retinal break(s) maximizes the height of the buckle for proper support of the break(s). The suture needle is placed at 1 to 2 mm from the margins of the silicone rubber (**Fig. 10.20**).

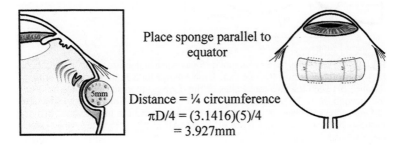

Place sponge parallel to equator

Distance = ¼ circumference
πD/4 = (3.1416)(5)/4
= 3.927mm

Fig. 10.19   To fit on the anterior slope of the buckle created by a circumferentially placed 5-mm sponge, the size of the tear needs to be within 4 mm (π × D/4 = 3.1416 × 5/4 = 3.927).

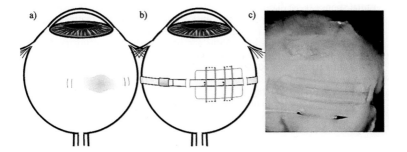

Fig. 10.20   The anchoring suture is placed at 1 to 2 mm from the margins of the circumferential solid silicone implant corresponding to the meridian of the retinal break to maximize the support of the break.

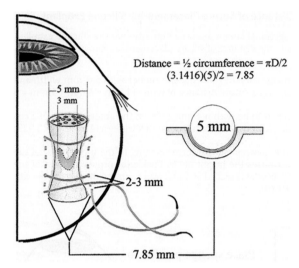

Fig. 10.21 When placing a radial sponge for a large tear, the size of the sponge should be 1 to 2 mm wider than the tear (e.g., 5-mm sponge for a 3-mm tear). The horizontal distance between the two radial bites of the double-armed suture should be 2 to 3 mm beyond the width of the sponge (e.g., 7 to 8 mm for a 5-mm sponge). The latter distance equals the half circumference of the sponge and can be calculated with the formula: Distance = ½ circumference = $\pi D/2$ = (3.416)(5)/2 = 7.85 mm. (Courtesy of Retina Consultants Ltd., St. Louis, MO.)

◆ Radial placement of a 5-mm sponge requires a suture distance of 7.85 or 8.0 mm. In general, the horizontal distance between the radial bites of the double-armed suture should be 2 to 3 mm beyond the width of the sponge (e.g., 7 to 8 mm for a 5-mm sponge). The precise calculation is half circumference of the radial sponge [½ (π diameter) or 3.1416 × 5/2 = 7.85 or 8.0 mm] (**Fig. 10.21**).

◆ For proper support of a retinal tear with a radial sponge, the mattress sutures need to be placed from 1 to 2 mm anterior to the anterior horns of the tear and 3 to 4 mm posterior to the apex of the tear. To achieve proper suture tension, the assistant holds the suture knot after the surgeon makes the first double throw of the suture knot (**Fig. 10.22**).

◆ For a large retinal tear, a 12-mm sponge or two 5-mm sponges are placed side by side. The proper horizontal distance between the two radial suture bites in the latter situation is calculated with the following formula: 7.85 mm + 5 mm – compression factor = 11.5 mm (**Fig. 10.23**).

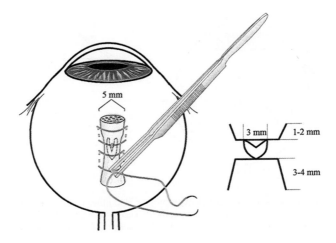

Fig. 10.22 For a radial sponge to support a large tear, the anterior mattress suture should start at 2 mm anterior to the anterior horn of the tear, whereas the posterior suture should extend 3 to 4 mm posterior to the apex of the tear. Achieving the proper tension on the suture may also require the assistant to hold the suture knot after the surgeon makes the first double throw of the suture knot.

Suture distance for 1 & 2 sponges

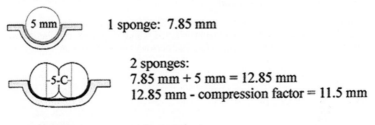

1 sponge: 7.85 mm

2 sponges:
7.85 mm + 5 mm = 12.85 mm
12.85 mm − compression factor = 11.5 mm

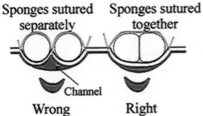

Fig. 10.23 For a very large tear, a 12-mm sponge or two 5-mm sponges may be placed side-by-side. The distance between the two radial bites of the mattress suture for two 5-mm sponges placed side-by-side can be calculated with the following formulas: distance across 2 sponges = 7.85 mm + 5 mm = 12.85 mm; 12.85 mm − compression factor = 11.5 mm. (Courtesy of Retina Consultants Ltd., St. Louis, MO)

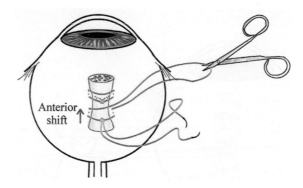

Fig. 10.24 If a large staphyloma is present along the course of an encircling band, it can be covered by a wider silicone groove-piece or tire under the band, which is then sutured on the thicker sclera outside of the staphyloma. (Courtesy of Retina Consultants Ltd., St. Louis, MO.)

◆ Anterior Shifting of Suture Tying for a Posterior Buckle

To ease tying of the suture knot for a radial buckle, the suture knot can be shifted from the posterior to the anterior portion of the mattress suture for tying (**Fig. 10.24**).

◆ Drainage of Subretinal Fluid

Drainage of subretinal fluid can be accomplished (1) via a radial scleral incision or (2) under a partial-thickness triangular-shaped scleral flap. The scleral cut-down is made by a no. 64 or 69 Beaver blade. Diathermy may be used to achieve hemo-

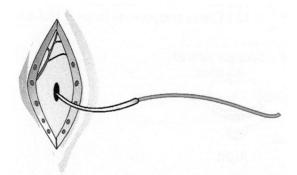

Fig. 10.25 A radial scleral drainage site is made with a 3- to 5-mm incision with a no. 64 or 69 Beaver blade. A 5–0 suture may be preplaced on the scleral edges and the edges may be diathermized. A tapered suture needle, a sharp diathermy electrode, a 27- or 30-gauge needle may be used for the transchoroidal penetration during drainage.

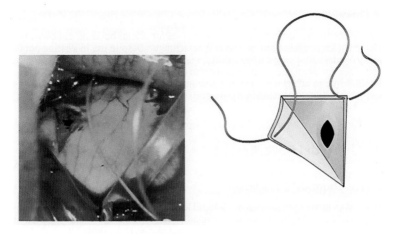

Fig. 10.26 A triangular scleral flap may also be made for a drainage site. A 5–0 nonabsorbable suture is preplaced on the apex of the scleral flap and the corresponding corner of the scleral bed. A minimal radial cut-down through the remaining thin scleral fibers of the drainage bed allows a quick exposure of the choroid for drainage.

stasis. The choroid is penetrated with a tapered needle (e.g., 6–0 silk C-1 needle), sharp diathermy tip, 27- or 30-gauge needle, or sharp knife. The alternative is the use of laser delivered by an endolaser probe or a laser indirect ophthalmoscope (**Figs. 10.25** and **10.26**).

Cotton applicators are used to gently compress the sclera adjacent to the drainage site (especially anterior to it) to enhance drainage of subretinal fluid. The appearance of small pigment clumps in the exiting fluid indicates the elimination of most of the subretinal fluid. Indirect ophthalmoscopy is performed to inspect the completeness of the fluid drainage and detect any complications associated with the drainage site (**Fig. 10.27**).

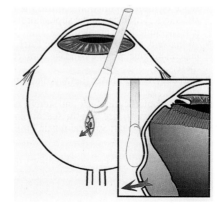

Fig. 10.27 Gentle traction of the edges of the sclerotomy and mild indentation of the sclera with a cotton-tipped applicator allow further drainage of the residual subretinal fluid.

◆ Conclusion

Adherence to the foregoing proper techniques for scleral buckling enhances the chance of successful repair of a retinal detachment. Despite the increasing popularity of alternative surgical procedures, scleral buckling remains a reliable surgical technique for repairing most primary and certain recurrent retinal detachments. Its vital role in achieving favorable anatomical and visual outcome for repairing retinal detachment persists in the modern era of vitreoretinal surgery.

◆ Choroidal Detachment

Serous Choroidal Detachment

◆ *Intraoperative or postoperative*: Wound leak, perforation of the sclera from a superior rectus, bridle suture, iritis, cyclodialysis cleft, leakage or excess filtration from a filtering bleb, or after laser photocoagulation or cryotherapy
◆ *Traumatic*: Often associated with a ruptured globe, rhegmatogenous retinal detachment, or after scleral buckling repair or a detachment

◆ Presentation

Patients present with decreased vision or are asymptomatic. There may be moderate to severe pain. Decreased vision may occur if the choroidal detachments (CDs) are touching ("kissing choroidals") or hemorrhagic. Smooth, bullous, orange-brown elevation of the retina and choroid usually extends 360 degrees around the periphery in a lobular configuration. Low intraocular pressure (IOP) (often less than 6 mm Hg), shallow anterior chamber with mild cell and flare, and positive transilluminations are associated findings.

◆ Differential Diagnosis

Melanoma of the ciliary body and RRD

◆ Management

◆ *Check history:* Gonioscopy, fundus examination of both eyes, B-scan, and absence of transillumination confirm the diagnosis. Cycloplegic, topical steroid, and surgical drainage of the suprachoroidal fluid are the treatment options. Repair the underlying problem.
◆ *Wound leak or leaky filtering bleb*: Patch for 24 hours, suture the site, use cyanoacrylate glue, place a bandage contact lens on the eye, or a combination of these.
◆ *Cyclodialysis cleft*: Laser therapy, diathermy, cryotherapy, or suture the cleft to close it.
◆ *Uveitis*: Topical cycloplegic and steroid as discussed previously
◆ *Inflammatory disease*: See the specific entity.
◆ *Retinal detachment*: Surgical repair. Proliferative vitreoretinopathy after repair is common.

Hemorrhagic or Expulsive Choroidal Detachment

Intraoperative or postoperative (from anterior displacement of the ocular contents and rupture of the short posterior ciliary arteries) is the most common cause.

◆ Presentation

Symptoms are the same as for serous choroidal detachment. Pain and red eye may be present more often. High IOP (if detachment is large), shallow anterior chamber with mild cell and flare, and absence of transillumination are features in which hemorrhagic CD differs from serous CD.

◆ Differential Diagnosis

Melanoma of the ciliary body and RRD

◆ Management

Check the history. Confirmation of the diagnosis depends on history, gonioscopy, fundus examination, B-scan, and absence of transillumination.

An anterior vitrectomy and drainage of the choroidal detachment is performed for severe cases with retina or vitreous to the wound. Otherwise use general treatment.

◆ Macular Hole

A macular hole is a round break involving the layers of the retina, either in a partial- or full-thickness manner, in the macular region. The lesion is found more commonly in women and is predominant in the fifth to seventh decades (**Fig. 10.28** and **10.29**).

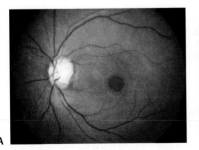
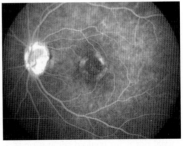

A   B

Fig. 10.28 **(A)** Color fundus photograph showing a well-circumscribed full-thickness macular hole with minimal surrounding fluid cuff. **(B)** Fundus fluorescein angiography of the same patient showing a fading fluorescence in the late phase indicating the window defect, the most common FFA finding in macular holes.

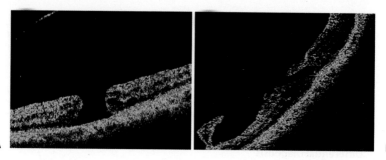

A   B

Fig. 10.29   Optical coherence tomography showing **(A)** a full-thickness and **(B)** lamellar macular hole.

◆ Presentation

Slit-lamp biomicroscopy of a full-thickness macular hole shows a well-circumscribed punched-out lesion that predominantly involves the fovea. A partial-thickness macular hole can be an outer lamellar hole or an inner lamellar hole, depending on the etiology behind it. It can be classified as follows:

- ◆ Full-thickness macular hole
- ◆ Outer lamellar hole
- ◆ Inner lamellar hole

Gass Classification for Stages of Idiopathic Macular Hole
- ◆ *Stage 1A*: Impending hole, foveal detachment with yellow spot
- ◆ *Stage 1B*: Impending hole, foveal detachment with yellow halo
- ◆ *Stage 2*: Full-thickness hole (central or eccentric) formation without vitreofoveal detachment or a PVD
- ◆ *Stage 3*: Full-thickness hole with focal vitreofoveal detachment but absence of a PVD
- ◆ *Stage 4*: Full-thickness hole with a PVD

◆ Differential Diagnosis

Various types of macular holes such as lamellar macular hole, pseudohole, myopic macular hole, microhole and macular hole associated with epiretinal membrane and retinal detachments, and pseudomacular hole

◆ Management

Observation
There are few studies describing stage 0 macular hole, which is a normal and healthy retinal morphology with altered vitreoretinal interface. Stage 0 macular hole is a clinically silent finding detected on optical coherence tomography where a parafoveal posterior hyaloid separation is present and a minimally reflective preretinal band is obliquely inserted at one end of the fovea. A similar finding when found in both the eyes is associated with a sixfold rise in the incidence of macular hole. Thus such cases must be followed closely and such patients must be counseled.

Surgical Management
Vitrectomy is the mainstay in the management of macular holes. Surgery for the treatment of macular hole revolves around two principles: (1) to relieve all vitreoretinal traction by meticulous removal of posterior cortical vitreous and (2) to use a tamponade to close the hole (**Fig. 10.30**).

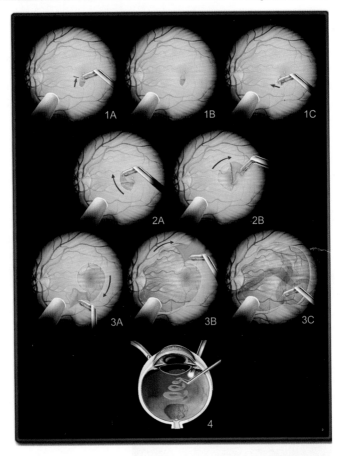

Fig. 10.30 "Apple peeling" technique for removal of the internal limiting membrane (ILM). (1A) The ILM is stained with indocyanine green (ICG) stain. The ILM is grasped with the ILM forceps 500–700 µm above or below the fovea, and a thin strip is peeled radially (*arrow*) almost to the fovea and released. (1B) This shows the extent of the initial peeled flap of ILM. (1C) The exposed edge is then grasped at its midpoint and a parafoveal strip of ILM is started with a circumferential movement (*arrow*) around the fovea. (2A) This parafoveal circumferential rhexis is continued (*arrow*), releasing and regrasping as necessary. (2B) The rhexis halfway around the fovea. (3A) The rhexis approaching a full circle around the fovea as an outward force vector (*arrow*) is then intentionally applied so that the ILM strip expands outwardly in a continuous fashion. (3B) Regrasping as necessary, this maneuver is continued (*arrow*) until the macular ILM has been removed in a single strip. (3C) The single-piece ILM strip ready for removal from the eye, avoiding the need for multiple forceps removals and reinsertions. (4) A conceptual view of the microforceps holding the single-piece removed ILM strip as removed from the retina. Note the unstained area of the retina from which this ILM strip was removed. Light is provided by an endofiberoptic and infusion via a separate infusion port. (Courtesy of *Highlights of Ophthalmology*, "Retinal and Vitreoretinal Surgery: Mastering the Latest Techniques" English Edition, 2002. Editor-in-Chief: Benjamin F. Boyd, MD, FACS; Co-Editor: Samuel Boyd, MD.)

◆ Idiopathic Epiretinal Membrane

Iwanoff was the first to describe idiopathic epiretin in 1865. It is commonly found in older age and has been called by various names:

◆ Macular pucker
◆ Preretinal macular fibrosis
◆ Epiretinal fibrosis
◆ Epiretinal gliosis
◆ Cellophane maculopathy
◆ Surface wrinkling retinopathy

Most of these epiretinal membranes (ERMs) are idiopathic and are called primary epiretinal membranes. When associated with some other ocular disorders, they are called secondary ERM (**Fig. 10.31**).

◆ Presentation

Patients complain of slow progressive loss of vision, mild to severe metamorphopsia, and monocular diplopia. Complaints usually progress over years. They may give some associated past or treatment history revealing the cause for the ERM.

Clinical characteristics vary with the grade of the ERM. An early ERM presents as an altered normal macular texture with a glistering shine on the surface. It is difficult to detect on ophthalmoscopic examination. A little more contractile membrane presents as fine retinal striae radiating from the center of the ERM.

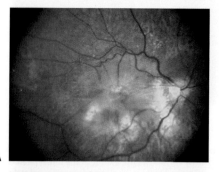

A

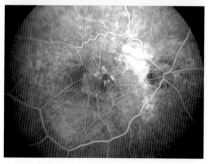

B

Fig. 10.31 **(A)** Fundus picture of patient showing gray-white epimacular membrane. Picture shows distortion of macular retinal vessels. **(B)** fundus fluorescein angiography (FFA) of the same patient.

The typical appearance of the blood vessels helps in the diagnosis. Dilated retinal veins and vascular tortuosity with tethering and straightening of the vessels are seen directed to the center of the contracting membrane. Foveal ectopia is a common finding. A wide range of other associated findings are noted, such as punctate hemorrhages, microaneurysms, profound vascular leakage and retinal edema, soft exudates, and retinal tear. Macular pucker usually develops after retinal detachments. They are opaque thick membranes with associated full-thickness retinal folds.

◆ Differential Diagnosis

Primary causes of ERM: idiopathic. Secondary causes of ERM: postocular inflammation, uveitis, retinal detachment, retinal vascular occlusions, macular holes, postintraocular surgeries, postretinal laser, cryopexy.

◆ Management

Vitrectomy is the only treatment for epiretinal membranes. After completing the vitrectomy, posterior hyaloid that is adherent to the retina is removed. Intravitreal triamcinolone can be used to facilitate this step. Then the membrane is peeled off the surface of the retina, preferably from the center to the periphery after finding an edge of the membrane. Recently intravitreal stains have been described. Trypan blue and indocyanine green are used to stain the epiretinal membrane and internal limiting membrane, respectively.

Ocular Neoplasms

Soosan Jacob, Santosh Hanovar, and Amar Agarwal

◆ Iris Tumors and Nodules

Iris Nevus

Iris nevus presents as a small (3 × 0.5mm), well-defined spot on the iris. It is commonly located in the stroma and presents either as a typical lesion (i.e., well-defined) or as a diffuse lesion. The lesion has to be differentiated from other pigmented lesions. Cogan-Reese syndrome is the common association.

◆ Presentation

Suspicion for malignant change is high when the nevus increases in size and changes color, increases in vascularity, rise in intraocular pressure (IOP), and there is pupil peaking, ectropion uveae, and iris splinting. Histopathological examination of the nevus shows proliferation of melanocytes, predominantly of spindle cells, though occasionally dendritic and balloon cells may occur.

◆ Differential Diagnosis

Iris freckle, iris melanoma, Lisch nodules, ocular melanocytosis

◆ Management

Management consists of reassurance of the patient regarding the benign nature of the lesion and simple observation for malignant change after careful photography and clinical documentation.

Iris Pigment Epithelial Cyst

Iris pigment epithelial cyst is rare and arises from the epithelium between layers of pigment epithelium. It presents differently depending on whether it is located in the epithelium or in the stroma.

◆ Presentation

When it is epithelial in location it can present as unilateral or bilateral as a solitary or multiple lesions. It is usually asymptomatic and obscures vision only when large. It is a globular lesion located at the papillary border or the midzone or the iris root. It is brown when iris epithelium is involved or transparent when the iridociliary epithelium is involved. It can get dislodged and float in the anterior chamber.

Lesions located in the stroma are usually smooth, unilateral, solitary translucent lesions presenting in the first year of life. When they increase in size they lead to secondary glaucoma, which in turn leads to corneal decompensation and pseudo-hypopyon.

◆ Differential Diagnosis

Iris and ciliary body melanoma

◆ Management

The nature of the lesion can be ascertained by either fine-needle aspiration or excision biopsy. If the tumor is large it can be treated with argon laser photocoagulation or by injecting ethanol into the lesion when it is recalcitrant.

Iris Melanoma

Iris tumors constitute 8% of uveal tumors presenting in the younger age group (40 to 50 years) with a slight female predilection. They usually have a better prognosis than other uveal melanomas.

◆ Presentation

The lesion can present as typical (spot), diffusely growing (diffuse color change), or tapioca melanoma (multiple surface nodules). Lesions are mostly asymptomatic, involving the inferior iris more commonly, but can present as a rise in IOP, hyphema, or cataract. Risk factor for malignant change is the same as that for iris nevus.

◆ Differential Diagnosis

Iridocorneal endothelial (ICE) syndrome, nevus, adenoma and ciliary body tumor, iris cyst, intraocular foreign body (IOFB), juvenile xanthogranuloma, and leiomyoma

◆ Management

B-scan and biopsy help to confirm the diagnosis. Biopsy can be fine needle aspiration cytology or incisional biopsy, either through a corneal or a limbal approach. The lesion can be observed until symptomatic or overt malignant changes occur for which excision (iridectomy or iridocyclectomy), proton-beam radiotherapy, or rarely enucleation have to be undertaken.

The prognosis is usually good when the lesion is small without ciliary body or extrascleral extension.

Juvenile Xanthogranuloma

Juvenile xanthogranuloma is a rare idiopathic granulomatous disease of childhood due to proliferation of non-Langerhans histiocytes. It can present either as cutaneous lesions or iris lesions. Iris infiltration is the most common ocular manifestation. It may also rarely involve the orbit, eyelids, cornea, episclera, ciliary body, choroid, and optic disk.

◆ Presentation

Cutaneous lesions present as yellowish papules with spontaneous regression. Iris lesions are either localized or diffuse. The patient may present as heterochromia of the iris. The lesions are usually associated with spontaneous hyphema. Anterior uveitis and glaucoma are other less common presentations.

◆ Differential Diagnosis

Retinoblastoma, sarcoid, leukemia, foreign body, meduloepithelioma

◆ Management

Treatment options include local corticosteroids, irradiation, and a combination of both and excision.

Leiomyoma (Uveal)

Leiomyoma is an extremely rare benign lesion arising from the smooth muscle. This is very similar to amelanotic melanoma, but generally it is not confined to the inferior iris only.

◆ Presentation

Patients typically present with a localized, flat to mildly elevated, lightly pigmented or nonpigmented, vascular lesion in the area of the iris sphincter. The lesion may also occur peripherally or in the anterior chamber angle.

◆ Differential Diagnosis

Amelanotic iris melanoma, metastatic iris lesions

◆ Management

Fine-needle aspiration cytology (FNAC) with electron microscopy and immunohistochemistry can diagnose and differentiate the condition from others. There is no known metastatic potential.

Leukemic Iris Nodules

Leukemic iris nodules are more common in chronic leukemias rather than in acute leukemia. Iris infiltration can present as iris nodules.

◆ Presentation

Iris involvement may be unilateral or bilateral. It is a vascularized lesion. It may be associated with anterior uveitis with or without hypopyon. Infiltration can also occur into the conjunctiva, orbit, and optic nerve. Glaucoma may be present due to blockage in the filtration from the trabecular meshwork. Leukemic retinopathy due to either direct infiltration or secondary to anemia has to be looked for.

◆ Differential Diagnosis

Retinoblastoma, uveitis, trauma

◆ Management

Workup involving an oncologist is preferred. Treatment consists of systemic chemotherapy with localized radiotherapy. Topical steroids cause quick but temporary resolution. Central nervous system (CNS) evaluation is must.

Melanocytosis

Ocular melanocytosis is an uncommon, congenital, premalignant condition. Nevus of Ota is the common variant followed by the limited dermal and ocular forms. This is more common in females and Asians.

◆ Presentation

Melanocytosis presents as unilateral hyperpigmentation of the face with ipsilateral iris hyperchromia, iris melanocytosis, glaucoma (10%), and lid pigmentation. The condition may be associated with pigmentation of the extraocular skin with ipsilateral uveal tract and meningeal involvement.

◆ Differential Diagnosis

Sturge-Weber syndrome, racial pigmentation

◆ Management

Because the hyperpigmented area has a predisposition to develop malignant melanoma, regular close follow-up every 6 to 12 months is required. Any suspicious lesion should be worked up accordingly for malignant melanoma.

Brushfield Spots (Down Syndrome)

Brushfield spots are seen in Down syndrome. They involve the peripheral stroma, can be multiple, and they occur as multiple, pale, benign lesions involving the peripheral iris stroma. The lesions appear as pale lesions. These can also be seen in normal individuals. Sarcoid nodules, iris nevus, or freckles must be ruled out. No treatment is required.

Lisch Nodules (Neurofibromatosis)

Lisch nodules are usually associated with neurofibromatosis. They are small and multiple. They appear similar to iris nevi, which are benign and bilateral. They are present in neurofibromatosis 1 in all patients after age 16 years. They consist of a collection of glial cells and melanocytes. They need to be differentiated from iris nevus. Clinical documentation and follow-up are required.

◆ Ciliary Body Tumors

Ciliary Body Melanoma

Ciliary body melanomas constitute ~12% of all malignancies and usually appear between the ages of 50 and 60 years.

◆ Presentation

Clinically they are asymptomatic, although they can produce visual symptoms occasionally. They are seen as ciliary body mass with sentinel vessels overlying. They can extend onto the iris or globe. Lens subluxation, angle-closure glaucoma, spontaneous hyphema, secondary cataract, and anterior uveitis are common associations.

Ciliary body melanomas are well detected by ultrasound and biopsy using FNAC.

◆ Differential Diagnosis

Ciliary body adenoma, ciliary body cyst, uveal effusion syndrome, meduloepithelioma, leiomyoma, and metastatic lesions

◆ Management

The tumors are amenable to excision when small. Radiotherapy, either as brachytherapy or proton beam therapy, is another option. Enucleation is done if other modalities are not possible. Prognosis is usually worse.

Medulloepithelioma (of the Ciliary Epithelium)

Medulloepithelioma arises from immature epithelial cells of the embryonic optic cup and are rare, slow-growing tumors that present in children younger than 10 years of age, with no sexual predilection. One third are benign and two thirds are malignant. They can be either teratoid or nonteratoid. They originate from the nonpigmented ciliary epithelium predominantly involving the iris and retina, though others can also be involved. Metastasis is rare.

◆ Presentation

Clinically patients can present with red eye and decreased vision or with an iris mass lesion with a change of color. Tumor may also be seen at the optic disk. Neovascular glaucoma, lens coloboma, or subluxation and cataract are the common complications.

◆ Differential Diagnosis

Persistent hyperplastic primary vitreous (PHPV), pars planitis, endophthalmitis, congenital glaucoma, retinoblastoma, malignant glaucoma

◆ Management

Ultrasound is useful in the diagnosis. Small, well-defined lesions of a benign nature are treated by iridocyclectomy, and enucleation is reserved for tumors not amenable to other treatment modalities.

◆ Choroidal Tumors

Choroidal Nevus

Choroidal nevus is a benign melanocytic tumor of the choroid and is found in 5 to 30% of white persons. These are usually found incidentally because they are asymptomatic and are the commonest of all intraocular malignancies.

◆ Presentation

Clinically they are asymptomatic but can present with a decrease in vision. Lesions close to the fovea can cause vision loss. They are small, gray-brown, homogeneous lesions. The lesion may be associated with lipofuscin deposits and drusen, or with subretinal fluid (SRF) is absent. These lesions gain importance in the fact that they have to be differentiated from malignant melanoma. Malignant transition is her-

Fig. 11.1 Choroidal nevus, fundus photograph shows a pigmented, placoid, well-demarcated choroidal mass with overlying drusen located temporal to the fovea.

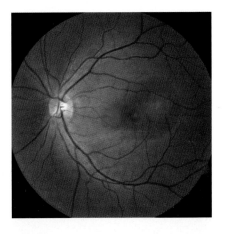

alded by the presence of symptomatic lesions, with increasing thickness, lesions with lipofuscin pigment and SRF, and an increase in IOP (**Fig. 11.1**).

◆ Differential Diagnosis

Choroidal melanoma, congenital hypertrophy of retinal pigment epithelium (RPE), combined hamartoma, hyperplasia of RPE, subretinal hemorrhage, choroidal hemangiomas, choroidal osteoma, and metastatic tumor.

◆ Management

Lesion must be investigated with fundus fluorescein angiography (FFA) and B-scan to rule out other lesions, especially malignant melanoma. Lesions should be closely monitored. Any changes in the morphology of the lesions should be alarming.

Choroidal Melanoma

Choroidal melanomas constitute ~80% of uveal melanomas presenting around 50 to 60 years of age. They are classified based on the size of the tumor as small (<10 mm), medium (10 to 15 mm), and large (>15).

◆ Presentation

They can present as a decrease in vision or field loss, or flashes of light may be the presenting features, but they are otherwise asymptomatic. They can present as an elevated sub-RPE mass and can be amelanotic. Lipofuscin deposits, exudative retinal detachment, and Bruch membrane rupture with vitreous hemorrhage are typical features of the lesion. Certain tumors are diffuse rather than being nodular. Patients at times may complain of blurry vision, visual-field loss, floaters, photopsia, and pain. Other associated findings can be retinal detachment, angle-closure glaucoma, rubeosis iridis, vitreous and subretinal hemorrhages, and lens subluxations (**Fig. 11.2**).

◆ **Differential Diagnosis**

Choroidal nevus, congenital hypertrophy of RPE, combined hamartoma, hyperplasia of RPE, subretinal hemorrhage, choroidal hemangiomas, choroidal osteoma, and metastatic tumor

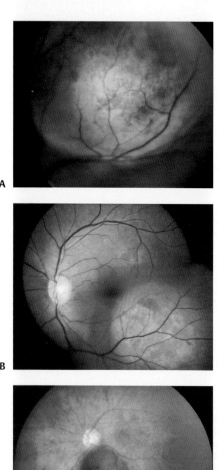

A

B

C

Fig. 11.2 (A) Choroidal melanoma, dome-shaped choroidal mass with moderate intrinsic pigmentation and subretinal fluid (SRF). **(B)** Choroidal melanoma, dome-shaped choroidal mass with mild intrinsic pigmentation. **(C)** Choroidal melanoma: wide-angle colored fundus photograph shows a dark-pigmented, dome-shaped choroidal mass with a smaller elevated nodule on its surface.

◆ Management

Choroidal melanomas can usually be picked up by ultrasound as acoustically hollow, low internal reflectivity solid tumors associated with choroidal excavation. Extraglobular extension is to be ruled out by computed tomography/magnetic resonance imaging (CT/MRI) along with a systemic workup for metastasis. FNAC is contraindicated.

Treatment guidelines are given by ocular melanoma study. Trans-pupillary thermotherapy can be tried when the lesion is away from the disk and the macula and when the lesion is pigmented. Radiotherapy either as plaque or as proton beam irradiation. Local resection can be used when the tumor is small and there is no metastasis. In advanced cases orbital exenteration is the option.

Choroidal Metastasis

Choroidal metastasis is the most common form of intraocular malignancy in adults, with more than 85% of metastatic uveal neoplasms being choroidal. It usually metastasizes from breast cancer in women and lung cancer in men. Less common sites of origin include the prostate, the kidney, the thyroid, and the gastrointestinal tract. Lymphomas and leukemias may also metastasize to the eye and the orbit. Metastases are usually bilateral, multiple lesions.

◆ Presentation

Most patients are asymptomatic or may complain of flashes, floaters, or metamorphopsia. Choroidal metastases are usually seen as solid, flat, plaquelike, mottled, yellow-brown lesions with or without associated serous retinal detachment (**Fig. 11.3**).

◆ Differential Diagnosis

Choroidal hemangioma, choroidal osteoma, exophytic retinal capillary hemangioma, other metastatic carcinomas, posterior scleritis, hemorrhagic RPE detachment, and amelanotic choroidal melanoma

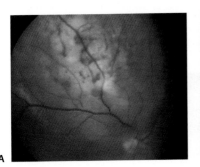 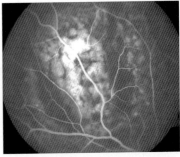

A   B

Fig. 11.3 **(A)** Choroidal metastasis, tallow pink smooth, dome-shaped juxtapapillary choroidal mass. **(B)** Choroidal metastasis. Fundus fluorescein angiography (FFA) shows hypofluorescence in the arterial and early venous phases.

◆ Management

A combined approach in consultation with the medical oncologist and radiation therapist is required. Though chemotherapy may be indicated in many cases, radiation therapy in the form of external beam radiotherapy is usually the more definitive treatment. Early treatment offers the best hope for preserving vision. Surgery is rarely required. If the primary is not readily identifiable, a biopsy may be required prior to treatment.

Cavernous Hemangioma of the Choroid

Cavernous hemangioma is a benign vascular hamartoma. Lesions can be localized or diffuse.

◆ Presentation

Cavernous hemangioma is congenital and asymptomatic until adulthood, at which time it can present with loss of vision. It can present either as an isolated, circumscribed lesion without systemic association or as a diffuse form along with other system or ocular abnormalities (Sturge-Weber syndrome). Circumscribed lesions are seen as an elevated, orange-red, choroidal mass. The diffuse form is seen as a deep red choroid, especially in the posterior pole compared with normal. Other features include fibrous change of RPE, tortuous retinal vessels, cystic change, or serous detachment of retina (**Fig. 11.4**).

◆ Differential Diagnosis

Choroidal nevus, congenital hypertrophy of RPE, combined hamartoma, hyperplasia of RPE, subretinal hemorrhage, choroidal melanoma, choroidal osteoma, and metastatic tumor

◆ Management

Ultrasonography is the common investigation and shows high internal reflectivity. Fundus fluorescein angiography (FFA) shows early hyperfluorescence due to intralesional vessels and later hyperfluorescence of the whole lesion. Indocyanine green (ICG) helps in delineating the lesion better than FFA. MRI helps in diffuse form. Brain and systemic workup to rule out hemangioma in other sites is essential. Histopathology reveals cavernous vascular channels (normal endothelial cells and supporting septa) and capillaries like vessels in the diffuse form.

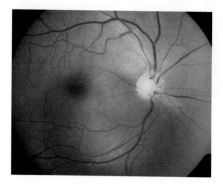

Fig. 11.4 Choroidal hemangioma, dome-shaped, juxtapapillary, reddish-orange choroidal mass.

Treatment options range from photodynamic therapy (PDT), TTT, and irradiation. A neurologist is to be consulted when there is CNS involvement.

Choroidal Osteoma

Choroidal osteoma is found more commonly in women in the second or third decade of life. It may be bilateral in 25% of cases.

◆ Presentation

Choroidal osteoma is seen as a well-demarcated, relatively flat (less than 2 mm thick), yellow-white lesion with clumps of black or brown pigment on the surface, generally near the optic nerve head. The choroidal osteoma impedes the circulation to the overlying retina and may be associated with adjacent RPE atrophy, subretinal neovascularization, subretinal fluid, and subretinal hemorrhage. Forty percent of cases enlarge on long-term follow-up. FFA shows early, patchy hyperfluorescence with intense late staining. Ultrasound shows intense reflectivity from the tumor with acoustic shadowing of the posterior orbital contents. CT scan shows a bonelike signal (**Fig. 11.5**).

◆ Differential Diagnosis

Choroidal nevus, congenital hypertrophy of RPE, combined hamartoma, hyperplasia of RPE, subretinal hemorrhage, choroidal melanoma, choroidal osteoma, and metastatic tumor

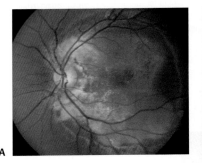

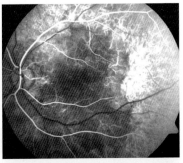

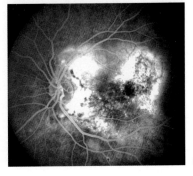

Fig. 11.5 (A) Choroidal osteoma: a well-defined, yellow-orange, placoid juxtapapillary choroidal mass with scalloped margins. **(B)** Choroidal osteoma: fundus fluorescein angiography (FFA) shows diffuse hypofluorescence in the arterial phase. **(C)** Choroidal osteoma: fluorescence intensifies diffusely in the late phase.

A

B

C

◆ Management

Management consists of periodic observation for growth and subretinal neovascularization. Subretinal neovascularization may be treated with laser.

◆ Retinal Pigment Epithelium Tumors

Congenital Hypertrophy of the Retinal Pigment Epithelium

Congenital hypertrophy of the RPE is generally discovered during routine eye screening and has an association with familial adenomatous polyposis and Gardner syndrome (intestinal polyposis, hamartoma of the skeleton, and multiple soft tissue tumors).

◆ Presentation

Lesions are generally seen in the periphery but may occasionally be seen near the disk. They occur as round, well-circumscribed, pigmented lesions, either solitary or multiple with flat or scalloped margins. They have a more distinct border and are darker than the choroidal nevus. There may be depigmented halos within the lesion. Rarely, there are multiple pigmented lesions in the same area (bear-track lesions) (**Fig. 11.6**).

◆ Differential Diagnosis

Chorioretinal scarring, choroidal melanoma, choroidal nevus, melanocytomas of the choroids, hyperplasia of the RPE, posthemorrhage hemosiderin deposits

◆ Management

Screening is performed by a gastroenterologist and is followed up by periodic ocular screening.

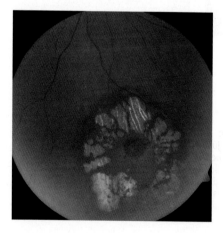

Fig. 11.6 Congenital hypertrophy of the retinal pigment epithelium, fundus photograph of the deeply pigmented, flat, well-circumscribed retinal lesion with characteristic halo and lacunae of depigmentation.

Fig. 11.7 Combined hamartoma of the retinal pigment epithelium and sensory retina, grayish juxtapapillary placoid mass with variable pigmentation and intrinsic vascularity. Note the altered configuration and dragging of retinal vessels with partial obscuration by fibroglial tissue.

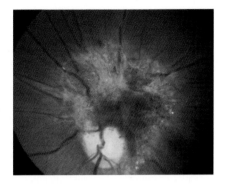

Combined Hamartoma of the Retinal Pigment Epithelium and the Retina

This rare, benign tumor is formed by a hamartomatous overgrowth of several constituents such as the RPE, vascular elements, and glial tissue of the retina to varying degrees.

◆ Presentation

Painless visual loss is the most common symptom. Retinal vascular tortuosity, hyperpigmentation, elevation of the lesion, and an epiretinal membrane may be found. Macular function may be affected secondary to tractional distortion of the retina. Combined hamartomas are most commonly located close to the optic disk followed by the macula and occur least commonly in the peripheral retina. It has been described to occur in neurofibromatosis 1 (**Fig. 11.7**).

◆ Differential Diagnosis

Pigmented fundus tumors, retinoblastoma, choroidal melanoma

◆ Management

Angiography may show vascular changes peripheral to the lesion referred to as "pseudoavascularity." Vitrectomy may be attempted in selected cases.

◆ Retinal Tumors

Retinoblastoma

Retinoblastoma is the most common primary ocular malignancy of childhood, with an incidence of 1 in 15,000 live births. It is caused by mutation in the long arm of chromosome 13q14, which codes for the *RB1* gene, a tumor suppressor gene. It affects the precursor cells that form the inner and outer retinal cells, leading to their malignant transformation.

The mode of inheritance may be heritable (germ-line mutation) or nonheritable (somatic mutation). In heritable mutation one allele of the *RB1* gene is mutated in all cells of the body. A "second hit" affects the second allele, leading to malignant transformation. These patients are predisposed to nonocular tumors such as pinealoma (trilateral retinoblastoma), osteosarcoma, and malignancies of the brain and lung.

◆ Presentation

In bilateral cases presentation is usually around age 1 year and in unilateral cases 2 years. Leukocoria (white pupillary reflex, cat's eye reflex) is the commonest sign. Strabismus, secondary glaucoma, proptosis, and inflammation secondary to tumor necrosis are other signs that can be seen. It can sometimes mimic uveitis in children, presenting as a masquerade syndrome.

Ocular examination by scleral indentation shows a white mass with calcification. It may be intraretinal or an endophytic tumor projecting and seeding into the vitreous or may be exophytic with a subretinal mass and overlying retinal detachment.

Histopathology shows the characteristic Flexner-Wintersteiner rosettes, Homer Wright rosettes, and fleurettes.

◆ Management

A thorough systemic and genetic evaluation is required. Ultrasonography and CT assess tumor size and calcification. MRI detects optic nerve, extraocular extension, and pinealoblastoma. Primary enucleation is advised for unilateral cases with advanced disease and large tumors, longstanding retinal detachments, neovascular glaucoma, or suspicion of optic nerve invasion/extrascleral extension. It is also used in bilateral cases for the more advanced eye. Treatment modalities available include photocoagulation, chemotherapy, transpupillary thermotherapy, cryotherapy for small tumors and external-beam radiotherapy (EBRT), and plaque brachytherapy for medium-sized tumors. EBRT may be associated with development of nonocular tumors in the irradiated field. Chemotherapy may be used prior to other treatment modalities to decrease the size of the tumor or in patients with systemic metastasis.

Capillary Hemangioma

This is a benign hamartoma of the retinal (or optic disk) vasculature, consisting of capillary-like vessels. Though most commonly diagnosed in young adults, it may present in any age. Isolated lesions are not associated with any systemic involvement, whereas von Hippel-Lindau disease presents with bilateral/multiple tumors.

◆ Presentation

Patients can be asymptomatic (diagnosed on family screening) or may present with a decrease in visual acuity. On examination it is seen as a red nodular lesion with tortuosity and dilatation of the feeding artery and draining vein with or without exudation, exudative retinal detachment, rubeosis/neovascular glaucoma, epiretinal membranes, tractional retinal detachment, and vitreous hemorrhage (**Fig. 11.8**).

Fig. 11.8 **(A)** Retinal capillary hemangioma: montage of fundus photographs shows a well-defined, intense, orange-red retinal lesion with prominent feeder and drainage vessels: **(B)** Retinal capillary hemangioma, higher magnification demonstrates intense vascularity of the lesion. **(C)** Optic disc capillary hemangioma: fiery red vascular mass located over the optic nerve head.

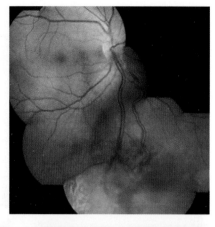

A

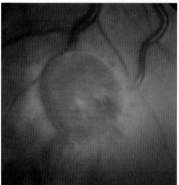

B

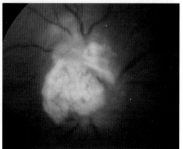

C

◆ Differential Diagnosis

Coats disease, racemose hemangioma, cavernous hemangioma, endophthalmitis, retinoblastoma, astrocytomas, familial exudative vitreoretinopathy (FEVR), sickle cell retinopathy, papilledema, and papillitis

◆ Management

FFA reveals rapid sequential filling of the feeder artery, hemangioma, and vein with extensive late leakage. Leakage into the vitreous may make late images hazy. Systemic disease needs multidisciplinary care. Ocular diseases can be managed with photocoagulation (<3 mm) with confluent burns including the feeder vessels. Cryotherapy, radiotherapy, and excision are other modalities of treatment.

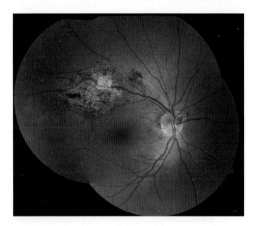

Fig. 11.9 Retinal cavernous hemangioma, fundus photograph shows a grapelike cluster of blood-filled secular spaces in the inner retinal layers.

Retinal Cavernous Hemangioma

This benign hamartoma of the retinal (or optic disk) vasculature consists of large-caliber vessels. It is isolated but can be bilateral in familial cases.

◆ Presentation

Patients are usually asymptomatic or can present with a decrease in visual acuity or floaters. Examination reveals a cluster of intraretinal blood-filled saccules with otherwise normal vasculature with or without vitreous hemorrhage (**Fig. 11.9**).

◆ Differential Diagnosis

Coats disease, racemose hemangioma, capillary hemangioma, endophthalmitis, retinoblastoma, astrocytomas, FEVR, sickle cell retinopathy, papilledema, and papillitis

◆ Management

FFA reveals slow filling that remains hyperfluorescent throughout without leakage. Treatment is usually noninterventional and is usually not necessary.

Fig. 11.10 Retinal arteriovenous malformation: fundus photograph shows abnormally dilated and tortuous retinal vessels with surrounding retinal edema, hemorrhage, and fibrous proliferation.

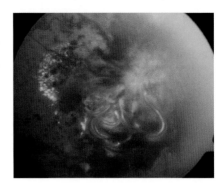

Arteriovenous Malformation

Congenital retinal arteriovenous malformation (AVM) (racemose hemangioma) is an anomalous artery to vein anastomosis.

◆ Presentation

AVM can present as a small, localized vascular communication near the disk, or it can present as a prominent tangle of large, tortuous blood vessels throughout most of the retina. It is usually asymptomatic or can present with a decrease in visual acuity. It can present as part of Wyburn-Mason syndrome (**Fig. 11.10**).

◆ Differential Diagnosis

Coats disease, racemose hemangioma, capillary hemangioma, cavernous hemangioma, endophthalmitis, retinoblastoma, astrocytomas, FEVR, sickle cell retinopathy, papilledema, and papillitis

◆ Management

There is no effective treatment, whereas intracranial AVM can be treated by surgery, radiotherapy, and embolization.

◆ Melanocytoma

Melanocytoma is a benign pigmented tumor. Optic nerve melanocytoma is thought to develop from dendritic uveal melanocytes present in the lamina cribrosa.

◆ Presentation

Tumors may grow deep in the optic nerve parenchyma, in the juxtapapillary choroid, or in the retinal nerve fiber layer. The most common position is on or adjacent to the optic nerve head. They are generally small and black and may grow, but they rarely transform into a malignancy (**Fig. 11.11**).

◆ Differential Diagnosis

Choroidal melanoma and other pigmented tumors

◆ Management

There is no treatment at present to prevent or stop optic nerve melanocytoma growth. Regular ocular examinations are done every 6 to 12 months with dilated ophthalmoscopy and visual-field examinations. The patient should be counseled regarding the risk of vision loss and compression-related vasculopathy and should be monitored for the rare possibility of malignant transformation.

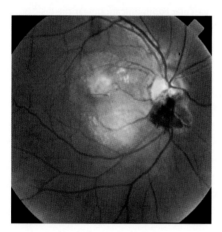

Fig. 11.11 Optic disc melanocytoma: fundus photograph shows a black lesion with irregular margins straddling the inferior aspect of the optic disk with subretinal fluid, exudates, and macular edema.

12 Strabismus

Federico G. Velez, Noa Ela-Dalman, and Arthur L. Rosenbaum

◆ Pseudostrabismus

Pseudostrabismus is a false appearance of strabismus caused by facial characteristics including a flat nasal bridge, eccentric position of the nose, wide epicanthal folds, wide interpupilar distance, and a positive or negative kappa angle (**Fig. 12.1**).

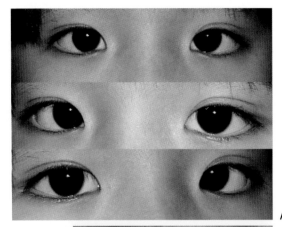

A

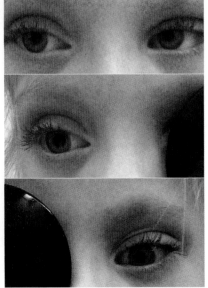

B

Fig. 12.1 **(A)** Pseudoesotropia. **(B)** Angle kappa.

◆ **Presentation**

In patients with pseudostrabismus, the corneal reflex is centered and symmetric bilaterally, and there is no manifest ocular deviation on covert testing. Patients with angle kappa have lateral (negative angle kappa) or medial (positive angle kappa) desentration of the corneal reflex, but there is no manifest deviation on cover testing.

◆ **Differential Diagnosis**

True horizontal or vertical deviation, orbital anomalies, and retinal abnormalities such as macular dragging in patients with retinopathy of prematurity

◆ **Management**

There is no treatment, but follow-up is indicated.

◆ **Infantile Esotropia**

Infantile esotropia is a convergent misalignment of the visual axes manifested by age 6 months (**Fig. 12.2**).

◆ **Presentation**

There is a large-angle esotropia associated with crossed fixation, limitation to abduction, latent nystagmus, pursuit asymmetry, dissociated vertical deviation, and inferior oblique overaction. Amblyopia is rare. Patients usually manifest a low degree of hyperopia.

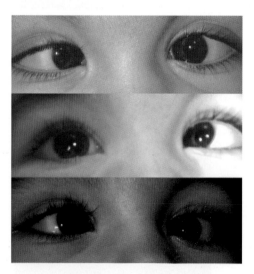

Fig. 12.2 Infantile esotropia.

◆ **Differential Diagnosis**

Sixth-nerve palsy, fibrosis syndrome, early accommodative esotropia, Duane syndrome

◆ **Management**

Bilateral medial rectus muscle recession is the initial usual treatment for infantile esotropia. Bilateral lateral rectus resection is used as a second procedure for undercorrection.

◆ **Accommodative Esotropia**

Convergent deviation of the visual axes is associated with activation of the accommodative reflex. The age of presentation averages 30 months, ranging from 6 months to several years (**Fig. 12.3**).

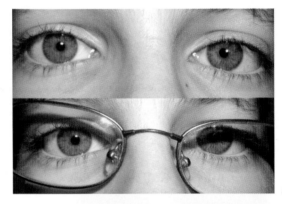

A

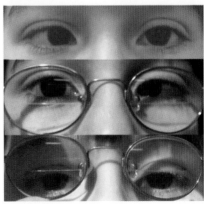

B

Fig. 12.3 **(A)** Refractive esotropia. **(B)** High accommodative convergence esotropia.

◆ Presentation

There is a moderate angle of esotropic deviation averaging 20 to 30 prism diopters. The condition progresses from intermittent to constant esotropia. The angle of deviation at near and at distance is usually similar unless there is a high accommodative convergence/accommodation (AC/A) ratio where the near angle of deviation is larger. The average hyperopic correction is +4.00 diopters. Accommodative esotropia is frequently associated with amblyopia.

Types
◆ *Refractive accommodative esotropia*: High hyperopia and normal accommodative convergence/accommodation. The angles of deviation at near and at distance are similar.
◆ *High accommodative convergence/accommodation esotropia*: Low hyperopia with a high accommodative convergence/accommodation. The angle of deviation at near is larger than the distance deviation.
◆ *Partially accommodative esotropia*: Combination of refractive and nonaccommodative esotropia. Hyperopic correction partially corrects the angle of deviation. Associated with a delay in correction of the accommodative there is an accommodative component.

◆ Differential Diagnosis

Basic nonrefractive nonaccommodative esotropia, infantile esotropia, acute esotropia associated with neurological disorders, cyclic esotropia, spasm of the near synkinetic reflex, nystagmus blockage syndrome

◆ Management

Management consists of full cycloplegic hyperopic correction. Bifocals are prescribed for patients with high accommodative convergence/accommodation if the eyes are straight at distance. Surgery corrects the nonaccommodative or decompensated component of the deviation.

◆ Intermittent Exotropia

Intermittent exotropia is intermittent divergent deviation of the visual axes. It is the most common deviation seen in the pediatric population (**Fig. 12.4**).

◆ Presentation

Onset is usually before age 5 years. The condition is aggravated by fatigue, sickness, and daydreaming. Patients frequently squint to recover alignment and eliminate diplopia, especially with exposure to bright sunlight. At the beginning it is usually seen only at distance, but it may progress to affect the near deviation. Amblyopia is rare. Patients usually manifest good stereopsis at near. Stereopsis at distance can decrease as a result of poor control.

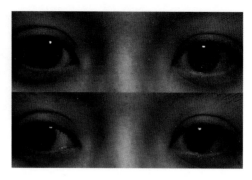

Fig. 12.4   Intermittent exotropia.

Intermittent exotropia can be divided into different types based on the differences between the near and distance angles of deviation:

◆ *Basic type*: The near and the distance angles of deviation are within 10 prism diopters.
◆ *Divergence excess*: The distance angle of deviation is larger than the near angle of deviation by 10 or more prism diopters. In patients with true divergence excess, the difference remains after monocular occlusion; if the difference disappears, the patient has simulated divergence excess.
◆ *Convergence insufficiency*: The angle of exotropia is 10 prism diopters or larger at near than at distance.

◆ **Differential Diagnosis**

Convergence insufficiency, dissociated horizontal deviation

◆ **Management**

Correction of any refractive error. Minus lenses induce accommodation. Patching of the nondeviating eye. Surgical indications include deterioration of control and stereoacuity, diplopia, and visual confusion. Surgery usually consists of bilateral lateral rectus muscle recession in patients with divergence excess, medial rectus muscle resection in convergence insufficiency, and medial rectus muscle resection combined with lateral rectus muscle recession in the basic type of intermittent exotropia.

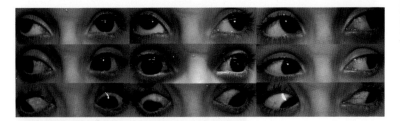

Fig. 12.5 Constant exotropia.

◆ Constant Exotropia

Constant exotropia is usually associated with a decrease in visual acuity, neurological disorder, disruption of binocular vision, previous strabismus surgery, or craniofacial abnormalities (**Fig. 12.5**).

◆ Presentation

Infantile exotropia is a constant exodeviation present before age 6 months, characterized by a large angle of deviation. This condition is usually associated with cerebral palsy, neurological abnormalities, or craniofacial disorders. Sensory exotropia is the result of disruption of binocularity and reduced visual acuity in one eye. Consecutive or secondary exotropia follows previous surgical correction of an exodeviation.

◆ Differential Diagnosis

Cranial third nerve palsy, slipped medial rectus muscle, Duane syndrome, deterioration of an intermittent exotropia

◆ Management

Always rule out neurological disorders, craniofacial syndromes, ocular abnormalities, or any abnormalities in the visual pathway associated with a decrease in vision. Treatment of amblyopia and correction of refractive errors are required. Surgery consists of unilateral or bilateral lateral rectus muscle recession combined with medial rectus muscle resection, depending on the angle of deviation.

◆ Pattern Strabismus

Horizontal change of alignment from the midline when the eyes are moved between a 25-degree upgaze, primary position and a 25-degree downgaze. The incidence of pattern strabismus is ~20%. Two principles have been advanced to explain the cause of the A and V patterns: (1) oblique muscle dysfunction or (2) rectus extraocular muscle overaction or weakness without oblique muscle dysfunction.

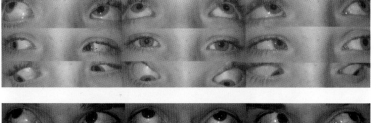

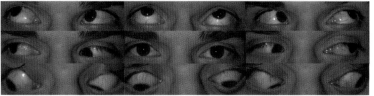

A

B

Fig. 12.6 **(A)** V pattern. **(B)** A pattern.

◆ Presentation

An A pattern is present when the eyes diverge 10 or more prism diopters between downgaze and upgaze. A V pattern is present when the eyes converge 15 or more prism diopters between upgaze and downgaze. Patients with pattern strabismus may present with anomalous head posture, ocular torsion, and overaction or underaction of the oblique muscles (**Fig. 12.6**).

◆ Differential Diagnosis

Craniofacial abnormalities, cyclovertical muscle weakness or overaction, horizontal rectus muscle overaction, pseudo A and V patterns in patients with accommodative esotropia, heterotopic or unstable rectus extraocular muscles

◆ Management

Tendon offsetting surgery of the horizontal rectus muscles is an effective operation for collapsing A and V pattern strabismus not associated with oblique muscle dysfunction with appropriate indications. The medial rectus muscle is always transposed toward the apex of the pattern (up for A pattern and down for V pattern). The lateral rectus muscle is transposed in the opposite direction. In the presence of oblique muscle dysfunction, appropriate oblique muscle weakening procedures are indicated.

◆ Inferior Oblique Overaction

Unilateral or bilateral over-elevation of the adducted eye is observed. Most cases of inferior oblique overaction are primary and not associated with other muscle weakness. Secondary inferior oblique overaction results from weakness of the ip-

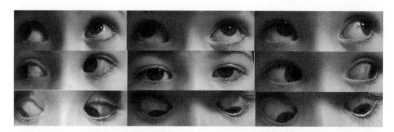

Fig. 12.7 Inferior oblique overaction.

silateral superior oblique muscle (antagonist muscle) or the contralateral superior rectus muscle (yoke muscle). Approximately 65% of patients with infantile esotropia will develop inferior oblique overaction (**Fig. 12.7**).

◆ Presentation

The primary and secondary overreactions of the inferior oblique muscles have different clinical presentations. In primary inferior oblique overaction, onset is usually after 1 year of age. It has the tendency to be bilateral and symmetric. It is frequently associated with a V pattern. Usually, there is neither vertical deviation in the primary position nor excyclotorsion, and the Bielschowsky head tilt test is negative. In contrast, secondary inferior oblique muscle overaction is associated with vertical deviation in the primary position and excyclodeviation and positive Bielchowsky head-tilt test.

◆ Differential Diagnosis

Secondary causes of inferior oblique overaction, heterotopic and unstable rectus extraocular muscles, orbital excyclotorsion, craniosynostosis

◆ Management

The treatment of an overacting inferior oblique muscle is a weakening procedure. Inferior oblique recession is the preferred surgical procedure.

◆ Dissociated Strabismus Complex

Dissociated strabismus complex is an intermittent or manifest deviation of the nonfixing eye. It is a dissociated movement that violates the Hering law; as opposed to true hypertropia, no compensatory movement of the fellow eye is seen when the fixing eye is covered. It may be characterized by one or more of these components: vertical, horizontal, and torsional (**Fig. 12.8**).

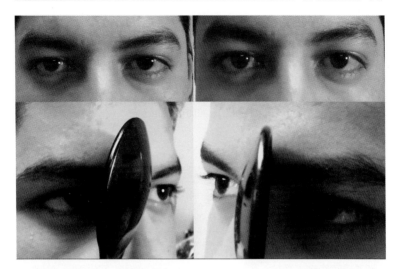

Fig. 12.8 Dissociated vertical deviation.

◆ Presentation

The most common clinical presentation is hyperdeviation, exodeviation, and ex-cyclodeviation of the nonfixing eye. The deviation may be comitant or incomitant, especially if associated with oblique muscle dysfunction. Suppression and visual confusion are common sensorial abnormalities. Other clinical manifestations may include nystagmus, torticollis, and oblique muscle dysfunction.

◆ Differential Diagnosis

Oblique muscle dysfunction

◆ Management

Surgical indications include decompensation, increase in magnitude and frequency, and torticollis. Bilateral surgery is always recommended unless there is strong evidence that the patient will never prefer fixation with the nonfixing eye. Large superior rectus muscle recession is the procedure of choice in patients with comitant deviations. Oblique muscle surgery is indicated in patients with incomitant deviation and overacting oblique muscles.

◆ Third-Nerve Palsy

Third-nerve palsy consists of isolated, multiple, or complete palsy or paresis of the structures innervated by the third cranial nerve

◆ **Presentation (Fig. 12.9)**

Complete third-nerve palsy is characterized by exotropia, hypotropia, and ptosis on the side of the affected nerve. The clinical presentation of the superior third-nerve-division palsy is hypotropia and ptosis of the side ipsilateral to the affected cranial nerve. Inferior third-nerve-division palsy presents with exotropia, hypertropia, and pupillary dilation. Third-nerve palsy can present as an isolated palsy of the medial rectus muscle, inferior rectus muscle, superior rectus muscle, inferior oblique muscle, levator muscle, and pupillary sphincter.

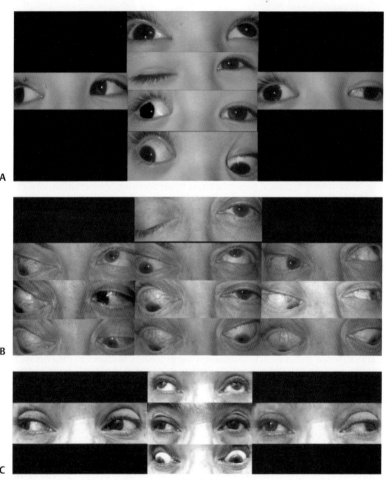

Fig. 12.9 **(A)** Complete third-nerve palsy. **(B)** Superior branch palsy. **(C)** Isolated medial rectus palsy.

Third-nerve palsy with pupillary involvement can be a clinical emergency. Workup is required to rule out supratentorial mass or basilar aneurysm. In cases without pupillary involvement one is required to rule out ischemia, compression, inflammatory process, neuropathy, and myoneuropathy.

In patients with congenital third-nerve palsy and those with palsy secondary to lesions in the cavernous sinus, aneurysms, meningioma, and trauma can develop aberrant innervation to the ciliary ganglia, levator muscle, and extraocular muscles.

◆ Differential Diagnosis

Restriction, Graves ophthalmopathy, orbital fracture, fibrosis of the extraocular muscles, myotoxicity, myasthenia, chronic progressive external ophthalmoplegia, congenital absence of the extraocular muscles

◆ Management

Cases secondary to diabetes, hypertension, or migraine usually completely resolve in 1 to 12 weeks. Nonsurgical treatment includes occlusion, prisms, and botulinum toxin. Surgical treatment depends on the deviation in the primary position and muscle function. Weakening of the ipsilateral lateral rectus muscle is necessary in cases of complete third-nerve palsy. Surgical treatment is challenging in cases with complete third-nerve palsy or when several extraocular muscles are affected.

◆ Fourth-Nerve Palsy (Superior Oblique Palsy)

Fourth-nerve palsy is a congenital or acquired paralysis of the superior oblique muscle. Congenital cases may be secondary to abnormalities of the tendon, including laxity, absence, or anomalous insertion. Acquired causes include trauma, compression, ischemia, infiltration, and hemorrhage. Tumors should always be suspected in patients with acquired bilateral superior oblique palsy (**Fig. 12.10**).

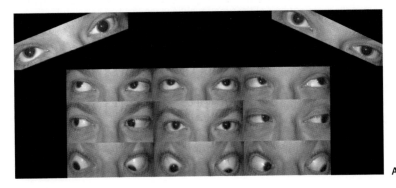

A

Fig. 12.10 **(A)** Unilateral superior oblique palsy. (*Continued on page 350*)

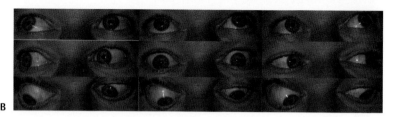

B

Fig. 12.10 (*Continued*) **(B)** Bilateral superior oblique palsy.

◆ Presentation

Unilateral superior oblique palsy is characterized by hypertropia in adduction, positive head-tilt test, V pattern, and excyclotropia. Other clinical signs include positive three-step test, large fusional amplitudes, and facial asymmetry with hypoplasia contralateral to the side of the palsy. Bilateral palsies are characterized by reverse hypertropia, positive head tilt test, V pattern, and excyclotropia larger than 10 degrees. Patients with symmetrical bilateral superior oblique palsy usually have little or no vertical deviation in the primary position.

◆ Differential Diagnosis

Skew deviation, Graves ophthalmopathy, and primary inferior oblique overaction

◆ Management

Many patients are able to compensate for the vertical deviation, especially those with long-standing superior oblique palsy. Surgical treatment depends on the amount of deviation in the primary position, the size of deviation in the vertical plane (upgaze and downgaze), and the ipsilateral gaze (field of action away from the affected superior oblique muscle) and degree of dysfunction of the superior oblique muscle. Patients with less than 15 prism diopters of vertical deviation in the primary position can be treated with surgery on one muscle. In patients with significant excyclotorsion, superior oblique muscle tucking or anterior lateralization of the anterior fibers of the superior oblique tendon may be helpful.

◆ Sixth-Nerve Palsy (Lateral Rectus Muscle Palsy)

Sixth-nerve palsy results in paralysis of the lateral rectus muscle.

◆ Presentation

Incomitant esotropia is larger in the abducted field of action of the affected lateral rectus muscle. Etiology includes trauma, compression, and infection. Newborns may present with a temporary paralysis (**Fig. 12.11**).

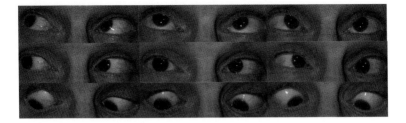

Fig. 12.11   Sixth-nerve palsy.

◆ Differential Diagnosis

Duane syndrome, fibrosis of the extraocular muscles, Möbius syndrome, inflammatory disorders, myasthenia gravis, infantile esotropia, horizontal gaze palsy, divergence palsy, and previous extraocular muscle surgery

◆ Management

Observe for the first 6 months. Complete resolution is seen in up to 90% of cases within the first 6 months after onset. Cases secondary to migraine and vascular lesion have the tendency to recur. Pediatric patients with a persistent palsy beyond 3 months and adult cases in whom the angle of deviation increases and those who develop neurological deficits require reevaluation. Rule out giant cell arthritis in patients older than 50 years.

Nonsurgical treatment includes occlusion, treatment of amblyopia, prism, and botulinum toxin

Surgical approach depends on the following variables: residual function of the lateral rectus muscle, ocular rotations, saccades, forced duction and forced generation test, deviation in primary position, anomalous head posture. Lateral rectus muscle resection in patients with residual lateral rectus muscle function and vertical rectus muscle transposition in patients with complete lateral rectus muscle palsy are the procedures of choice in these patients. Many cases require ipsilateral medial rectus muscle recession.

◆ Duane Syndrome

Duane syndrome involves misinnervation of the lateral rectus muscle associated with absence or hypoplasia of the sixth cranial nerve. Most frequently fibers of the third cranial nerve going to the medial rectus muscle are redirected to the lateral rectus muscle. The lack of normal innervation from the sixth nerve to the lateral rectus muscle results in limitation of abduction. The misinnervation of the lateral rectus muscle with fibers from the third cranial nerve results in abnormal contraction of the lateral rectus muscle in attempted adduction (**Fig. 12.12**).

◆ Presentation

Duane syndrome occurs more frequently in females than in males, and it most commonly involves the left eye. The majority of patients with Duane syndrome have straight eyes. Bilateral involvement is seen in 20% of the cases. The most characteristic clinical presentations are unilateral limitation of abduction associated with globe retraction and narrowing of the palpebral fissure in attempted adduc-

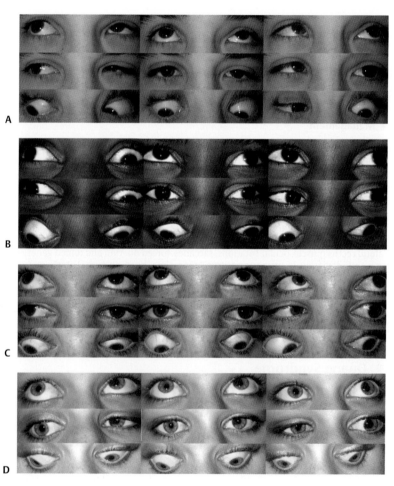

Fig. 12.12 **(A)** Duane type 1. **(B)** Duane type 2. **(C)** Duane type 3. **(D)** Bilateral Duane.

tion. Other manifestations include anomalous head posture, limitation to adduction, strabismus in the primary position, and anomalous vertical movements.

Classically three types of Duane syndrome have been described. Type 1 is characterized by esotropia in the primary position with limitation to abduction, globe retraction, and palpebral fissure narrowing in adduction. Type II is characterized by exotropia in the primary position and limitation to adduction. Type III is characterized by exotropia or esotropia with limitation to abduction and adduction.

Duane syndrome may be associated with systemic manifestations, including hearing loss, Klippel-Feil syndrome, Goldenhar syndrome, Holt-Oram syndrome, atrial septal defect, hand anomalies, crocodile tears, and cleft palate.

◆ Differential Diagnosis

Sixth-nerve palsy, infantile esotropia, fibrosis of the extraocular muscles, congenital misinnervation syndromes

◆ Management

Indications for surgery include strabismus in the primary position, diplopia, and anomalous head posture. The surgical approach is based on the alignment in the primary position, limitation to ocular rotations, severity of retraction, and the presence of anomalous vertical movements. In general, medial rectus recession and vertical rectus muscle transpositions are the procedures of choice in patients with esotropia in the primary position. Lateral rectus muscle recession is the procedure of choice in patients with exotropia in the primary position. Y splitting of the lateral rectus muscle may be added in patients with up/downshoot.

◆ Brown Syndrome

Brown syndrome is a congenital or acquired limitation to elevation in adduction.

◆ Presentation

The patient's inability to elevate the eye in adduction is worse than in the midline or abduction. There is a V pattern, minimal superior oblique overaction, widening of the palpebral fissure in adduction, overdepression in adduction ("downshoot" of the affected eye in adduction), anomalous head posture, and hypotropia of the affected eye. The inability to elevate the eye in adduction on forced duction testing is confirmatory of Brown syndrome. Patients with acquired Brown syndrome may present with a trochlear tenderness and click (**Fig. 12.13**).

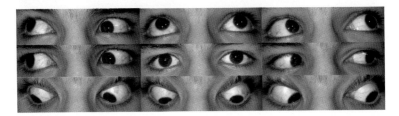

Fig. 12.13 Brown syndrome.

◆ Differential Diagnosis

Monocular elevation deficiency, fibrosis of the extraocular muscles, inferior oblique muscle palsy, orbital floor fracture, thyroid ophthalmopathy, and heterotopic or dynamic displacement of the rectus muscles

◆ Management

Acquired Brown syndrome is frequently inflammatory. Spontaneous resolution is common. Medical treatment includes local and systemic corticosteroids. Indications for surgical correction include disruption of the binocular vision in a congenital Brown syndrome, anomalous head posture, hypotropia in primary position, diplopia, and downshoot in adduction. Ipsilateral superior oblique muscle weakening is the procedure of choice in Brown syndrome.

◆ Monocular Elevation Deficiency

Monocular elevation deficiency is a supranuclear or infranuclear limitation to elevation frequently associated with ptosis or pseudoptosis (**Fig. 12.14**).

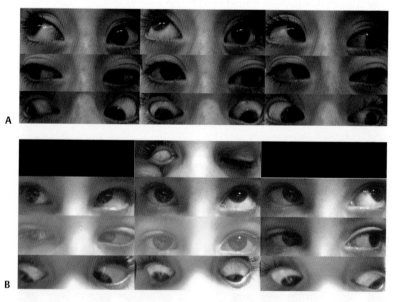

Fig. 12.14   **(A)** Monocular elevation deficiency. **(B)** Supranuclear palsy.

Presentation

Limitation to elevation in the primary position and lateral gaze is greater in upgaze. Ptosis or pseudoptosis is present in ~50% of the cases. Pupillary abnormalities are usually seen in acquired cases. An anomalous chin elevation head posture is frequently seen. Congenital causes include supranuclear abnormalities, superior rectus muscle weakness, and inferior rectus muscle restriction. Acquired monocular elevation deficiency may result from central nervous system tumor, inflammation, infection, or stroke.

Differential Diagnosis

Brown syndrome, Duane syndrome, fibrosis of the extraocular muscles, third-nerve palsy, Graves disease, myasthenia gravis, orbital floor fracture, myositis, myotoxicity, cerebellar tumors

Management

Management consists of treatment of amblyopia. The goal of surgery is alignment in the primary position and improvement of elevation. The surgical approach is based on the presence of restriction, weakness, or a combination of both factors and includes inferior rectus recession, superior rectus muscle resection, or horizontal rectus muscles transposition.

◆ Graves Ophthalmopathy

Proptosis, eyelid retraction, and extraocular muscle motility disorders associated with hyperthyroidism or inflammatory disease of the thyroid gland are characteristic of Graves ophthalmopathy. Many patients are euthyroid at presentation (**Fig. 12.15**).

Presentation

Patients present with proptosis, conjunctival injection, chemosis and lid edema, eyelid retraction, and lid lag on downgaze. Graves ophthalmopathy occurs more frequently in women (3:1), with two peaks, one at age 40 and one at age 60. Restriction to ocular movements more commonly affects the inferior rectus muscle,

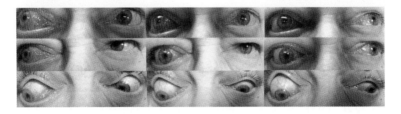

Fig. 12.15 Graves disease.

followed by the medial rectus muscle, superior rectus muscle, lateral rectus muscle, and the oblique muscles. Orbital imaging demonstrates the typical extraocular muscle enlargement sparing the tendons at the muscle insertion.

◆ Differential Diagnosis

Orbital inflammatory disease, myositis, lymphoma, sarcoidosis, amyloidosis, orbital tumors, vascular lesions, high myopia

◆ Management

Treatment of the hyperthyroidism. Systemic steroids, immunosuppressants, and radiation therapy are used during the acute phase of the disease. Strabismus surgery should be delayed until the inflammatory phase is resolved and the strabismus is stable. The primary surgical approach includes recession of the extraocular muscle involved.

◆ Myasthenia Gravis

This is an autoimmune disorder, more common in women, characterized by weakness and fatigability of striated muscles (**Fig. 12.16**).

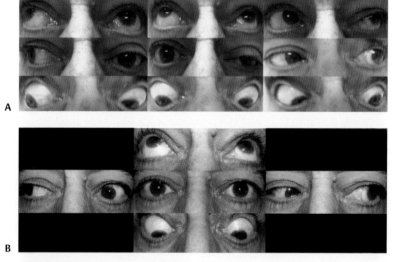

Fig. 12.16   **(A)** Myasthenia gravis. **(B)** Myasthenia gravis post ice-pack test.

◆ **Presentation**

Myasthenia gravis can be congenital, juvenile, or adult onset. Ocular myasthenia is localized to the extraocular muscles. Systemic myasthenia involves other skeletal and bulbar musculature. The most common ocular manifestation is ptosis followed by underaction of the extraocular muscles. Pharmacological testing with anticholinesterases is the standard diagnostic test for myasthenia.

◆ **Differential Diagnosis**

Chronic external ophthalmoplegia, medications interfering with neuromuscular transmission, central nervous system tumors

◆ **Management**

Management includes thymectomy, oral anticholinesterases, steroids, prism, botulinum toxin, and strabismus surgery.

◆ **Congenital Fibrosis of the Extraocular Muscles**

Ptosis and restricted limitation of ocular rotations secondary to myopathic and neurogenic abnormalities lead to fibrosis of the extraocular muscles. The condition may include one or multiple extraocular muscles. Gene mutations have been identified for CFEOM type 1 (*KIF21A* gene), CFEOM type 2 (*PHOX2A*), and CFEOM type 3 (*FEOM3*) (**Fig. 12.17**).

◆ **Presentation**

Presentation includes unilateral or bilateral blepharoptosis, fibrosis of the extraocular muscles, chin-up posture, limitation to elevation and horizontal ocular rotations, and absence of Bell phenomenon. The condition is sometimes associated with optic nerve and retinal abnormalities.

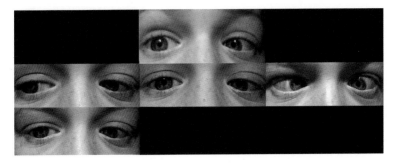

Fig. 12.17 Fibrosis syndrome.

◆ Differential Diagnosis

Monocular elevation deficiency, third-nerve palsy, Brown syndrome, chronic pro-gressive external ophthalmoplegia, Möbius syndrome, myasthenia gravis, orbital fracture, atypical Duane syndrome

◆ Management

Management consists of treatment of amblyopia and lubricants to avoid corneal dryness due to poor Bell's phenomenon and eyelid closure. Strabismus surgery consists of large recession of involved muscle.

13 Neuro-Ophthalmology

Soosan Jacob and Amar Agarwal

◆ Cranial Nerve Palsies

Isolated Oculomotor (Third) Nerve Palsy

The common causes of oculomotor nerve palsy include neoplasms, trauma, aneurysms, ischemic lesions, and ophthalmoplegic migraine. Oculomotor nerve palsy could be congenital due to a hereditary cause. The mode of transmission could be either autosomal dominant or recessive.

◆ Presentation

Total third-nerve paresis may be central, sparing the pupil, or peripheral with pupillary involvement. If the pupil is spared, the most likely cause is a vascular lesion. If the pupil is involved, it is most likely due to an aneurysm. The patient has a large exotropia with hypotropia. A fixed, dilated pupil is seen. On attempted adduction, the eye intorts as the superior oblique would be normal. One can also get partial paresis as the third nerve divides into superior and inferior division. If the superior division of the third nerve is involved, generally other cranial nerves are also involved. One can get an isolated involvement of the inferior division of the third cranial nerve (**Figs. 13.1A,B,C**).

Nuclear Third-Nerve Paresis
This is extremely rare. Following are the important points about this lesion:

◆ Each superior rectus is innervated by the contralateral third-nerve nucleus; if there was nuclear third-nerve palsy on one side then there would be a paresis of the contralateral superior rectus.
◆ Both levator palpebrae superioris are innervated by one subnuclear structure, the central caudal nucleus. Therefore, nuclear third-nerve palsy leads to bilateral ptosis.

Third-Nerve Fascicle Syndromes
In these cases the third nerve has already left the nucleus, so the lesions affect only one side. There are various syndromes that can occur, depending on the site of lesion. They are due generally to an ischemic, infiltrative (tumor) or rarely to an inflammatory lesion.

Nothnagel Syndrome
In this case the lesion is in the area of the superior cerebellar peduncle. As the lesion involves the superior cerebellar peduncle the patient has an ipsilateral third-nerve paresis with cerebellar ataxia.

Benedikt Syndrome
In Benedikt syndrome the lesion is in the area of the red nucleus. This leads to contralateral hemitremor with ipsilateral third-nerve paresis.

Claude Syndrome
This syndrome has features of both Nothnagel and Benedikt syndromes.

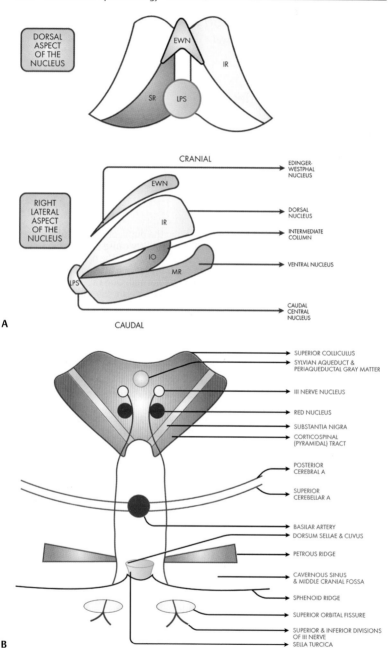

DORSAL
ASPECT
OF THE
NUCLEUS

EWN

IR

SR LPS

CRANIAL

→ EDINGER-
WESTPHAL
NUCLEUS

RIGHT
LATERAL
ASPECT
OF THE
NUCLEUS

EWN

IR

→ DORSAL
NUCLEUS

→ INTERMEDIATE
COLUMN

IO

MR

→ VENTRAL NUCLEUS

LPS

→ CAUDAL
CENTRAL
NUCLEUS

A

CAUDAL

→ SUPERIOR COLLICULUS
→ SYLVIAN AQUEDUCT &
PERIAQUEDUCTAL GRAY MATTER

→ III NERVE NUCLEUS

→ RED NUCLEUS

→ SUBSTANTIA NIGRA
→ CORTICOSPINAL
(PYRAMIDAL) TRACT

→ POSTERIOR
CEREBRAL A

→ SUPERIOR
CEREBELLAR A

→ BASILAR ARTERY
→ DORSUM SELLAE & CLIVUS

→ PETROUS RIDGE

→ CAVERNOUS SINUS
& MIDDLE CRANIAL FOSSA

→ SPHENOID RIDGE

→ SUPERIOR ORBITAL FISSURE

→ SUPERIOR & INFERIOR DIVISIONS
OF III NERVE
→ SELLA TURCICA

B

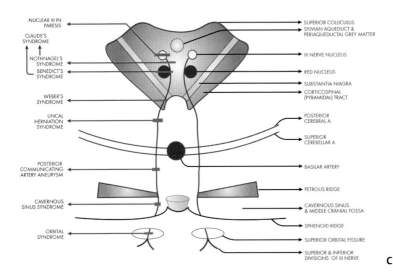

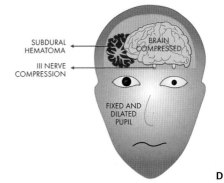

Fig. 13.1 (A) Oculomotor nerve nuclei. (B) Oculomotor nerve anatomy. (C) Syndromes of the oculomotor nerve. (D) Hutchinson pupil. (E) Posterior communicating artery aneurysm.

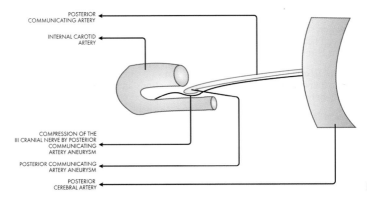

Weber Syndrome

In Weber syndrome the lesion is in the area of the corticospinal (pyramidal) tract. This leads to an ipsilateral third-nerve paresis with contralateral hemiparesis.

Uncal Herniation Syndrome

As the third cranial nerve goes toward the cavernous sinus, it rests on the edge of the tentorium cerebelli. A supratentorial space-occupying mass located anywhere in or above this cerebral hemisphere may cause a downward displacement and herniation of the uncus across the tentorial edge, thereby compressing the third nerve. This leads to a dilated and fixed pupil. This is called the Hutchinson pupil and is the first indication that altered consciousness is due to a space-occupying intracranial lesion (**Fig. 13.1D**).

Posterior Communicating Artery Aneurysm

As the third cranial nerve moves toward the cavernous sinus, it travels alongside the posterior communicating artery. If there is an aneurysm of the posterior communicating artery it can lead to compression of the third nerve. This leads to an isolated third-nerve paresis with the pupil becoming involved (**Fig. 13.1E**).

Cavernous Sinus Syndrome

In cavernous sinus syndrome, there would be third-nerve paresis with involvement of other nerves, such as cranial nerves IV, V, and VI. These patients have painful ophthalmoplegia, possibly due to trauma, neoplasms, aneurysms, or inflammations. This syndrome can lead to aberrant regeneration of the third cranial nerve.

Orbital Syndrome

Proptosis can be an early sign. The fifth cranial nerve can also be involved, but this would involve only the ophthalmic division.

Pupil-Sparing Isolated Third-Nerve Paresis

The pupillomotor fibers travel in the third nerve in the outer layers and are therefore closer to the nutrient blood supply enveloping the nerve. This is the reason why the pupillomotor fibers are generally spared in ischemic third-nerve paresis but are affected in compressive lesions such as tumors. Ocular myasthenia can mimic a pupil-sparing third-nerve palsy, so one can perform the Tensilon test to differentiate the two.

◆ Differential Diagnosis

Other causes of paralytic and restrictive squints

◆ Management

Occlusion

One can occlude the paretic eye until the healing occurs and the third-nerve paresis is cured.

Medical Treatment

One can give the patient multivitamin injections and tablets and treat the cause, like diabetes or hypertension.

Surgical Treatment

The surgical management of a complete third-nerve paralysis is a difficult job. At the very best, the surgeon will succeed only in moving the paretic eye into the primary position without restoring adduction, elevation, or depression to a significant degree. A very good method to treat this condition is to do a tenotomy of the lateral rectus and the superior oblique combined with a transposition of the vertical recti muscles to the insertion of the medial rectus muscle. Even though the treated eye will continue to be immobile, it will at least be centered, and this operation should be considered, especially in patients who fixate with the paralyzed eye. For the ptosis one should perform a frontalis muscle sling operation. This can be done as a second step.

If the patient has a partial palsy with slight medial rectus movement one can perform a maximal recession of the lateral rectus muscle (at least 12 mm) and resection of the medial rectus (at least 7 mm) with upward transposition of the tendons in case of an associated hypotropia. This may restore a small but useful field of vision even though double vision will persist in upward and downward gaze.

Isolated Trochlear (Fourth) Nerve Palsy

The trochlear nerve (fourth cranial nerve) is the thinnest and also has the longest intracranial course (~75 mm). This is the only cranial nerve that emerges from the dorsal aspect of the brainstem. It is also the only cranial nerve that crosses completely to the opposite side. In other words, the trochlear nerve arises from the contralateral nucleus.

◆ Presentation

Depending on the level of the lesion, various syndromes can occur as a result of damage to the trochlear nerve. They are as follows (**Figs. 13.2A,B**):

Nuclear Fascicular Syndrome
It is difficult to distinguish between nuclear and fascicular lesions because of the short course of the fascicles within the midbrain. The nuclear fascicular syndrome could be due to hemorrhage trauma or demyelination. It is seen with contralateral Horner syndrome because the sympathetic pathways descend through the dorsolateral tegmentum of the midbrain adjacent to the trochlear fascicles.

Subarachnoid Space Syndrome
As the fourth nerve emerges from the dorsal surface of the brainstem, it can be injured easily. When bilateral fourth-nerve palsies occur, the site of injury is likely to be in the anterior medullary velum. Contracoup forces transmitted to the brainstem by the free tentorial edge may injure the nerves at this site. Other causes could be tumors, such as pinealoma or tentorial meningiomas.

Cavernous Sinus Syndrome
If the lesion is in the cavernous sinus, other cranial nerves in close association with the fourth cranial nerve can also be involved.

Orbital Syndrome
In orbital syndrome other cranial nerves close to the fourth cranial nerve are also involved. Other orbital signs such as proptosis, chemosis, and conjunctival injection are also seen. This could be due to trauma, inflammation, or tumors.

Isolated Fourth-Nerve Palsy
Isolated fourth-nerve palsy could be due to a congenital cause or it could be acquired. The features of a fourth-nerve palsy are as follows:

◆ *Hyperdeviation*: The involved eye is higher as a result of the weakness of the superior oblique muscle. One should perform the Bielschowsky head-tilting test because when the head is tilted toward the ipsilateral shoulder the hyperdeviation becomes more obvious.

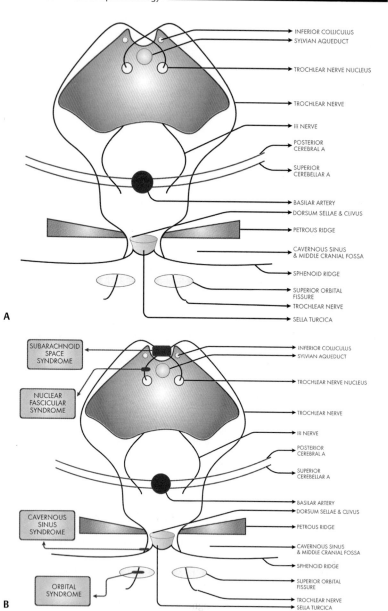

INFERIOR COLLICULUS
SYLVIAN AQUEDUCT

TROCHLEAR NERVE NUCLEUS

TROCHLEAR NERVE

III NERVE

POSTERIOR
CEREBRAL A

SUPERIOR
CEREBELLAR A

BASILAR ARTERY
DORSUM SELLAE & CLIVUS
PETROUS RIDGE

CAVERNOUS SINUS
& MIDDLE CRANIAL FOSSA

SPHENOID RIDGE

SUPERIOR ORBITAL
FISSURE
TROCHLEAR NERVE

SELLA TURCICA

A

SUBARACHNOID
SPACE
SYNDROME

INFERIOR COLLICULUS
SYLVIAN AQUEDUCT

TROCHLEAR NERVE NUCLEUS

NUCLEAR
FASCICULAR
SYNDROME

TROCHLEAR NERVE

III NERVE

POSTERIOR
CEREBRAL A

SUPERIOR
CEREBELLAR A

BASILAR ARTERY
DORSUM SELLAE & CLIVUS
PETROUS RIDGE

CAVERNOUS
SINUS
SYNDROME

CAVERNOUS SINUS
& MIDDLE CRANIAL FOSSA

SPHENOID RIDGE

ORBITAL
SYNDROME

SUPERIOR ORBITAL
FISSURE

TROCHLEAR NERVE
SELLA TURCICA

B

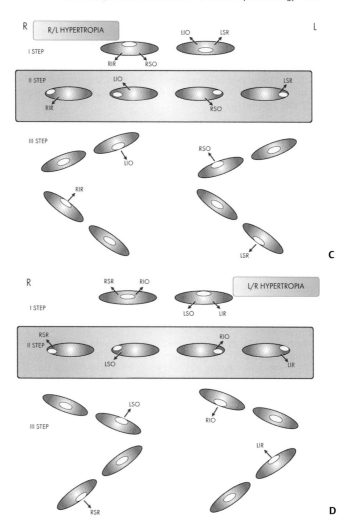

Fig. 13.2 **(A)** Trochlear nerve anatomy. **(B)** Lesions of the trochlear nerve. **(C)** Biel-schowsky's head tilting test for R/L (right/left) hypertropia. **(D)** Bielschowsky's head tilting test for L/R (left/right) hypertropia. LIO, left inferior oblique; LSR, left superior rectus; RIR, right superior rectus; RSO, right superior oblique.

◆ *Ocular movements*: Depression is limited in adduction. Intorsion is also limited. Homonymous vertical diplopia occurs on looking downward. Usually the vision is single as long as the eyes look above the horizontal plane. The patient especially notices diplopia when walking down the stairs.

◆ *Abnormal head posture*: To avoid diplopia, the head takes an abnormal posture toward the action of the superior oblique muscle (i.e., the face is slightly turned to the opposite side, the chin is depressed, and the head is tilted toward the opposite shoulder).

Checking Fourth-Nerve Function in the Setting of a Third-Nerve Paresis

The problem with checking the fourth cranial nerve function if a patient also has a third cranial nerve paresis is that the involved eye cannot be adducted well because of third cranial nerve involvement. Because the eye cannot be adducted, one cannot test the vertical action (depression) of the superior oblique muscle.

To solve this problem, first of all we should note a limbal or conjunctival landmark, such as a blood vessel or pterygium. The patient, on being asked to look down, will not be able to do so as the eye is abducted and not adducted (because of third-nerve involvement). But the eye will intort as the superior oblique muscle works. We should then check from the conjunctival landmark if the eye is intorting. If the conjunctival landmark is moving, the eye is intorting, and that means the fourth nerve is intact.

Bielschowsky Head-Tilting Test

The Bielschowsky head-tilting test can diagnose which muscle is paralyzed. Let us first look at a case of R/L hypertropia in which the right eye is at a higher position than the left eye (**Figs. 13.2C,D**).

R/L Hypertropia

If the patient has an R/L hypertropia, then it could mean that the right eye is hypertropic, in which case the depressors are paralyzed like the right inferior rectus (RIR) or the right superior oblique (RSO). It could also mean that the right eye is in the normal position but the left eye is hypotropic. This could be due to the elevators of the left eye being paralyzed like the left inferior oblique (LIO) and the left superior rectus (LSR). This is the first step of the test. We have thus narrowed down the diagnosis to four of the extraocular muscles.

Now we perform the second step of the test. In this we ask the patient to perform dextroversion or levoversion. This means we ask the patient to look to the right and to the left. If we ask the patient to look to the right, the right eye could be higher than the left eye. If the right eye is higher on dextroversion, then it could mean that the RIR is involved or it could mean that the left eye is hypotropic. This would be due to an LIO paralysis. In levoversion if the right eye is higher, it could be due to an RSO paralysis. Alternately, it could mean that the left eye is hypotropic, and this would be due to LSR paralysis. Thus we have narrowed down the muscles from four to two.

Finally, we perform the third step in which we tilt the patient's head to the right and then to the left. If we tilt the head to the right, the right eye will intort and the left eye will extort. This is because nervous impulses will be sent from the semicircular canals to keep the eyes in a straight position. *Remember, the superiors are intorters.* So if the right eye intorts, it means the superiors in that eye (RSR and RSO) work, and if the left eye extorts it means the inferiors of that eye (LIO and LIR) work. When this happens in the right eye the RIR will not be used at all because it is an extorter, and in the right eye extortion is not taking place. But in the left eye, extortion will take place and the LIO and LIR will work. Now as the LIO is paralyzed, only the LIR acts in that eye. As a balance is not be maintained between these two muscles, the left eye moves down as the LIR is also a depressor. Thus, one can diagnose a patient with LIO paralysis.

If we ask the patient to tilt the head to the left, the left eye will intort and the right eye will extort. In the right eye the extorters will be the RIR and right inferior oblique (RIO). Now the RIR is paralyzed, and so only the RIO will work and the right eye will move upward.

Similarly, we can differentiate between the RSO and the LSR in the third step. If we tilt the head to the right the right eye will intort, and the muscles that will work are the RSO and RSR. Because the RSO is paralyzed only the RSR will work, and the right eye will move upward.

If we tilt the head to the left, the left eye will intort, and the muscles that will work are the LSR and LSO. If the LSR is paralyzed the LSO will work and the left eye will move down.

L/R Hypertropia

If we now work on the same principle and get the muscle involved in an L/R hypertropia. If the patient has an L/R hypertropia, then it indicates that the depressors are paralyzed like the LIR and the LSO. It could also mean that the left eye is in the normal position but the right eye is hypotropic. This could be due to the elevators of the right eye, namely, the RIO and the RSR, being paralyzed. This is the first step of the test. Of the extraocular muscles we have narrowed the diagnosis of extraocular muscle paralysis to four muscles, the two depressors of the right eye, or the two elevators of the left eye.

Next, we perform the second step of the test. In this we ask the patient to perform dextroversion or levoversion. This means we ask the patient to look to the right and to the left. If we ask the patient to look to the right, the left eye could be higher than the right eye. If the left eye is higher on dextroversion, then it could mean that the LSO is involved or it could mean that the right eye is hypotropic. This would be due to an RSR paralysis. In levoversion if the left eye is higher it could be due to an LIR paralysis. Alternately, it could mean that the right eye is hypotropic, which would be due to RIO paralysis. Thus we have narrowed down the muscles from four to two.

Finally, we perform the third step, in which we tilt the patient's head to the right and then to the left. If we tilt the head to the left, the right eye will extort and the left eye will intort. This is because nervous impulses will be sent from the semicircular canals to keep the eyes in a straight position. Remember that the superiors are intorters. So if the right eye extorts, it means the inferiors in that eye (LIO and LIR) work, and if the left eye intorts it means the superiors of that eye (RSO and RSR) work. When this happens, in the left eye the LSO and LSR should work. Now the LSO is paralyzed and so cannot work. Therefore, only the LSR will work to intort the eye. And because the balance will not be maintained between these two muscles, the left eye will move up given that the LSR is also an elevator. Thus one can diagnose the case of LSO.

If we ask the patient to tilt the head to the right, the left eye will extort and the right eye will intort. In the right eye the intorters will be the RSR and RSO. Since the RSR is paralyzed, only the RSO will work. This will cause the right eye to move downward.

Similarly, we can differentiate between the LIR and the RIO in the third step. If we tilt the head to the left, the right eye will extort and the muscles that will work are the RIO and RIR. Because the RIO is paralyzed only the RIR will work to extort the eye, thereby moving the right eye downward.

If we tilt the head to the right, the left eye will extort and the muscles that will work are the LIR and LIO. If the LIR is paralyzed the LIO will work and the left eye will move up.

◆ Differential Diagnosis

Primary inferior oblique over action

◆ Management

Occlusion
When double vision is restricted to downward gaze as in fourth-nerve paralysis, one can occlude the lower third of the spectacle lens in front of the paretic eye with semiopaque tape. This can be performed if the medical condition is not suitable for surgery.

Surgery
Depending on the class of superior oblique (SO) paralysis, the surgical treatment is based on the class of paralysis as described by von Noorden (**Table 13.1**).

Table 13.1   Treatment of Superior Oblique Paralysis Based on Class

Class of SO Paralysis	Surgical Treatment
Class 1	Inferior oblique myectomy
Class 2	Superior oblique tuck (8–12 mm); recession of contralateral inferior rectus as a secondary procedure
Class 3	Hypertropia of < 25 prism diopters; inferior oblique myectomy; if there is hypertropia of < 25 prism diopters; inferior oblique myectomy with superior oblique tuck
Class 4	As in class 3 plus recession of ipsilateral superior rectus or contralateral inferior rectus
Class 5	Superior oblique tuck with recession of ipsilateral superior rectus or recession of contralateral inferior rectus
Class 6	As in classes 1–5 but bilateral surgery
Class 7	Explore trochlea

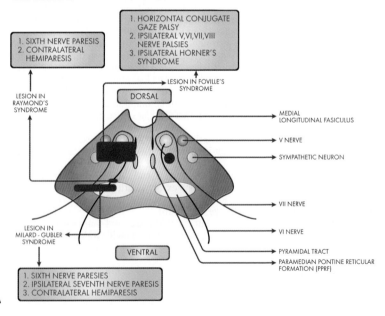

A

Abducens (Sixth) Nerve Palsy

The abducent (sixth cranial) nerve is a small, entirely motor nerve that supplies the lateral rectus of the eyeball (**Figs. 13.3A,B**).

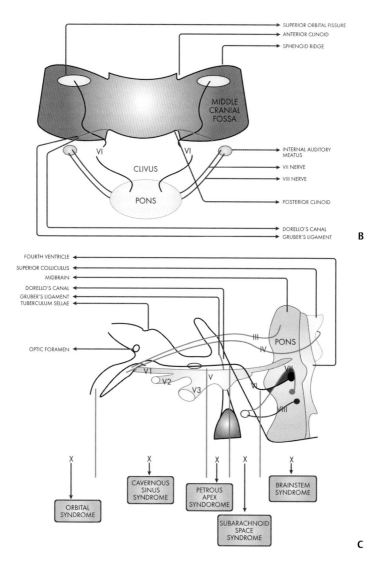

Fig. 13.3 **(A)** Nucleus of the abducent nerve and the brainstem syndromes. **(B)** Course of the abducent nerve. **(C)** Lesions of the abducent nerve.

◆ Presentation

In the primary position the eyeball is converged because of the unopposed action of the medial rectus muscle. Abduction is limited due to weakness of the lateral rectus muscle. Uncrossed horizontal diplopia occurs, which becomes worse toward the action of the paralyzed muscle. The face is turned toward the action of the paralyzed muscle to minimize diplopia.

Lesions
Various lesions of the abducent nerve in its course can produce various syndromes as described in the following sections (**Fig. 13.3C**).

The Brainstem Syndrome
A brainstem lesion of the sixth nerve may also affect the fifth, seventh, and eighth cranial nerves and also the cerebellum. The sixth-nerve nucleus also has connections via the medial longitudinal fasciculus with the third-nerve nucleus, and so a lesion here produces a gaze palsy. Three syndromes can occur in the brainstem:

1. *Millard-Gubler syndrome*: In this the lesion is ventral and involves the facial nerve and the pyramidal tract. Thus there is a sixth-nerve paresis, ipsilateral seventh-nerve paresis, and contralateral hemiparesis.
2. *Raymond syndrome*: In this syndrome the lesion involves only the sixth cranial nerve and the pyramidal tract. Thus the patient has a sixth-nerve paresis and contralateral hemiparesis.
3. *Foville syndrome*: In this the lesion is dorsally. Because the lesion is dorsal the areas affected are the medial longitudinal fasciculus, the pontine paramedian reticular formation, the fifth nerve, and the sympathetic neurons. Thus the patient has horizontal conjugate gaze palsy and palsies of the ipsilateral fifth, sixth, seventh, and eighth nerves with ipsilateral Horner syndrome.

Subarachnoid Space Syndrome
Elevated intracranial pressure may result in downward displacement of the brainstem, with stretching of the sixth nerve, which is tethered at its exit from the pons and in the Dorello canal. This gives rise to nonlocalizing sixth-nerve palsies of raised intracranial pressure. Thirty percent of patients with pseudotumor cerebri have sixth nerve paresis, besides papilledema and its visual field changes.

Petrous Apex Syndrome
The sixth nerve passes under the Gruber ligament in the Dorello canal. This makes the nerve liable to paralysis due to a lesion of the petrous apex.

Gradenigo Syndrome
Gradenigo syndrome is due to a localized inflammation or extradural abscess of the petrous apex following complicated otitis media. This lesion can lead to the following:

◆ Sixth-nerve palsy
◆ Ipsilateral decreased hearing (eighth-nerve involvement)
◆ Ipsilateral facial pain in the distribution of the fifth nerve
◆ Ipsilateral facial paralysis

Pseudo-Gradenigo Syndrome
This syndrome is seen in two conditions:

◆ *Nasopharyngeal carcinoma*: This may cause serous otitis media due to obstruction of the eustachian tube, and the carcinoma may subsequently invade the cavernous sinus, causing sixth-nerve paresis.

◆ *Cerebellopontine angle tumor*: This may cause sixth-nerve paresis with decreased hearing (eighth nerve), seventh-nerve palsy, fifth-nerve palsy, ataxia, and papilledema.

Cavernous Sinus Syndrome
In this syndrome other nerves (e.g., the third, fourth, fifth nerves) in the cavernous sinus are also involved.

Orbital Syndrome
In this syndrome proptosis is an early sign, and the optic nerve may appear normal or demonstrate atrophy or edema. The ophthalmic division of the fifth nerve is involved. The third, fourth, and sixth nerves are also involved. It occurs due to trauma, tumors, or inflammations.

Isolated Sixth-Nerve Palsy
Isolated sixth-nerve paralysis can also be seen in the absence of any other associated signs.

◆ Differential Diagnosis

Thyroid eye disease, myasthenia gravis, Duane syndrome type 1, spasm of the near reflex, medial wall orbital blow-out fracture with restrictive myopathy, break in fusion of a congenital esophoria

◆ Management

Occlusion
One can perform occlusion when double vision is present in lateral gaze in patients with mild sixth-nerve paresis.

Treatment of the Cause
One should determine the cause and treat it.

Surgery
A maximal recession-resection procedure suffices in most instances of incomplete abducens paralysis to restore a useful field of single binocular vision and to eliminate the head turn. If there is a complete paralysis of the lateral rectus muscle, one can perform a transposition of the superior and inferior rectus muscles to the insertion of the lateral rectus muscle. This is called the Hummelsheim operation. In this surgery, half of the thickness of the superior rectus (SR) and inferior rectus (IR) are transposed to the insertion of the lateral rectus (LR). Recession of the medial rectus (MR) is also done. In Jensen's operation also, the transposition is done with recession of the medial rectus. In this operation, the LR is split as are the SR and inferior rectus (IR). Then the split portions of the SR and IR are sutured to the split portions of the LR (**Figs. 13.4** and **13.5**).

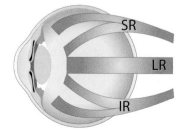

Fig. 13.4 Hummelsheim operation. Half the superior rectus (SR) and inferior rectus (IR) are transposed to the area of the lateral rectus (LR). This is also combined with a recession of the MR.

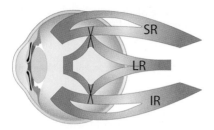

Fig. 13.5 Jensen operation. The superior rectus (SR), lateral rectus (LR), and the inferior rectus (IR) are split. The superior half of the split MR is sutured to one half of the split SR, and the inferior half of the LR is sutured to one half of the split IR. The MR is also done.

Botulinum Toxin Injection

Temporary paralysis of an extraocular muscle can be used in conjunction with the transposition procedures or in isolation. To determine the state of recovery of the LR following a sixth-nerve palsy, a tiny dose of botulinum toxin is injected into the belly of the overacting medial rectus muscle. This paralyzes the medial rectus and so the horizontal forces on the globe are more balanced and the esotropia reduced or eliminated.

Facial (Seventh) Nerve Palsy

The facial nerve is the seventh cranial nerve, and it is both a motor as well as a sensory nerve. The seventh cranial nerve has three nuclei:

◆ *Main motor nucleus*: Lies in the lower part of the pons. The part of the nucleus that supplies the muscles of the upper part of the face receives corticonuclear fibers from both cerebral hemispheres. The part of the nucleus that supplies the muscles of the lower part of the face receives corticonuclear fibers from the opposite cerebral hemisphere only.
◆ *Parasympathetic nuclei*: Include the superior salivatory and lacrimatory nuclei. The former supplies the submandibular and sublingual glands and the latter the lacrimal gland.
◆ *Sensory nucleus*: Situated in the upper part of the medulla oblongata

◆ Presentation

The lesions of the facial nerve are shown in **Figure 13.6** and are described in the following sections.

Supranuclear Lesion

If the lesion is supranuclear only the lower half of the face is involved, and if it is a lower motor neuron lesion the whole half of the face is involved. This is because the upper half of the face has a bilateral innervation.

Cerebellopontine Angle Tumor

The seventh nerve may be affected by a cerebellopontine angle tumor as it exits the brain. The presenting signs include:

◆ Total ipsilateral facial weakness (seventh-nerve involvement)
◆ Decreased tearing (lacrimation involved)
◆ Hyperacusis (nerve to stapedius involved)

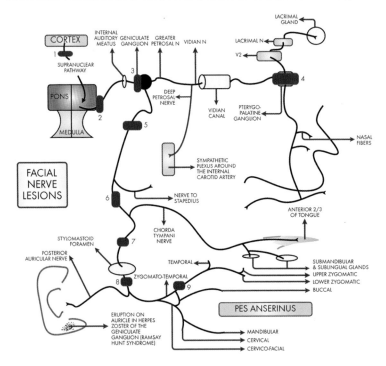

Fig. 13.6   Lesions of the facial nerve: 1, supranuclear lesion; 2, cerebellopontine angle tumor; 3, geniculate ganglionitis (Ramsay-Hunt syndrome); 4, isolate ipsilateral tear deficiency; 5, lesion before nerve to stapedius; 6, lesion after nerve to stapedius; 7, lesion after chorda tympani nerve; 8, Bell palsy—isolated total ipsilateral facial palsy; 9, isolated partial ipsilateral facial palsy.

◆ Decreased taste from the anterior two thirds of the tongue (chorda tympani nerve involved)
◆ Fifth, sixth, and eighth nerve involved with cerebellar dysfunctions

Geniculate Ganglionitis
Geniculate ganglionitis is known as the Ramsay-Hunt syndrome and is characterized by the following features:

◆ Same findings as in cerebellopontine-angle tumors except no associated neurological deficits
◆ There may be zoster vesicles on the tympanic membrane, external auditory canal, or external ear.

Isolated Ipsilateral Tear Deficiency
Isolated ipsilateral tear deficiency occurs in nasopharyngeal carcinomas, which affect the vidian nerve or the pterygopalatine ganglion.

Lesion before Nerve to Stapedius
Lacrimation is normal. The other findings are as follows:

◆ Hyperacusis (nerve to stapedius involved)
◆ Decreased taste from the anterior two thirds of the tongue (chorda tympani nerve involved)
◆ Total ipsilateral facial weakness (seventh-nerve involvement)

Lesion after Nerve to Stapedius
◆ Decreased taste from the anterior two thirds of the tongue (chorda tympani nerve involved)
◆ Total ipsilateral facial weakness (seventh-nerve involvement)

Lesion after Chorda Tympani Nerve
Only total ipsilateral facial weakness (seventh-nerve involvement)

Bell Palsy
Only total ipsilateral facial weakness (seventh-nerve involvement)

Isolated Partial Ipsilateral Facial Palsy
In this condition only certain branches of the seventh-nerve are affected.

◆ Differential Diagnosis

Parkinsonism, basal ganglia lesion

◆ Management

Work up and treat according to cause.

Multiple Cranial-Nerve Palsies (Cavernous Sinus Syndrome and Orbital Apex Syndrome)

Causes of multiple cranial-nerve palsies can be traumatic, vascular (internal carotid artery aneurysm, posterior cerebral artery aneurysm, direct or indirect carotid cavernous fistulas, thrombosis, etc.), neoplasms (may be primary cranial tumors or metastasis), inflammations, and infections such as herpes zoster, syphilis, tuberculosis, mucormycosis.

◆ Presentation

Patients present with periorbital or epicranial pain, ipsilateral ocular motor nerve palsies, oculosympathetic paralysis, and sensory loss in the ophthalmic and maxillary division of the trigeminal nerve. Orbital apex syndrome occurs owing to a similar cause at the apex of the orbit and is distinguished by involvement of the optic nerve in it.

◆ Management

Management is directed toward the cause.

◆ Pupillary Abnormalities

When light is shone in one eye, both the pupils constrict. Constriction of the pupil to which light is shone is called *direct light reflex* and that of the other pupil is called *consensual (indirect) light reflex*. If both pupils are illuminated simultaneously, the response summates. This means the constriction of each pupil is greater than the constriction noted when only one pupil is illuminated. Rods and cones initiate the light reflex (**Fig. 13.7**).

Anisocoria

Unequal size of pupils with differences in the diameter of 0.3 mm or more is referred to as *anisocoria*. Causes include the following:
◆ *Sympathetic paralysis*: Miosis of the affected pupil. Degree of inequality increases in the dark.
◆ *Parasympathetic paralysis*: Mydriasis of the affected pupil. Degree of inequality increases in light.
◆ *Central anisocoria*: Occurs in 20% of normal individuals. Normal reaction is seen with dim light and near target. Degree of inequality also decreases in light.

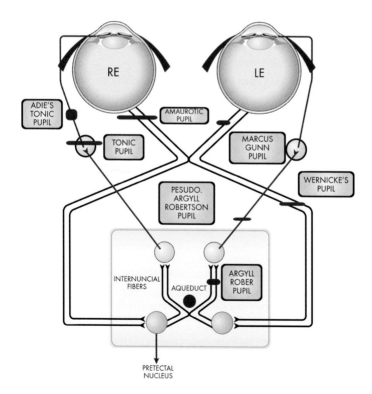

Fig. 13.7 Lesions of the pupil.

(Relative) Afferent Pupillary Defect

Common causes include optic nerve involvements (optic neuritis, compression of optic nerve, anterior ischemic optic neuropathy, etc.), dense media opacity, retinal causes (e.g., RD, central retinal vein occlusion or branch retinal vein occlusion, central serous retinochoroidopathy, etc.) Also called Marcus Gunn pupil.

◆ Presentation

The condition can be detected by the swinging flashlight test. The test can be performed in corneal opacity, third-nerve palsy, or an atropinised pupil as it is not related to visual acuity. Since relative afferent pupillary defect occurs in conditions where there is a relative decrease in the conduction of the optic nerve as compared to normal, it is absent in bilateral symmetrical optic nerve or retinal lesions.

To perform the swinging flashlight test the examiner shines a bright light into the normal eye while the patient is fixing on a distance target. The light is kept 3 to 5 cm from the eye just below the visual axis. The speed and extent of constriction are observed. A normal direct and consensual light reflex can be observed. Light is then shifted briskly to the contralateral eye. Each eye is illuminated for ~1 second and pupillary reaction is observed. The affected eye shows paradoxical dilatation instead of contraction.

◆ Differential Diagnosis

Other pupillary abnormalities

Horner Syndrome

Horner syndrome occurs in lesions involving the sympathetic pupillomotor pathway.

◆ Presentation

Patients present with miosis, normal pupillary reaction to light, and near, increased anisocoria in dim conditions, ptosis, ipsilateral anhidrosis (in lesions proximal to carotid bifurcation), enophthalmos, loss of ciliospinal reflex (in lesions distal to the ciliospinal center of Budge), hypochromic anisocoria (eye with Horner syndrome is light in color) (**Fig. 13.8**).

◆ Differential Diagnosis

Central anisocoria

◆ Management

Investigations include the following pharmacological tests:

◆ *Cocaine test*: Cocaine (4%) is instilled in both eyes. The Horner pupil will not dilate (>0.8 mm anisocoria significant). Noradrenalin reuptake is blocked by cocaine causing dilatation. In Horner syndrome no noradrenalin is present at the nerve endings.
◆ *Hydroxyamphetamine test*: Hydroxyamphetamine (1%) is instilled in both eyes. In preganglionic lesions both pupils will dilate and in postganglionic lesions the Horner pupil will not dilate. Noradrenaline release is potentiated by Paredrine (hydroxyamphetamine) causing dilatation. In postganglionic lesions neurons are destroyed so no dilatation is seen.

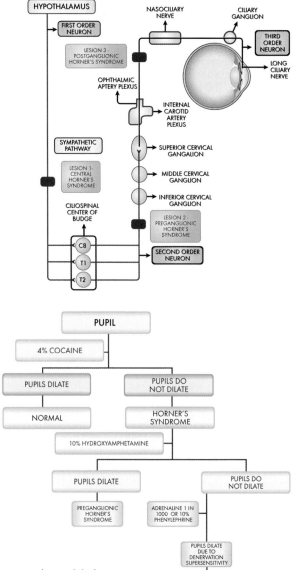

Fig. 13.8 **(A)** Horner syndrome. **(B)** Pharmacological tests to localize Horner syndrome.

♦ *Adrenaline test*: Adrenaline 1:1000 is instilled in both eyes. No dilatation is seen in preganglionic lesions, but dilatation of a Horner pupil is present in postganglionic lesions because adrenaline is not broken down because of the absence of monoamine oxidase (MAO) inhibitor in destroyed nerve endings. This is due to "denervation hypersensitivity" to adrenergic neurotransmitter.

♦ *Other investigations*: Magnetic resonance imaging (MRI) of the brain/spinal cord/orbit; computed tomography (CT) of the thorax; Doppler of the carotid; ear, nose, and throat (ENT) assessment; chest x-ray. Treatment depends on the exact cause and site of the lesion. The patient is referred to a suitable specialist.

Argyll-Robertson Pupil

This condition is usually seen in patients suffering from syphilis. It shows a bilateral and asymmetrical involvement. Lesions usually affect the neurons of the pretectal area.

♦ Presentation

Signs include bilateral, miotic, irregular pupil with asymmetrical response to light and near stimulus for accommodation. Light reflex is absent and accommodation is retained. The main associated causes are tertiary syphilis, diabetes mellitus, Wernicke encephalopathy, encephalitis, hereditary neuropathies, midbrain tumors, herpes zoster ophthalmicus, and chronic alcoholism.

♦ Management

Management addresses the underlying cause.

Adie Pupil/Tonic Pupil

Adie tonic pupil results from damage to the postganglionic parasympathetic nerve supply to the sphincter pupillae. This is seen in young adults and is unilateral in 80%.

♦ Presentation

Signs include a large, regular pupil with poor light reaction and exaggerated, slow, sustained near response (tonic) with characteristic vermiform movements of the pupillary border on slit lamp. Light-near dissociation is present. In chronic cases, the pupil becomes poor and poorly dilating.

This condition is associated with diminished deep tendon reflexes (Adie syndrome) and patchy hypohidrosis (Ross syndrome).

♦ Management

Investigations include pharmacological tests (e.g., instillation of 0.125% pilocarpine in both eyes). An Adie pupil constricts, whereas the normal pupil does not because of parasympathetic denervation supersensitivity. Reassure the patient about any obvious aniscoria and accommodative dysfunction. Pilocarpine (0.1%) helps in reducing the mydriatic blurring. Glasses also help with accommodative dysfunction.

Fig. 13.9 Arterial loop. Color photograph shows a tortuous vessel above the optic disk. (Courtesy of Robin D. Hamilton, A.M. Hamilton)

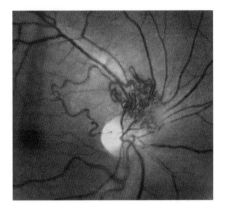

◆ Developmental Optic Nerve Anomalies

Prepapillary Vascular Loop

These blood vessels project from the optic disk into the vitreous and return to the optic disk to continue their usual course; 80 to 90% are arterial in origin (**Fig. 13.9**).

◆ Presentation

Prepapillary vascular loop is an incidental finding.

Optic Nerve Hypoplasia

This condition is characterized by a decreased number of optic nerve axons and normal mesodermal and glial supporting tissue.

◆ Presentation

Visual acuity may range from 20/20 to perception of light. Ophthalmoscopically the disk appears small and pale. A peripapillary halo surrounded by a pigment ring (double-ring sign) is always present.

De Morsier syndrome is a combination of optic nerve hypoplasia, absence of septum pellucidum, and agenesis or partial development of the corpus callosum. Coexistent hemispheric abnormalities and absence of pituitary infundibulum with or without postpituitary ectopia may be present. Pituitary hormone deficiency may be present.

◆ Management

Management consists of neurological and endocrinological evaluations with supplementation of required hormones.

Optic Nerve Pit

Optic nerve pit is herniation of rudimentary neuroectodermal tissue into a pocket-like depression within the nerve substance with unknown pathogenesis.

◆ **Presentation**

A round or oval gray-white or yellowish depression is seen in the optic disk, preferably at the temporal margin. Associated visual field defects may be present, most commonly paracentral arcuate scotoma. There is a 45% risk of serous retinal detachment.

◆ **Differential Diagnosis**

Acquired depression in the optic disc in normal tension glaucoma patients, optic nerve coloboma, central serous retinopathy (CSR), age-related macular degeneration, pigment epithelium detachment

◆ **Management**

Patients should be given regular follow-up. Laser photocoagulation is performed at the peripapillary retina adjacent to the pit if serous retinal detachment is present. Internal gas tamponade is recommended for retinal detachment.

Optic Disk Coloboma

Optic disk coloboma is a sporadic or autosomal dominant condition arising from faulty closure of the embryonic optic cup.

◆ **Presentation**

Visual acuity is variably affected. There is visual-field defect depending on the nerve fiber involvement. An enlarged, white, glistening, bowl-shaped disk with central excavation, which may extend to the retina and choroid. Microophthalmia may present.

Associations include CHARGE syndrome (coloboma of iris or retinochoroid, heart anomaly, choanal atresia, retardation, genital anomalies, ear anomalies), Goltz focal dermal hypoplasia, Walker-Warburg syndrome, linear nevus sebaceous syndrome, and Goldenhar syndrome. Optic disk coloboma is rarely associated with transsphenoidal encephalocele (**Fig. 13.10A**).

◆ **Management**

Visual-field testing must be done. Observation is needed.

Morning Glory Syndrome

Morning glory syndrome is due to a funnel-shaped expansion of the distal portion of the optic stalk, which is due to normal closure but abnormal progression of closure of the embryonic fissure in the distal portion of the optic stalk. It is sporadic in occurrence (**Fig. 13.10B**).

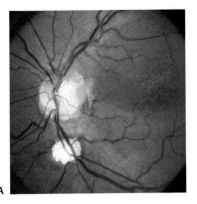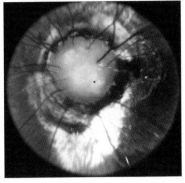

A   **B**

Fig. 13.10 **(A)** Coloboma of the optic disk. **(B)** Morning glory syndrome. (Courtesy of Robin D. Hamilton, A.M. Hamilton)

◆ Presentation

Visual acuity may be variably affected. Ophthalmoscopy reveals an enlarged, pink disk situated in a funnel-shaped excavation with overlying glial tissue. Retinal blood vessels are increased in number, arise from the disk periphery, and run an abnormally straight course with acute branching. The macula may be incorporated in the postglial excavation (macular capture). There is an increased risk of retinal detachment. Associations include transsphenoidal encephalocele, ipsilateral intracranial vascular hypoplasia, hypopituitarism, and facial abnormalities-hypertelorism, depressed nasal bridge, and midline upper lip notch cleft palate.

◆ Management

Management consists of regular follow-up and patient assurance.

Tilted Disk

Tilted disk is bilateral, nonhereditary, presumably due to ectasia of the inferonasal fundus.

◆ Presentation

Patients present with an obliquely placed disk with a posteriorly displaced inferonasal portion and situs inversus of the vessels. Bilateral hemianopia that does not respect the vertical meridian is seen. Myopic astigmatism is present. The condition is associated with visual-field defects. It may be associated with congenital suprasellar tumor.

◆ Management

Management consists of correction of the refractive error and patient assurance.

◆ Optic Disk Pathology

Optic Neuritis

Inflammation of the optic nerve may be a retrobulbar neuritis with normal optic disk (most frequently multiple sclerosis, young adults), papillitis where the disk is swollen (most commonly in children), or neuroretinitis-associated inflammation of retinal nerve fibers with macular star formation.

Demyelinating optic neuritis is due to phagocytosis of the myelin nerve sheaths and subsequent lay-down of fibrous plaques. It affects the white matter tracts, brainstem, and spinal cord, but the peripheral nerves are spared.

◆ Presentation

Presentation is usually at age 20 to 30 years and is subacute and unilateral. There is decreased vision, pain exacerbated by eye movements, and tiny flashes of light (phosphenes). Visual acuity usually varies between 20/60 (6/18) to 20/200 (6/60) in retrobulbar neuritis and papillitis. Afferent pupillary defect, dyschromatopsia (not proportional to visual loss), diminished light and brightness appreciation, and decreased contrast sensitivity are present. There is diffuse depression of the central 30 degrees of the visual field.

Demyelinating diseases causing ocular involvement include the following:

- *Multiple sclerosis:* Most common. MRI shows periventricular plaques.
- *Devic disease (neuromyelitica optica):* Bilateral optic neuritis with transverse myelitis. Severe bilateral diminished visual acuity with paraplegia.
- *Schilder disease:* Onset before 10 years and death within 1 to 2 years. Bilateral, progressive optic neuritis.

◆ Differential Diagnosis

Compressive optic lesions, sarcoidosis, vasculitis (e.g., systemic lupus erythematosus), syphilis, anterior ischemic optic neuropathy (AION), Leber's hereditary optic neuropathy (LHON), toxic or nutritional neuropathies, postviral demyelination

◆ Management

◆ Presentation

Presentation is usually at age 20 to 30 years and is subacute and unilateral. Diagnosis is usually clinical. There is decreased vision, pain exacerbated by eye movements, and tiny flashes. In the case of an atypical presentation, progressive optic neuropathy needs to be ruled out.

Investigations required include MRI, chest x-ray, serological tests antinuclear antibody (ANA), erythrocyte sedimentation rate, syphilis, antineutrophil cytoplasmic antibodies (ANCA), and cerebrospinal fluid (CSF) analysis. Typical white matter plaques in MRI with oligoclonal bands in CSF suggest a demyelinating cause. Treatment modalities include intravenous methylprednisolone 1 g daily for 3 days followed by oral prednisolone 1 mg/kg/day for 11 days, then tapered over 3 days. The results of the ONTT (optic neuritis treatment trial) show that the above regimen hastens visual recovery, but does not affect long term visual outcomes. Intramuscular interferon β-1a at the first episode delays the development of multiple sclerosis.

Band Optic Atrophy

Also called bowtie atrophy, this is a kind of primary optic atrophy seen with chiasmal syndrome with bitemporal hemianopic field defects in the ipsilateral eye, and optic tract lesions in the contralateral eye.

◆ Presentation

Optic disk pallor is seen primarily at the nasal and temporal portions of the optic disk. Superior and inferior portions are not involved because of sparing of the superior and inferior bundles of arcuate fibers.

◆ Differential Diagnosis

Other causes of optic atrophy

◆ Management

MRI and neurological evaluations are a must. Treatment is in collaboration with a neurologist and neurosurgeon.

Papilledema

Papilledema is bilateral disk swelling due to raised intracranial tension (ICT), which is transmitted along the subarachnoid space via nerve sheaths to block the axoplasmic flow. Causes include intracranial tumors, pseudotumor cerebri, subdural and epidural hematomas, subarachnoid hemorrhage, brain abscess, sagittal sinus thrombosis, and posterior fossa tumors (in children).

◆ Presentation

Patients present with transient visual obscurations of a few seconds, which may be accentuated with posture or straining, headache, nausea, vomiting, double vision, and decreased vision. Bilateral asymmetric disk swelling, disk hyperemia with dilated capillaries, dilated veins, loss of spontaneous venous pulsations, splinter hemorrhages, cotton-wool spots, obscuration of the blood vessels entering and leaving the disk, and concentric retinal folds (Paton line) form the hallmarks of the acute papilledema.

Elevation of the disk without hemorrhages (champagne cork disks), decreased venous dilatation, and eventual atrophy of the disk with a decrease in the disk elevation over a period of 6 weeks is characteristic of chronic papilledema. Enlargement of a blind spot is seen in field examination (**Fig. 13.11**).

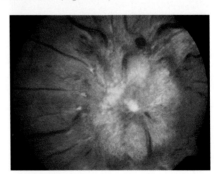

Fig. 13.11   Papilledema.

◆ Differential Diagnosis

Intracranial space-occupying lesions (tumors, hemorrhage, abscess, etc.), infiltrative (leukemia, lymphoma), inflammatory (optic neuritis, scleritis, etc.), granulomatous (sarcoidosis, tuberculosis, etc.), and vascular causes (AION, diabetic papillopathy, etc.) of disk swelling and pseudopapilledema

◆ Management

Fundus fluorescein angiography (FFA) shows leakage from dilated disk capillaries, and late pooling of the dye is evident. Magnetic resonance venography is done to check the cerebral sinuses and lumbar puncture for CSF analysis. Treatment is directed toward the underlying cause; neurosurgery may be required. Regular ophthalmic follow-up with disk status, vision, color vision, and field changes is required.

Pseudopapilledema

Anomalies resemble papilledema but are not due to raised ICT. They can instead be due to disk drusen, tilted disks, hyperopic disks, myopic disks, and myelinated peripapillary nerve fibers. Disk drusen is autosomal dominant, bilateral lumpy disk with absent cup and centrally emerging vessels with an abnormal branching pattern. Visual acuity is usually normal but associated field defects are usually present. Diagnosis is by autofluorescence, B-scan, ultrasonography, and CT scan.

Similarly myopic disks may be elevated nasally and may leak on FFA. Hyperopic disk is crowded and elevated and thus can lead to confusion. Tilted disks are elevated superotemporally (**Fig. 13.12**).

Pseudotumor Cerebri

Pseudotumor cerebri is usually a benign, self-limiting disease of unknown etiology characterized by signs and symptoms of raised intracranial pressure with normal CSF, papilledema, and normal nervous system imaging. It can be idiopathic and is known to be associated with vitamin A intoxication, tetracycline therapy, steroid withdrawal, nalidixic acid, impairment of central venous drainage, and systemic lupus erythematosus.

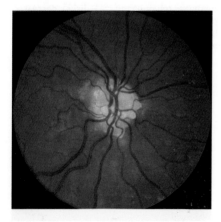

Fig. 13.12 Optic nerve head drusen. (Courtesy of Robin D. Hamilton, AM Hamilton)

◆ **Presentation**

Presenting and diagnostic features of pseudo tumor cerebri are holocranial headache, monocular or binocular blackouts of vision (due to microcirculations disturbance at the temporal lobe), sixth-nerve palsy with diplopia, tinnitus, papilledema, arcuate scotomas in the nasal region, and relative afferent pupillary defect (RAPD).

◆ **Differential Diagnosis**

Brain tumors (most commonly glioma), arteriovenous malformations, infectious diseases such as viral encephalitis, and anomalous optic nerve with headache

◆ **Management**

Asymptomatic patients should be followed up regularly. Carbonic anhydrase inhibitors (inhibit the CSF production), corticosteroids, oral hypoglycemic agents, lumboperitoneal shunt, and optic nerve sheath decompression (ONSD) are other treatment modalities.

Arteritic Ischemic Optic Neuropathy (Giant Cell Arteritis)

This infarction of the optic disk is associated with giant cell arteritis (GCA). Twenty percent of cases do not have any systemic signs of GCA at the time of presentation (occult GCA).

◆ **Presentation**

The patient presents with sudden, profound, unilateral visual loss with periocular pain (preceded by transient visual loss and flashes of light unlike nonarteritic ischemic optic neuropathy. Altitudinal field defect is common in these patients. Patients may experience associated symptoms such as headache, neck pain, jaw pain with claudication, scalp tenderness, fevers, weight loss, and myalgias.

The age of the patient is more than 55 years. Palpable and tender temporal artery, elevated erythrocyte sedimentation rate, and coexisting anemia are also present.

◆ **Differential Diagnosis**

Nonarteritic ischemic optic neuropathy, optic neuritis, optic nerve compression, optic neuropathy, central retinal vein occlusion (CRVO).

◆ **Management**

ESR, C-reactive protein (CRP), and total blood count-raised platelets are the blood investigations required to diagnose and follow up with the patient. Temporal artery biopsy shows granulomatous inflammation with a grossly narrow lumen. FFA shows severe hypoperfusion of choroid.

Patients are treated with intravenous methylprednisolone 1 g/day with 80 mg oral prednisolone for 3 days. After 3 days, 60-mg and 50-mg oral dose each for 1 week followed by gradual reduction of 5 mg each week till 10 mg/day, which is the maintenance dose. Azathioprine has been tried in patients intolerant of steroids. Prognosis is poor in spite of early start of steroids, and it worsens with time and subsequent episodes.

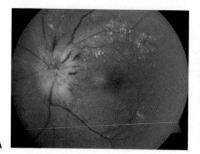
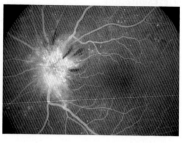

A

B

Fig. 13.13 **(A)** Nonarteritic ischemic optic neuropathy (diabetic), color picture. **(B)** Nonarteritic ischemic optic neuropathy (diabetic), fundus fluorescein angiography.

Nonarteritic Ischemic Optic Neuropathy

This neuropathy occurs because of occlusion of the short posterior ciliary arteries. It is most common in elderly patients, with structural crowding of the optic nerve head due to a small or absent physiological cup. Systemic hypertension, hypercholesterolemia, diabetes mellitus, hypercoagulation states, and sildenafil intake are some of the predispositions for the condition.

◆ Presentation

Patients have a sudden unilateral painless visual loss, particularly after awakening, associated with color vision abnormalities (proportional to visual loss) and inferior altitudinal field defects. Late stages present with optic atrophy following chronic vision loss.

Disk pallor with disk edema (diffuse or sectoral) with peripapillary splinter hemorrhages is the typical presentation (**Fig. 13.13**).

◆ Differential Diagnosis

AION, optic neuritis, optic nerve compression, optic neuropathy, and CRVO

◆ Management

Lipid profile, blood glucose, complete blood count, antinuclear antibody, fluorescein treponema antibody (FTA)/venereal disease research laboratory test, ESR, and C-reactive protein (to rule out GCA) must be done for all patients. FFA shows early disk hyperfluorescence, which increases in intensity in the late stages. Intermittent blocked fluorescence is seen owing to splinter hemorrhages. Treatment consists of managing the underlying medical condition. Prognosis is favorable with maintenance of good visual acuity in most patients.

Toxic or Nutritional Optic Neuropathy

This condition is also referred to as tobacco-alcohol amblyopia because it is prevalent in heavy drinkers and chronic pipe or cigar smokers who neglect their diet. Other etiologies include thiamine and vitamin B_{12} deficiency, methanol, ethambutol, chloramphenicol, isoniazide, rifampicin, lead, and digitalis.

◆ Presentation

Presentation includes insidious, progressive, bilateral visual impairment with dyschromatopsia. The optic disk may be normal or temporal pallor with splinter hemorrhages around the disk. Centrocecal scotoma (better appreciated by red target instead of white) is present.

◆ Differential Diagnosis

Bilateral AION, hypotensive shock, radiation injury, infiltrative optic neuropathy, Leber optic neuropathy, and bilateral compressive optic neuropathy

◆ Management

Blood investigations might reveal an associated pernicious anemia and vitamin B_{12} deficiency. Weekly injections of 1000 units of hydroxycobalamin for 10 weeks along with multivitamins are the mainstay of the treatment. Abstain from drinking and smoking. Prognosis is good with treatment in the early stages.

Leber Optic Neuropathy

Leber optic neuropathy is a maternally transmitted trait arising from point mutations (most commonly 11778 mutation) in mitochondrial DNA. It typically affects men (3:1) in their twenties or thirties. It is unilateral initially with subsequent involvement of the other eye.

◆ Presentation

Patients present with painless unilateral gradual loss of vision. The other eye is involved subsequently. Dyschromatopsia is present. There is a mildly edematous, hyperemic disk with telangiectatic vessels in the peripapillary retina. The late stage presents with optic atrophy. Dense central or paracentral scotoma is seen. The condition may be associated with spasticity and gait disturbances owing to the inability to detoxify cyanide.

◆ Differential Diagnosis

Bilateral AION, hypotensive shock, radiation injury, infiltrative optic neuropathy, nutritional optic neuropathy, and bilateral compressive optic neuropathy

◆ Management

A detailed history helps in ruling out other causes of optic neuropathy. CT scan and MRI scan help to rule out a compressive lesion. Consider a blood test to detect mitochondrial chromosomal mutations. Genetic counseling helps.

Compressive Optic Neuropathy

Compressive optic neuropathy results from compression of the pregeniculate portion of the optic nerve. Common causes include Graves thyroid ophthalmopathy, meningiomas, orbital space-occupying lesion, pseudotumor, craniopharyngioma, and pituitary tumors.

◆ **Presentation**

Visual acuity, color vision, and contrast sensitivity are usually affected. Initially disk swelling is present, followed by atrophy in the late stages. Afferent pupillary defect and central and arcuate scotomas are common findings. Proptosis may or may not be associated.

◆ **Differential Diagnosis**

Bilateral AION, hypotensive shock, radiation injury, infiltrative optic neuropathy, nutritional optic neuropathy, and Leber optic neuropathy

◆ **Management**

CT scan and MRI of the orbit and brain are performed to note the compressive lesion and its extent. Treatment is directed toward the underlying cause of compression.

Infiltrative Optic Neuropathy

Infiltration of the optic nerve can be by neoplastic or inflammatory cells from lymphomas, leukemias, sarcoidosis, syphilis, tuberculosis (TB), fungal infection, or metastasis from lung or breast carcinoma.

◆ **Presentation**

Patients present with progressive, bilateral, severe vision loss. Initially the disk is normal ophthalmoscopically but later may become swollen due to infiltration at the optic nerve head.

◆ **Differential Diagnosis**

Bilateral AION, hypotensive shock, radiation injury, compressive optic neuropathy, nutritional optic neuropathy, and Leber optic neuropathy

◆ **Management**

MRI of the orbit and brain, CSF analysis, and screening tests for granulomatous disorders and blood-related disorders are required to confirm the cause. Palliative radiotherapy for infiltrative neoplasms and corticosteroids or antimicrobials for infiltrative or infectious disorders are advocated forms of treatment.

Radiation Optic Neuropathy

The neuropathy is usually delayed by 2 years after standard doses of radiation but may be seen many years after the treatment. The optic nerve can be affected by radiation to the eye, orbit, sinus, nasopharynx, or brain.

◆ **Presentation**

Bilateral decreased visual acuity is the presenting symptom.

◆ **Differential Diagnosis**

Bilateral AION, hypotensive shock, infiltrative optic neuropathy, compressive optic neuropathy, nutritional optic neuropathy, and Leber optic neuropathy

◆ **Management**

The history is significant. CT and MRI are done to evaluate the optic nerve. No treatment is available.

◆ Tumors of Neural Origin

Optic Nerve Glioma

Low-grade, pilocytic astrocytoma can involve optic nerve and chiasm; 30% are associated with neurofibroma type 1 (NF-1) and have a better prognosis.

◆ **Presentation**

Optic nerve glioma usually presents in the first decade with gradual visual loss associated with proptosis (<3 mm, axial, nonpulsatile, nonreducible). Strabismus and nystagmus can also be the presenting complaints. Other features include relative afferent papillary defect, optic atrophy, optic disk swelling, optociliary shunts, and CRVO. In chiasmal lesions, hypothalamic and pituitary dysfunction symptoms and symptoms of increased intracranial pressure may be present. Optic nerve glioma in adults is rare, but if present it tends to be aggressive and fatal.

CT scan shows a fusiform enlargement of the nerve, kinking or irregular nerve, and regions of low intensity within the nerve. There is no calcification or hyperostosis. MRI reveals hypointense areas on T1-weighted images and hyperintense areas on T2-weighted images. It may show intracranial extension.

Histology shows spindle-shaped astrocytes with deeply eosinophilic large cell processes known as Rosenthal fibers with associated degenerative foci and reactive hyperplasia of meninges.

◆ **Differential Diagnosis**

Other neoplasms (meningioma, lymphangioma, hemangioma, rhabdomyosarcoma), acute ethmoiditis, hyperthyroidism, craniostenosis, and trauma

◆ **Management**

The treatment line consists of observation for small tumors with good vision. Surgical excision with globe preservation is recommended for large tumors confined to the orbit. Radiochemotherapy is used for intracranial extension.

Neurofibroma and Schwannoma

NF is a benign tumor derived from glial cells of peripheral nerves. Endoneural cells and axons may also be involved in NF. Schwannomas tend to be singular and encapsulated, whereas NFs are more likely to be multiple and encapsulated and are more likely to undergo malignant transformation. Plexiform NFs (another type) are almost always associated with autosomal dominant neurofibromatosis type 1 (NF-1, von Recklinghausen NF) linked to chromosome 17, which usually presents in early childhood.

◆ Presentation

Patients can present with a subcutaneous lump around the eye or with double vision, decreased vision, and proptosis in cases with intraorbital tumor. Multiple neurofibromas (NF-1) are associated with pigmented skin lesions, osseous lesions, café-au-lait spots, S-shaped deformity of the lid, Lisch nodules in the iris, and hypertrophy of periocular tissue, which on palpation has a "bag of worms" feeling.

◆ Differential Diagnosis

Other neoplasms (optic nerve glioma, lymphangioma, hemangioma, rhabdomyosarcoma), acute ethmoiditis, hyperthyroidism, craniostenosis, and trauma

◆ Management

Ophthalmic workup includes a complete medical history, assessment of visual acuity, ocular movements, displacement, exophthalmometry, tonometry, dilated fundus examination, CT scan, MRI, and ultrasonography. Symptomatic tumors need excision.

Orbital surgery should not be done because the tumor is related to important orbital structures.

Meningioma

Middle-aged females are affected. Presentations vary with the site of the lesion.

◆ Presentation

Optic nerve sheath meningiomas are benign proliferations of meningoepithelial cells presenting with progressive monocular vision loss, optic atrophy, and optociliary shunts. Tuberculum sellae meningioma compresses the junction of the optic chiasm with the optic nerve causing ipsilateral central scotomas with contralateral junctional scotoma. Sphenoidal ridge tumors will compress the optic nerve, and similarly olfactory lesions will cause compression of the optic nerve and loss of the sense of smell.

CT shows diffuse tubular enlargement of the optic nerve seat, tram track or railroad sign, and calcification. MRI reveals isointense or hyperintense lesion on T1 and T2. CT or MRI with contrast is more helpful.

◆ Differential Diagnosis

Other intraocular tumors, metastasis, mucocele, and lymphoma

◆ Management

Patients with progressive field loss require treatment by a neurosurgeon. Treatment requires surgery followed by radiotherapy.

◆ Blepharospasm

Blepharospasm is a type of facial dystonia, mainly affecting females (2:1) and associated with tonic spasms of orbicularis oculi (**Fig. 13.14**).

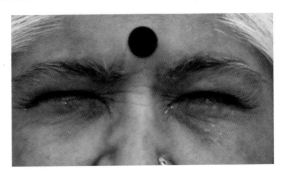

Fig. 13.14 Blepharospasm.

Benign (Essential) Blepharospasm

Blepharospasm can be a very disabling condition in terms of vision and social life.

◆ Presentation

Blepharospasm more commonly affects women in the older age group. This is a type of facial dystonia in which there is idiopathic tonic contraction of the orbicularis oculi. If it is secondary to any ocular pathology (corneal or conjunctival foreign body, trichiasis, blepharitis, dry eyes) then it is called secondary blepharospasm. There is a bilateral involuntary lid closure that may be precipitated by stress, fatigue, or social interactions. This is always bilateral. It disappears during sleep. Secondary ocular changes like ptosis or entropion can occur.

This can be differentiated from hemifacial spasm, which does not disappear during sleep.

◆ Differential Diagnosis

Hemifacial spasm, facial myokymia, trigeminal neuralgia, Parkinson disease, progressive supranuclear palsy, multiple sclerosis, stroke, Tourette syndrome, and tardive dyskinesia

◆ Management

Botulinum toxin is given as multiple injections on the upper and lower lid. The effect generally lasts for 3 months. In cases of secondary blepharospasm, treat the underlying cause that is precipitating the blepharospasm.

Other treatment options are medical (e.g., benzodiazepine) or surgical (e.g., myectomy).

Hemifacial Spasm

This is a tonic clonic spasm of the musculature that occurs even during sleep.

◆ Presentation

The condition usually affects the younger age group. It is thought to be caused by irritation of the root of the seventh cranial nerve by a compressive lesion. MRI of the cerebellopontine angle should be obtained to rule out tumor.

◆ Differential Diagnosis

Blepharospasm, facial myokymia, trigeminal neuralgia, Parkinson disease, progressive supranuclear palsy, multiple sclerosis, stroke, Tourette syndrome, and tardive dyskinesia

◆ Management

Management includes observation, botulinum toxin injection, or neurosurgical decompression of the seventh nerve (Jannetta procedure).

◆ Myasthenia Gravis

Myasthenia results from dysfunction of the neuromuscular junction caused by autoimmunity. It is a chronic autoimmune disorder associated with a reduced number of acetylcholine receptors neuromuscular junctions resulting in weakness and fatigability of muscle. Ocular myasthenia most commonly presents with diplopia, ptosis, or both, which are variable and characteristically worse toward the end of the day. Serum antibodies to acetylcholine receptors are detected in 90% of the patients with generalized myasthenia, but only 50% will be detected in ocular myasthenia. Neonatal forms of myasthenia gravis occur in 10 to 15% of children born to mothers with myasthenia gravis because of the placental transfer of antibodies to Ach (Acetylcholine) receptor.

The impairment of the neuromuscular conduction causes weakness and fatigue of the skeletal musculature but not of cardiac and involuntary muscles. The disease affects females twice as commonly as males and may be ocular, bulbar, or generalized.

◆ Presentation

Myasthenic signs and symptoms are variable and tend to worsen with fatigue and stress.

- ◆ *Fatigability*: During testing for lid fatigue, the patient is asked to look up without blinking at the examiner's hand for 1 to 2 minutes. Lid fatigue on prolonged upgaze is perhaps the most frequently elicited sign (**Fig. 13.15**).
- ◆ *Peek sign*: When the patient is asked to close the lids gently, one or both inadvertently open slightly or peek.
- ◆ *Absent Bell's Phenomenon*: There can an absence of Bell phenomenon.
- ◆ *Cogan lid twitch*: After prolonged downgaze refixation to the primary position results in overshooting of the upper lid.
- ◆ *Upper lid hop*: Hop of the upper lid occurs on looking to the side.
- ◆ *Myasthenic ptosis*: When unilateral is associated with contralateral lid retraction.
- ◆ *Oscillatory movements*: If one eyelid is elevated manually as the patient looks up, the fellow eyelid will show fine oscillatory movements.
- ◆ *Ice pack test*: The degree of ptosis improves after the ice pack is placed on the eyelid for 2 minutes. The test is negative in nonmyasthenic ptosis.

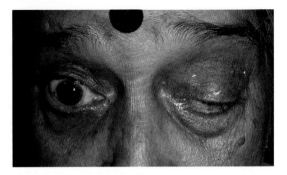

Fig. 13.15 Myasthenia gravis.

◆ *Diplopia*: This is very frequently vertical, although any of the muscles can be involved. The pupil is not involved. A pseudointernuclear ophthalmoplegia can occur.
◆ *Saccadic abnormalities*: Abnormalities such as hypometric large saccades, hypermetric small saccades, quiver movements, and hyperfast saccades can occur.

◆ Differential Diagnosis

Isolated or combined palsies of the third, fourth, sixth, or seventh cranial nerves; decompensated strabismus; thyroid disease; Eaton-Lambert myasthenic syndrome; botulism; chronic progressive ophthalmoplegia; myotonic dystrophy

◆ Management

Tensilon test
Intravenous injection of edrophonium is the gold standard for the diagnosis of ocular myasthenia. Edrophonium is a short-acting anticholinesterase that increases the amount of acetylcholine available at the neuromuscular junction. In myasthenia this results in transient improvement of symptoms and signs such as weakness, ptosis, and diplopia. Uncommon complications include bradycardia, loss of consciousness, and even death. Lacrimation, salivation, and abdominal cramps are mentioned as common minor side effects. The test should be done with a resuscitation trolley in hand in case of sudden cardiorespiratory arrest.

◆ Objective baseline measurement of ptosis or diplopia with a Hess chart should be taken.
◆ Intravenous injection of atropine 0.3 mg is given to minimize muscarinic side effects.
◆ Intravenous dose of 0.2 mL containing 2 mg of edrophonium hydrochloride is given. If definitive improvement is noted the test can be terminated.
◆ If no response then the remaining 0.8 mL of 8 mg is injected after 60 seconds if there is no adverse reaction. The response lasts only for 5 minutes.
◆ Perverse reaction such as worsening of the strabismus or a paradoxical response such as right hypertropia becoming a left hypertropia after the injection is considered positive by some.

Neostigmine Test
◆ Intramuscular injection of neostigmine is useful in children. The effect lasts for 15 minutes to peak and lasts for only 30 minutes.
◆ Presence of acetylcholine receptor antibodies is virtually diagnostic of myasthenia gravis.
◆ On electromyography, repetitive stimulation of a single muscle fiber will show a decremental response.

Sleep Test
◆ Useful in neonates and infants. There will be improvement after sleep.
◆ Imaging the chest with CT or MRI for the presence of thymoma

Optical Treatment
◆ Because of the variability of signs and symptoms, it is difficult to treat. For binocular diplopia occlusion of one eye can help, but it forces the patient to view monocularly.
◆ Fresnel prism can be tried if the ocular deviation is stable for weeks.
◆ Crutch glasses are helpful in the case of ptosis.

Medical Treatment
◆ Anticholinergic drugs such as pyridostigmine (60 mg) three times a day. One must be aware of cholinergic crisis if too much of pyridostigmine is given. The patient should be told to stop if bulbar symptoms or generalized weakness occurs.
◆ Corticosteroids are used along with pyridostigmine. The patient should be maintained on steroids for months before tapering slowly tapering. When the patient is maintained on a low dose of steroids, there can be a relapse or unmasking of generalized myasthenia.
◆ Immunosuppressant azathioprine is effective against myasthenia at a dose of 2 to 3 mg/kg/day.
◆ Cyclosporine A, plasmapheresis, mycophenolate, and intravenous gamma globulin can also be used in generalized myasthenia.

Surgical Treatment
◆ Thymectomy is very effective for ocular myasthenia. The results of thymectomy for generalized myasthenia are very favorable, with ~35% entering complete remission and 50% improving.
◆ Eyelid surgery or ptosis and eye muscle surgery for diplopia are considered only if it is stable for a few months and as a last resort.
◆ Antibodies to acetylcholine receptors are the etiology behind the disorder.

◆ Eye Movement Disorders

Nystagmus

Nystagmus is a rhythmic to-and-fro oscillation of the eyes. In nystagmus, generally the movement in slow phase is in one direction and the fast phase is in the opposite direction. The fast phase of nystagmus is mediated by the saccadic system under all conditions. One or more of the other systems will mediate the slow phase. It is important to remember that *nystagmus is given its direction based on the fast phase.* This means that if we say a nystagmus is to the right, the fast phase of the nystagmus is to the right. But actually, the important point of nystagmus is the slow phase. So actually, *nystagmus should be given its direction depending on the slow phase—but this is not done.* An abnormality in the slow phase is more significant. But by convention the direction of nystagmus is described by the fast phase (**Fig. 13.16A**). The null zone is the field of gaze in which the intensity of nystagmus is minimal, whereas in the neutral zone a reversal of direction of jerky nystagmus occurs and any of several bidirectional waveforms, pendular nystagmus, or no nystagmus may be present.

Latent nystagmus is not normally present when both eyes are open but is elicited on covering either eye. In the classic case the nystagmus appears on closing one eye. Bilateral jerky nystagmus is seen with the fast phase toward the uncovered eye. Another condition, called manifest latent nystagmus, occurs in patients with amblyopia or strabismus who, although viewing with both eyes open, are fixing monocularly. Again the fast phase is toward the direction of the intended viewing eye. The phenomenon of latent nystagmus is particularly evident when the visual acuities of the two eyes are unequal. Sometimes if one eye has very poor vision, on covering the better eye, instead of nystagmus a conjugate deviation of both eyes occurs toward the side of the closed eye. This is called the *latent deviation of Kestenbaum.* The cause of latent nystagmus is unknown. It could be due to lack of coordination of the supranuclear centers. It could also be due to the fact that the nystagmus was latent but kept in check by convergence so that abolition of the impulse to binocular convergence allowed it to become manifest.

◆ Presentation

Types of Nystagmus

- ◆ *Pendular nystagmus*: This condition consists of an undulatory movement of equal speed and amplitude in both directions.
- ◆ *Jerky nystagmus*: Jerky nystagmus demonstrates a biphasic rhythm wherein a slow movement in one direction is followed by a rapid saccadic return to the original position. Jerky nystagmus usually increases in amplitude with gaze in the direction of the fast component. This is called *Alexander's law.*
- ◆ *Micronystagmus*: Micronystagmus a nystagmus that is subclinical; it is incapable of being detected with ordinary clinical tests because of its extremely small amplitude. The diagnosis is apparent by the fixation pattern, which shows a regular jerky type of nystagmus with fast and slow phases of extremely small amplitude within the parafoveal areas so that it may be revealed only by a careful examination with the visuoscope or direct ophthalmoscope.

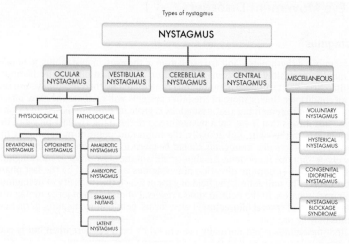

A

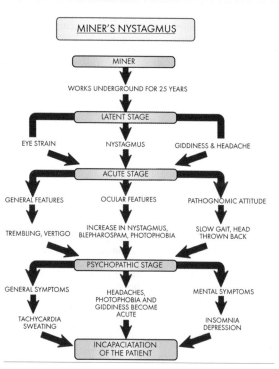

B

Fig. 13.16 **(A)** Types of nystagmus. **(B)** Miner's nystagmus.

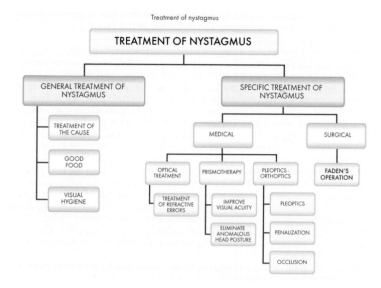

Treatment of nystagmus

C

Fig. 13.16 (*Continued*) **(C)** Methods to treat nystagmus.

Grades of Nystagmus
Nystagmus is divided into three grades:

◆ *Grade I*: Jerky nystagmus is evident only in the direction of the fast phase (i.e., on conjugate deviation to one side).
◆ *Grade II*: When in addition, it is evident in the primary position.
◆ *Grade III*: Evident in all positions of the eyes.

Pathological Ocular Nystagmus
◆ *Amaurotic nystagmus*: Nystagmus of pendular or rarely jerky type may occur in those who have been blind for a long time. The nystagmus is sometimes constant, and at other times it appears only when attention is aroused.
◆ *Amblyopic nystagmus*: This is due to a defect in central vision in both eyes, which precludes the normal development of the fixation reflex.
◆ *Spasmus nutans*: In this the nystagmus occurs with head nodding. It is also called *Dunkel syndrome*. It generally occurs within the first year of life. The cause appears to be difficulty in maintaining fixation, which is frequently associated with inadequate light. There is also insufficient control due to instability of the motor cortical centers in early life.
◆ *Miner's nystagmus*: This is an acquired occupational disease of the nervous system with special manifestations in the ocular motor apparatus, occurring in workers in coal mines (**Fig. 13.16B**). Basically it is due to lack of illumination. In the early latent stage there is a mild nystagmus. The acute stage is characterized by trembling of the head and hands, with marked nystagmus, and a pathognomic posture of the head being thrown back. The late psychopathic stage is characterized by cramps, headaches, tremors, and insomnia. The nystagmus

is generally pendular in type in the primary position but frequently changes to the jerky type on lateral gaze. The treatment of this condition is to give the patient surface work and improve the general health.

◆ *Vestibular nystagmus*: The semicircular canals are three fine tubes arranged in the ear. The lateral semicircular canal is tilted up 30 degrees. Normally the eyes at rest are in the primary position. Impulses go from each semicircular canal to the respective vestibular nuclei. From here, the impulse goes to the opposite pontine gaze center, which in turn connects to the same side sixth-nerve nucleus and opposite side third-nerve nucleus. The impulses thus reach the medial and lateral recti and the eyes are balanced and in the primary position.

◆ *Cerebellar nystagmus*: The exact mechanism of cerebellar nystagmus is not known. When nystagmus occurs it is opposite that found in a vestibular lesion. In a right-sided vestibular lesion, the slow phase of the nystagmus is to the right and the fast phase to the left. This means the nystagmus is to the left, in other words opposite the side of the lesion. In cerebellar disease, the fast phase of the nystagmus is on the same side of the lesion. So, if there is a right-sided cerebellar lesion, the fast phase of the nystagmus is toward the right side. This could be due to the flocculo-oculomotor pathway, which works in the reverse of the vestibular pathway. The left vestibular pathway pushes the eyes to the right, whereas the left flocculo-oculomotor pathway from the left cerebellum pushes the eyes to the left.

◆ *Central nystagmus*: In central nystagmus, the nystagmus is of the jerky type. It is occasionally present when the eyes are at rest but usually develops only when they are deviated to one or the other direction. The nystagmus is symmetrical. This means that the movement starts at the same angle of eccentricity and has approximately the same excursion whether the gaze is directed to one or the other side.

◆ Differential Diagnosis

Voluntary eye movements, dysmetria, flutter, opsoclonus, myoclonus, spasmus nutans, optic nerve glioma, superior oblique myokymia, myasthenia gravis (quiverlike movements), ocular bobbing

◆ Management

Management can consist of treating the cause, use of prisms, or surgery in which the Faden operation is performed. The methods to treat nystagmus are shown in **Figure 13.16C**. The treatment can be general, where the cause is treated, or specific, which can be medical or surgical. In medical treatment one can improve the visual acuity by using prisms, base out, to simulate fusional convergence. One can use prisms to eliminate anomalous head postures also. For a head turn to the left, the neutral zone is in dextroversion and a prism base out before the right eye and base in before the left eye will shift the eyes conjugately along with the neutral zone toward the primary position. One can also use occlusion, in which partial occlusion of the sound eye with a neutral density filter decreases visual acuity in the fixating eye to a level below that of the amblyopic eye but not dark enough to elicit the nystagmus. Surgically one can perform the Faden operation, in which the required muscle creating the nystagmus is sutured to the sclera at the equator.

Internuclear Ophthalmoplegia

Lesions affecting the pathways by which the various ocular nuclei are linked together [i.e., lesions of the medial longitudinal fasciculus (MLF) or medial longitudinal bundle] produces internuclear ophthalmoplegia. The MLF connects the third-nerve and the sixth-nerve nuclei. If a lesion occurs in this there is prevention of the harmonious coordination of these nuclei in producing conjugate movements. So one eye carries out a voluntary movement of gaze, whereas the other eye does not, thus leading to failure of the conjugate movement (i.e., both eyes moving in the same direction). This leads to a misalignment of the eyes and thus to diplopia. This feature differentiates the internuclear palsies from the other supranuclear lesions.

Depending on whether the lesion is unilateral or bilateral, various causes of internuclear ophthalmoplegia are present. The common causes are vascular lesions or multiple sclerosis (**Fig. 13.17A**).

◆ Presentation

Internuclear ophthalmoplegia (INO) may present as three types as enumerated below:

◆ *Type I*: In this type, the lesion is near the third cranial nerve nuclei, including the convergence area (**Fig. 13.17B**). Essentially there is paralysis of both medial recti. The impulses coming from the pontine gaze center go to the sixth-nerve and third-nerve nuclei. Because the connections to the sixth-nerve nuclei are not affected no disturbance is present in lateral rectus movements. The eyes are divergent owing to bilateral involvement of the medial recti and there is loss of convergence. It occurs in hypertensive brainstem lesions and multiple sclerosis. Divergence may be complicated by skew deviation of the eyes in which one eye may be up and out and the other eye looks down and out. There may be a see-saw nystagmus present in which the eyes jerk up and down alternately.
◆ *Type II*: In this relatively common variety of INO, the MLF is damaged and the medial recti fail to move synchronously with the lateral recti (**Fig. 13.17C**) on attempted lateral gaze to either side. Yet when each eye is tested alone, the medial recti function is evident but incomplete. Test this by covering the abducting eye and making the adducting eye follow the finger. In type II INO convergence is normal because the convergence area is not affected. This occurs in multiple sclerosis, pontine glioma, or encephalitis
◆ *Type III*: The third variety of INO occurs in multiple sclerosis. In this type of INO (**Figs. 13.17D,E**), none of the eye abducts completely, whereas adduction is complete. The relay to the sixth cranial nerve nuclei is affected on both sides. If you test the eye individually by closing the other eye, the eye would abduct, differentiating this from an infranuclear lesion (sixth-nerve palsy).

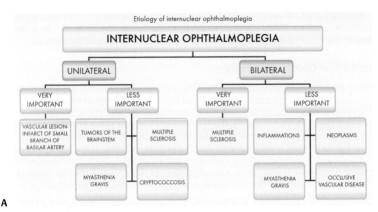

Etiology of internuclear ophthalmoplegia

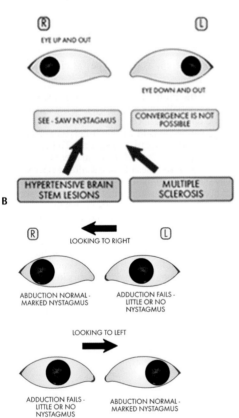

Fig. 13.17 **(A)** Causes for internuclear ophthalmoplegia (INO). **(B)** Type I INO. **(C)** Type II INO.

◆ Differential Diagnosis

Myasthenia gravis, orbital disease, other supranuclear movement disorders

◆ Management

Work up and manage according to the cause.

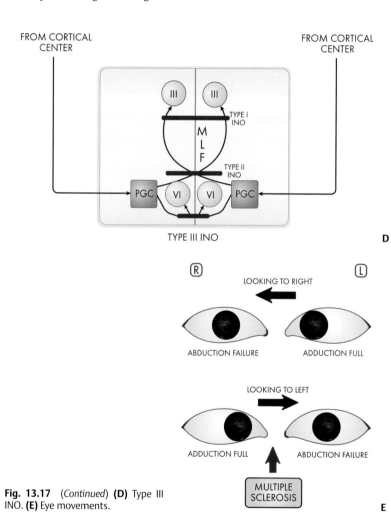

Fig. 13.17 (*Continued*) **(D)** Type III INO. **(E)** Eye movements.

One-and-a-Half Syndrome

One-and-a-half syndrome is also known as *paralytic pontine exotropia.*

◆ Presentation

In the primary position the eye that is opposite the side of the lesion is exotropic. The eye on the same side of the lesion looks straight ahead. The lesion is in the pontine paramedian reticular formation (pontine gaze center) or sixth-nerve nucleus and ipsilateral medial longitudinal fasciculus (**Fig. 13.18A**). From the figure one will understand that only the sixth nerve on the side opposite the side of the lesion will work. The patient is not able to gaze with either eye toward the side of the lesion and is not able to adduct the eye on the side of the lesion (**Fig. 13.18B**). This is why this is called one-and-a-half syndrome, because on one side gaze is absent and on the other side only half the gaze movement is present.

◆ Differential Diagnosis

Myasthenia gravis, orbital disease, other supranuclear movement disorders

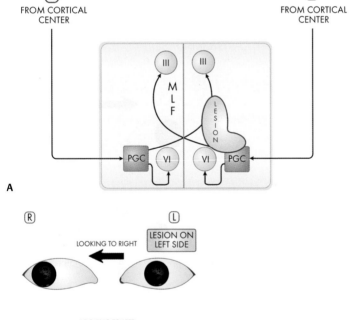

A

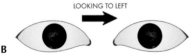

B

Fig. 13.18 (A) One-and-a-half syndrome. (B) One-and-a-half syndrome. MLF, medial longitudinal fasciculus; PGC, pontine gaze center.

◆ **Management**

Work up and manage according to the cause.

Progressive Supranuclear Palsy

In progressive supranuclear palsy there is loss of nerve cells, vascular degeneration, and glial reactions in the basal ganglia and midbrain.

◆ **Presentation**

The first manifestation of progressive supranuclear palsy is an inability to make vertical saccades, particularly downward saccades. At this point, the patients bang their shins, eat off only the top part of their plates, and complain of being unable to read (they cannot look down). As the disease progresses, horizontal fast movements become involved as well. Eventually, occular movements cease to be smooth and rapid. Pursuit movements become characteristically cogwheel.

◆ **Differential Diagnosis**

Chronic progressive external ophthalmoplegia, myasthenia gravis, brainstem lesions, cavernous sinus syndrome

◆ **Management**

No treatment is available except supportive care.

Parinaud Syndrome

There are several manifestations of lesions in the collicular area. The signs are thought to be caused by pressure and distortion of underlying structures in the midbrain and not by damage to specific pathways traversing the colliculi. The general name for the clinical picture produced is known as *Parinaud syndrome*.

◆ **Presentation**

Any combination of impaired upward gaze, impaired downward gaze, pupillary abnormalities, or loss of accommodation reflex can occur. In general, loss of upward gaze associated with dilated pupils that are fixed to light suggests a lesion at the level of the superior colliculus. Loss of downward gaze, normal pupillary reactions to light, and loss of convergence suggest that the lesion is slightly lower in the area of the inferior colliculus. It could be due to lesions of the pineal gland, multiple sclerosis, vascular diseases, or Wernicke encephalopathy.

A special type of nystagmus, retractory nystagmus, is present. This is a very rare sign of disease in the collicular area and consists of an inward and outward movement of both eyes when the patient attempts to look upward. Presumably, it is produced by all the extraocular muscles acting simultaneously—jerking the globe back into the orbit or attempted upward gaze—in an attempt to overcome the inability to look upward.

◆ **Differential Diagnosis**

Thyroid orbitopathy, cavernous sinus syndrome, myasthenia gravis

◆ **Management**

Work up and manage according to the cause.

Chronic Progressive External Ophthalmoplegia

◆ Presentation

The clinical features are the involvement of the upgaze and then the lateral movements and may later be affected in all gaze resulting in a fixed globe. Because the muscle involvement is symmetrical, diplopia does not usually occur. There is also slowly progressive bilateral ptosis.

Kearns-Sayre syndrome is a mitochondrial cytopathy inherited from the mother. It is characterized by pigmentary retinopathy with coarse granularity. Conduction defects of the heart can occur. Heart block may result in sudden death. Other features are short stature, muscle weakness, cerebellar ataxia, neurosensory deafness, mental handicap, and delayed puberty.

◆ Differential Diagnosis

Other causes of paralytic and restrictive strabismus, myopathies, myasthenia gravis, supranuclear palsies

◆ Management

Treat the associated conditions. Use lubricants for the exposure keratopathy and base-down prisms within reading glasses if the downgaze is restricted. Pacemaker may be required for the cardiac condition. In oculopharyngeal dystrophy, dysphagia, and recurrent aspirations may warrant cricopharyngeal surgery. Genetic counseling is needed.

14 Ophthalmic Pharmacology

James M. Hill, Jean T. Jacob, Lori Vidal Denham, Blake A. Booth, Duncan A. Friedman, Jeffery A. Hobden, Andrea T. Murina, Marie D. Acierno, Jean T. Jacob, Herbert E. Kaufman, and Donald R. Bergsma

Two generalizations can be made about pharmacological agents. First, all drugs have more than one effect. Second, all drugs can be toxic. Certainly, most drugs have a primary mechanism of action, and many drugs are safe and well tolerated. However, everyone should be aware of the possible unintended consequences of any pharmacological agent. Although most ophthalmic drugs are administered through topical application, even with this type of drug delivery, both topical and systemic toxicity can occur. This review highlights the most frequent and most severe toxicities but does not give an exhaustive listing of all side effects of these ophthalmic drugs. The generic name and the primary trade name of the drugs are given. When appropriate, we have based the review on the class of the drug and have selected agents that are most used to be included in this review. Finally, this review is not meant to be an exhaustive review of all ophthalmic drugs but outlines the most important and most frequently used agents.

◆ Antibacterial Agents

Topical Antibacterial Agents

Treatment of ocular infectious diseases (**Fig. 14.1**) involves either topical administration of antimicrobial agents (for corneal, conjunctival, and lid margin infections) or direct injection of therapeutic agents into the eye itself (for posterior eye infections).

Table 14.1 lists commercially available antibacterial agents used topically as prophylaxis for surgical procedures or for treating corneal ulcers, conjunctivitis, or marginal lid disease. Most of these antibiotics are broad spectrum, covering both gram-positive and gram-negative pathogens, yet some are more active against one group versus the other. Antibiotics such as polymyxin B, which is effective only

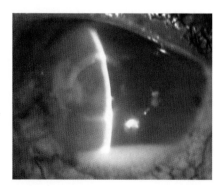

Fig. 14.1 Bacterial corneal ulcer with hypopyon. (Courtesy of Nibaran Gangopdhyay)

Table 14.1 Topical Antibacterial Agents

Trade Name	Antibacterial Agent	Chemical Class	Formulation
Bleph-10	Sulfacetamide sodium	Sulfonamide	10% solution
Sulamyd			10% ointment
Generic	Bacitracin	Peptide	500 Units/g ointment
Generic	Erythromycin	Macrolide	0.5% ointment
Genoptic	Gentamicin	Aminoglycoside	0.3% solution
Garamycin			0.3% ointment
Tobrex	Tobramycin	Aminoglycoside	0.3% solution
			0.3% ointment
Ciloxan	Ciprofloxacin	Second-generation fluoroquinolone	0.3% solution
			0.3% ointment
Ocuflox	Ofloxacin	Second-generation fluoroquinolone	0.3% solution
Quixin	Levofloxacin	Third-generation fluoroquinolone	0.5% solution
Zymar	Gatifloxacin	Fourth-generation fluoroquinolone	0.3% solution
Vigamox	Moxifloxacin	Fourth-generation fluoroquinolone	0.5% solution

against gram-negative bacteria, are combined with other antibiotics to increase the spectrum of coverage (**Table 14.2**). Some of these antibiotics are formulated as aqueous drops or ointment. Others combine antiinflammatory agents to reduce a host inflammatory response that can be as damaging to ocular tissues as bacterial proteases and toxins (**Table 14.3**).

Table 14.2 Combinations of Antibacterial and Antiinflammatory Drugs with Polymyxin B

Trade Name	Antibacterial Agent(s)	Chemical Class	Formulation
Polysporin	Bacitracin	Peptide	500 Units/g ointment
Neosporin ointment	Neomycin + bacitracin	Aminoglycoside + peptide	3.5 mg/g ointment 400 Units/g ointment
Neosporin solution	Neomycin + gramicidin	Aminoglycoside + peptide	10,000 Units; 1.75 mg/mL solution 0.025 mg/mL solution
Terramycin	Oxytetracycline	Tetracycline	5 mg/g ointment
Polytrim	Trimethoprim	Diaminopyrimidine	1 mg/mL solution

Table 14.3 Combination Antibacterial/Antiinflammatory Agents

Trade Name	Antibacterial Agent	Antiinflammatory Agent	Formulation
Blephamide	Sulfacetamide sodium (10%)	Prednisolone acetate (0.2%)	Suspension
Blephamide S.O.P.	Sulfacetamide sodium (10%)	Prednisolone acetate (0.2%)	Ointment
FML-S	Sulfacetamide sodium (10%)	Fluorometholone (0.1%)	Suspension
Vasocidin	Sulfacetamide sodium (10%)	Prednisolone sodium phosphate (0.25%)	Solution
Pred-G	Gentamicin (0.3%)	Prednisolone acetate (1%)	Suspension
Pred-G S.O.P.	Gentamicin (0.3%)	Prednisolone acetate (0.6%)	Ointment
Tobrasone	Tobramycin (0.3%)	Fluorometholone (0.1%)	Suspension
Tobradex	Tobramycin (0.3%)	Dexamethasone (0.1%)	Suspension
Tobradex	Tobramycin (0.3%)	Dexamethasone (0.1%)	Ointment
Zylet	Tobramycin (0.3%)	Loteprednol etabonate (0.5%)	Suspension
Maxitrol (generic)	Neomycin (3.5 mg/mL), polymyxin B (10,000 units/mL)	Dexamethasone (0.1%)	Suspension
AK-Trol (generic)	Neomycin (3.5 mg/mL), polymyxin B (10,000 units/mL)	Dexamethasone (0.1%)	Ointment
Cortisporin (generic)	Neomycin (3.5 mg/mL), polymyxin B (10,000 units/mL)	Hydrocortisone (1%)	Suspension
AK Spore HC (generic)	Neomycin (3.5 mg/mL), polymyxin B (10,000 units/mL), bacitracin (400 units/g)	Hydrocortisone (1%)	Ointment
Poly-Pred	Neomycin (0.35 mg/mL), polymyxin B (10,000 units/mL)	Prednisolone acetate (0.5%)	Suspension

Table 14.4   Injectable Antibacterial Agents

Antibacterial Agent	Chemical Class	Trade Name	Dosage	Route of Injection
Gentamicin	Aminoglycoside	Garamycin	20 mg/0.5 mL	Subconjunctival
Amikacin	Aminoglycoside	Amikin	250 µg/0.1 mL	Intravitreal
Vancomycin	Glycopeptide	Vancocin	2 mg/0.2 mL	Intravitreal
			25 mg/0.5 mL	Subconjunctival
Ceftazidime	Third-generation cephalosporin	Fortraz	2.2 mg/0.1 mL	Intravitreal

Injectable Antibacterial Agents

Bacterial infections of the posterior portion of the eye (endophthalmitis) are treated with antibiotics injected subconjunctivally or intravitreally. Current antibiotic treatment regimens are listed in **Table 14.4**. Dosage recommendations for these antibiotics should not be exceeded to avoid inducing retinal toxicity. Administration of these antibiotics is contraindicated where there is a known hypersensitivity to these agents.

◆ Ocular Antivirals

More than 45 years ago, Kaufman first reported the use of idoxuridine (Herplex) for the treatment of herpes simplex virus (HSV) epithelial keratitis (**Fig. 14.2**). Since then, 50 antivirals have been licensed in the United States; 10 new antivirals and combinations have been introduced in the last 10 years. Acyclovir (ACV) (Zovirax) has been called the "penicillin of antivirals." There are three antivirals that have purine structures similar to ACV: valacyclovir (Valtrex), famciclovir (Famvir), and ganciclovir (Cytovene, Vitraset). Idoxuridine (Herplex) and trifluorothymidine (Viroptic) have very similar pyrimidine structures. Viroptic is the drug of choice for HSV patients. **Table 14.5** is a summary of the most important antivirals and their therapeutic use in viral infections of the eye.

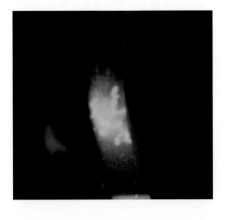

Fig. 14.2 Herpes simplex viral keratitis with large dendrite in late untreated stage.

Table 14.5 Ophthalmic Antiviral Medications

Ophthalmic Disease	Generic Name (Abbreviation)	Trade Name	Route of Administration	Principal Mechanism of Action	Dosage
HSV epithelial keratitis	Idoxuridine (IDU)	Herplex	Topical	Abnormal base results in false mRNA and faulty viral proteins	1.0%
	Trifluridine (TFT)	Viroptic	Topical	Similar to IDU	1.0%
	Acyclovir (ACV)	Zovirax	Oral	Abnormal sugar results in DNA chain termination	400 mg 5 times daily for 7–14 days, 400 mg twice daily for prophylaxis
CMV retinitis	Ganciclovir (GACV)	Vitrasert	Intravitreal	Abnormal sugar results in DNA chain termination	4.5-mg insert (sustained drug delivery)
	Ganciclovir (GACV)	Cytovene	Intravenous, oral		IV 5 mg/kg every 12 h for 14–21 days Maintenance: 5 mg/kg daily for 7 days or 6 mg once daily 5 days a week; Oral: 1000 mg 3 times daily with food or 500 mg 6 times daily every 3 h
	Foscarnet (PAA)	Foscavir	Intravenous	Blocks viral DNA polymerase	Controlled infusion: either central line or peripheral vein induction 60 mg/kg given over 1 h for every 8 hours for 14–21 days; maintenance: 90–120 mg/kg given over 2 h once daily
	Fomiversen	Vitravene	Intravitreal	Antisense to CMV mRNA	330 mg every other week for 4 doses, then every 4 weeks
VZV ophthalmicus	Acyclovir (ACV)	Zovirax	Oral		800 mg 5 times daily for 10 days
	Valacyclovir (VACV)	Valtrex	Oral	Similar to ACV	1 g 3 times daily for 7 days
	Famciclovir (FACV)	Famvir	Oral	Similar to ACV	500 mg 3 times daily for 7 days

Abbreviations: IDU, idoxiuridine; HSV, herpes simplex virus; CMV, cytomegalovirus; VZV, varicella zoster virus.

Table 14.6   Antifungal Agents to Treat Fungal Keratitis and Endophthalmitis

Antifungal Agent	Chemical Class	Trade Name	Dosage	Route of Administration
Natamycin	Polyene	Natacyn	5% suspension	Topical
Amphotericin B	Polyene	Fungizone	0.1–0.5% solution	Topical
			0.8–1.0 mg	Subconjunctival
			5 μg	Intravitreal
Miconazole	Imidazole	Micatin	1% solution	Topical
			5–10 mg	Subconjunctival
			10 μg	Intravitreal
Voriconazole	Triazole	Vfend	1% solution (made from IV solution; dosing ranges from hourly to twice a day as determined by clinician.	Topical
			200 mg twice daily	Oral
			3–6 mg/kg every 12 h	IV*

*Because of potential side effects and toxicity, the practitioner should consult the *Physicians' Desk Reference* for possible dosage adjustments and warnings.
Abbreviations: IV, intravenous.

◆ Antifungal Agents

There is only one commercially available topical antifungal drug (**Table 14.6**): natamycin (Natacyn). The remaining antifungal agents in **Table 14.6** must be extemporaneously compounded for topical, subconjunctival, or intravitreal use. All of these agents are effective against yeast and filamentous fungi. Because of poor penetration, all of these antifungal agents administered topically for corneal infections are dosed at hourly or 2-hour intervals for the first 2 or 3 days. The dosing schedule may be extended to a drop six to eight times a day, depending on how the infection is resolving. Drug penetration into corneal tissue improves if the epithelium is absent. Adverse reactions to topical antifungal agents are limited to local hypersensitivity reactions (e.g., conjunctival chemosis and hyperemia, foreign body sensation).

◆ Antiparasite Agents

Exogenously acquired parasite infections of the eye are caused primarily by amoeba of the genus *Acanthamoeba*. There are no chemotherapeutic agents approved by the United States Food and Drug Administration specifically for the treatment of *Acanthamoeba* keratitis. However, an over-the-counter aromatic diamidine available in the European Union, propamidine isethionate (Brolene), has been shown to be effective when combined with the antibacterial drug neomycin. Propamidine isethionate is available as a 0.1% solution or as an ointment (0.15%).

◆ Antiinflammatories

An inflammatory response results when cells are damaged by microbes, physical agents, or chemical agents and can be characterized by redness, pain, heat, and swelling (**Fig. 14.3**).

Corticosteroids

Corticosteroids commonly used in ophthalmic practice are shown in **Table 14.7**, and are divided into subtypes (short-acting, intermediate-acting, and long-acting) based on their duration of action.

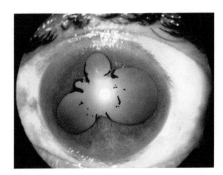

Fig. 14.3 Antiinflammatories are given to suppress inflammation in patients with uveitis.

Table 14.7 Topical Corticosteroids

Generic Name and Preparation	Concentration	Trade Name	Typical Adult Dosage
Dexamethasone sodium phosphate solution	0.1%	Generic	1–2 drops every hour during the day and every 2 h during the night
Dexamethasone ophthalmic suspension or ointment	0.1%	Maxidex	Mild disease: 1–2 drops 4–6 times per day. Severe disease: apply drops hourly
Fluorometholone acetate suspension	0.1%	Flarex	1–2 drops 2–4 times daily
Fluorometholone ophthalmic suspension	0.1%	FML and available generically	1 drop 2–4 times daily
	0.25%	FML Forte	1 drop 2–4 times daily
Fluorometholone ophthalmic ointment	0.1%	FML S.O.P.	$\frac{1}{2}$-inch ribbon into the conjunctival sac 1–3 times/day
Loteprednol etabonate suspension	0.5%	Lotemax	1–2 drops 4 times daily
	0.2%	Alrex	1 drop 4 times daily
Medrysone ophthalmic suspension	1%	HMS	1 drop every 4 h
Prednisolone acetate ophthalmic suspension	1%	Pred Forte and available generically	1–2 drops 2–4 times daily
	1%	Econopred Plus	2 drops 4 times daily
	0.125%	Econopred	2 drops 4 times daily
	0.12%	Pred Mild	1–2 drops 2–4 times daily
Prednisolone sodium phosphate ophthalmic solution	1.0%	Inflamase Forte and available generically	1–2 drops up to every hour
	0.125%	Inflamase Mild and available generically	1–2 drops up to every hour
Rimexolone ophthalmic suspension	1%	Vexol	1–2 drops 4 times daily

Periocular injections are also used to deliver corticosteroids when inflammatory conditions are unresponsive to topical treatments. The main indications for periocular injections are treatment of intermediate or posterior uveitis and cystoid macular edema. The corticosteroids typically used are methylprednisolone (Depo-Medrol), triamcinolone acetonide (Kenalog-40), betamethasone (Celestone Soluspan), dexamethasone (Decadron Phosphate), or available generic equivalents as shown in **Table 14.8**.

Table 14.8   Injectable Corticosteroids

Generic Name and Preparation	Concentration	Trade Name
Betamethasone sodium Phosphate and betamethasone acetate injectable suspension	6 mg/mL	Celestone Soluspan
Dexamethasone sodium phosphate injection	4 mg/mL	Decadron and available generically
Methylprednisolone acetate injectable suspension	40 mg/mL and 80 mg/mL	Depo-Medrol and available generically
Triamcinolone acetonide injectable suspension	40 mg/mL	Kenalog-40

Topical Nonsteroidal Antiinflammatory Drugs (NSAIDs)

Topical NSAIDs currently used in ophthalmology are shown in **Table 14.9** and can be classed as acetic acids, propionic acids, and a prodrug arylacetic acid.

Table 14.9   Topical Nonsteroidal Antiinflammatory Drugs

Generic Name and Preparation	Trade Name	Indication	Dosing/ Concentration
Bromfenac sodium solution	Xibrom	Postoperative inflammation in patients who have undergone cataract extraction	One drop twice a day/0.09%
Diclofenac sodium solution	Voltaren	Postoperative inflammation following cataract extraction and for the temporary relief of pain and photophobia following corneal refractive surgery	One drop four times a day/ 0.1%
Flurbiprofen sodium solution	Ocufen and generic	Inhibition of interoperative miosis	One drop every ½ hour 2 h prior to surgery/0.03%
Ketorolac tromethamine solution	Acular and generic	Postoperative inflammation in patients who have undergone cataract extraction and for relief of ocular itching due to seasonal allergic conjunctivitis	One drop four times a day/ 0.5%
	Acular PF	Reduction of ocular pain and photophobia following incisional refractive surgery	One drop four times a day/ 0.5%
	Acular LS	For the reduction of ocular pain and burning/stinging following corneal refractive surgery	One drop four times a day/ 0.4%
Nepafenac ophthalmic suspension	Nevanac	For pain and inflammation associated with cataract surgery	One drop three times a day/ 0.1%

◆ Drug Combinations (Corticosteroids/Antibiotics)

The combination treatments are multiple-dose suspensions, solutions, and ointments for topical application that include corticosteroids combined with antibiotics such as gentamicin, polymyxin B, neomycin, tobramycin, and sulfacetamide. The various corticosteroid/antibiotic combinations are shown in **Table 14.10.**

◆ Mydriatics and Cycloplegics

Mydriatic and cycloplegic agents have been used in the practice of ophthalmology since the mid-nineteenth century. Trade names, strengths, and dosages are shown in **Table 14.11**.

◆ Glaucoma

Medications can prevent vision loss due to glaucoma by slowing or preventing intraocular pressure (IOP)-related damage to the optic nerve (**Fig. 14.4**). The majority of glaucoma agents were developed for the more common, insidious form of the disease, primary open-angle glaucoma (POAG). IOP plays an important role in the neuropathology of POAG. Prevalence and incidence of POAG increase as IOP increases. Therefore, if patients with increased IOP or signs of optic nerve damage are started early on medications that decrease IOP, vision can often be preserved in the long term. Seven classes of glaucoma drugs are used; the names, administration, and concentrations are listed in **Table 14.12**.

Table 14.10 Combinations of Topical Corticosteroids and Antibiotics

Generic Name and Preparation	Trade Name	Dosing
Dexamethasone 0.1%, tobramycin 0.3% suspension and ointment	TobraDex and available generically	Suspension: 1–2 drops every 4–6 h Initial 24–48 h: 1–2 drops every 2 h Ointment: Apply small amount ($\frac{1}{2}$-inch ribbon) into the conjunctival sac 3–4 times/day
Dexamethasone 0.1%, neomycin sulfate 3.5 mg base/mL, polymyxin B sulfate 10000 units/mL suspension	Maxitrol suspension and available generically	Suspension: 1–2 drops every 3–4 h
Dexamethasone 0.1%, neomycin sulfate 3.5 mg base/g, polymyxin B sulfate 10000 units/g ointment	Maxitrol ointment and available generically	Ointment: Apply small amount into the conjunctival sac 3–4 times/day
Fluorometholone 0.1%, sulfacetamide sodium 10% ophthalmic suspension	FML-S	Instill 1 drop 4 times/day
Fluorometholone acetate 0.1%, tobramycin 0.3% suspension	Tobrasone	Instill 1–2 drops every 4–6 h Initial 24–48 hours: If necessary, 1–2 drops every 2 hours
Hydrocortisone 1%, neomycin sulfate 3.5 mg base/g, polymyxin B sulfate 10000 units/g suspension	Cortisporin ointment and available generically	Suspension: 1–2 drops every 3–4 h
Hydrocortisone 1%, neomycin sulfate 3.5 mg base/g, polymyxin B sulfate 10000 units/g, bacitracin zinc 400 units/g ointment	Cortisporin ointment and available generically	Ointment: Apply the ointment in the affected eye every 3–4 h, depending on condition severity
Loteprednol etabonate 0.5%, tobramycin 0.3% ophthalmic suspension	Zylet	Shake vigorously before using; instill 1–2 drops every 4–6 h Initial 24–48 hours: If necessary, 1–2 drops every 2 h

(Continued on page 416)

Table 14.10 (*Continued*) **Combinations of Topical Corticosteroids and Antibiotics**

Generic Name and Preparation	Trade Name	Dosing
Prednisolone acetate 1.0%, gentamicin sulfate (equivalent to 0.3% gentamicin base) suspension	Pred-G	Suspension: Instill 1 drop 2–4 times/day; initial 24–48 h: If necessary, 1–2 drops/hour
Prednisone acetate 0.6%, gentamicin sulfate (equivalent to 0.3% gentamicin base) ointment	Pred-G S.O.P.	Ointment: Apply small amount ($\frac{1}{2}$-inch ribbon) into the conjunctival sac 1–3 times/day
Prednisolone acetate 0.5%, neomycin sulfate (equivalent to 0.35%, neomycin base), polymyxin B sulfate 10,000 units/mL ophthalmic suspension	Poly-Pred	To treat the eye: Instill 1–2 drops every 3 or 4 h or more frequently as required; acute infections may require 30-min dosing To treat the lid: Instill 1–2 drops every 3–4 h, close eye, and rub the excess on the lids and lid margins
Prednisolone acetate 0.2%, sulfacetamide sodium 10% ophthalmic suspension	Blephamide	Suspension: Shake well before using instill 2 drops every 4 h during the day and at bedtime
Prednisolone acetate 0.2%, sulfacetamide sodium 10% ophthalmic ointment	Blephamide S.O.P.	Ointment: Apply small amount ($\frac{1}{2}$-inch ribbon) into the conjunctival sac 3–4 times/day and once or twice at night
Prednisolone sodium phosphate 0.25% sulfacetamide sodium 10% solution	Vasocidin and generic	Instill 2 drops every 4 h

Table 14.11 Mydriatic and Cycloplegic Agents

Generic Name	Trade Name	Strength	Dosage	Time to Mydriasis	Duration of Action	Time to Cycloplegia
Phenylephrine	Ak-Dilate, Ak-Nefrin, Dilatair, I-Phrine, Isopto Frin, Mydfrin, Ocu-Phrin, Ocugestrin, Phenoptic, Prefrin	2.5% 10%	Refraction: 1 drop 2.5% solution repeat in 5–10 min Uveitis: 1 drop 2.5% three times a day	20–60 min	4–6 h	
Atropine	Atropine Care 1% Atropisol Isopto Atropine Ocu-Tropine	0.5%, 1%, 2%, and 3%	Refraction: 1 drop 1% twice a day 1–2 days prior to exam (Children—use 0.5%) Uveitis: 1–2 drops 1% up to 4 times daily	30–40 min	7–10 days	60–90 min
Tropicamide	Mydriacyl, EyeMycl, Opticyl, Tropicacyl, Ocu-Tropic	0.5% and 1%	Refraction: 1–2 drops 1% solution; repeat in 5–10 min	20–40 min	4–8 h	20–30 min
Phenylephrine and tropicamide	Diophenyl-T, Phenyltrope	Phenylephrine 5%, Tropicamide 0.8%	Refraction: 1–2 drops, repeat in 5–10 min			
Cyclopentolate and phenylephrine	Cyclomydril	Cyclopentolate 0.2% Phenylephrine 1%	Refraction: 1 drop every 5–10 min for up to 3 doses			

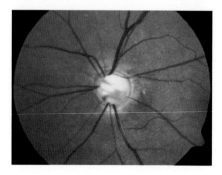

Fig. 14.4 Cupping of the disk in glaucoma.

Beta-Adrenergic Blocking Agents

◆ Mechanism

A disruption in the physiological production of aqueous humor naturally results in fluctuations in IOP. The major site of aqueous humor production is in the ciliary body and is partially controlled by β-adrenergic receptors. Activation of these receptors causes an increase in the production of aqueous humor within the ciliary body. A β-antagonist reduces the formation of aqueous humor resulting in a lower IOP.

◆ Indications

This agent is used as a first-line treatment of POAG. Primary angle closure glaucoma (PACG) is also an indication, but the agents that suppress aqueous humor formation may be less effective in this form of glaucoma because the ciliary body may be ischemic, rendering the β-receptors nonfunctional. Nevertheless, β-antagonists are still indicated in PAC because of the reduction in IOP-enhancing relaxation of the anterior chamber angle.

◆ Contraindications/Adverse Effects

The same β-adrenergic receptors in the ciliary body are found in other organs, and systemic side effects may include decreased heart rate, decreased blood pressure, and exacerbation of intrinsic bronchial asthma and chronic obstructive pulmonary disease due to bronchospasm. This topical medication should be used with caution in patients with cardiac or lung disease. Betaxolol is a cardioselective β-1-adrenergic antagonist developed to avoid the pulmonary complication of timolol, the nonselective classic topical β-adrenergic antagonist. The selective antagonist may be as effective in lowering IOP as the nonselective, but pulmonary side effects have occasionally been noted. Therefore, because of the severity of pulmonary complications in the use of this class of glaucoma agent, caution should be used when considering this drug in the patient with excessive impairment of pulmonary function. Also, the effects of systemic medications such as β-blockers, digitalis, and reserpine can be enhanced with the use of topical β-adrenergic antagonists.

Table 14.12 Antiglaucoma Agents

Agent Type	Generic Name	Trade Name	Route of Administration	Concentration
Beta-adrenergic blockers	Betaxolol	Betoptic-S	Topical	0.25%, 0.5%
	Carteolol	Ocupress	Topical	1%
	Levobunolol	Betagan	Topical	0.25%, 0.5%
	Metipranolol	OptiPranolol	Topical	0.3%
	Timolol	Betimol	Topical	0.25%, 0.5%
Miotics	Carbachol	Isopto Carbachol	Topical	0.75%, 1.5%, 3%
	Pilocarpine hydrochloride	Isopto Carpine	Topical	0.25%, 1%, 2%, 4%, 8% according to PDR
		Pilocar		0.5%, 1%, 2%, 4%, 6%
		Pilopine-HS gel		4%
		Piloptic		0.5%, 1%, 2%, 3%, 4%, 6%
Sympathomimetic	Dipivefrin	Propine	Topical	0.1%
	Epinephrine	Epifrin	Topical	0.5%, 1%, 2%
Alpha₂ selective agonists	Apraclonidine	Iopidine	Topical	0.5%, 1%
	Brimonidine	Alphagan P	Topical	0.1%, 0.15%
		Generic		0.15%, 0.2%
Prostaglandins	Bimatoprost	Lumigan	Topical	0.03%
	Latanoprost	Xalatan	Topical	0.005%
	Travoprost	Travatan	Topical	0.004% (PDR)
	Unoprostone	Rescula	Topical	0.005%
Combination agent	Dorzolamide and timolol	Cosopt	Topical	2% dorzolamide/0.5% timolol
Carbonic anhydrase inhibitors	Acetazolamide	Diamox	Oral	500-mg (timed-release) capsules
		Generic		125-mg, 250-mg tablets (PDR)
	Brinzolamide	Azopt	Topical	1%
	Dorzolamide	Trusopt	Topical	2%
	Methazolamide	Generic	Oral	25, 50-mg tablets

Abbreviations: PDR, *Physicians' Desk Reference.*

Prostaglandin Analogues

◆ Mechanism

The prostaglandin class of glaucoma agents attempts to alter the IOP by enhancing the outflow of aqueous humor. The classic route of aqueous outflow is through the trabecular meshwork into the canal of Schlemm. The prostaglandins also take advantage of a supplemental route of aqueous outflow through the uveoscleral pathway by increasing the portion of aqueous that the pathway normally drains.

◆ Indications

Latanoprost was the first synthetic prostaglandin analogue that formed a new class of drugs developed specifically for glaucoma. A single daily dose has been shown to be more effective in reducing IOP than timolol 0.5% administered twice daily, establishing the prostaglandin class as a first-line treatment for POAG. The prostaglandins are administered topically only.

◆ Contraindications/Adverse Effects

There have been no major systemic toxic effects of topical prostaglandin analogue use in glaucoma thus far, but these drugs are well known for some common, unique ocular effects. Patients frequently acquire permanent darkening of the iris, conjunctival hyperemia, conjunctival flushing, red eye, and a hypertrichosis of the eyelashes that remits when the medication is stopped. There are rare adverse effects including cystoid macular edema, damage to the blood–retinal barrier, and a periocular pigmentation of cosmetic concern.

Carbonic Anhydrase Inhibitors

◆ Mechanism

Like the β-adrenergic blocking agents, this class suppresses aqueous humor production. The mechanism involves decreasing the formation and secretion of aqueous at an intracellular level. Carbonic anhydrase inhibitors (CAIs) are the only class of glaucoma medications that utilize a systemic route of delivery through oral medications. A topical form, dorzolamide, is also available and is more commonly used than the systemic form.

◆ Indications

Oral CAIs are usually used to supplement various topical agents when IOP is not being adequately lowered. Because of their systemic effects and inability to lower IOP independently, CAIs are usually not used as a first-line or sole primary treatment of glaucoma. A combination of dorzolamide and topical timolol, a β-antagonist, is available (Cosopt).

◆ Contraindications/Adverse Effects

The possible adverse effects of the systemic CAIs, acetazolamide, methazolamide, and dichlorphenamide, include paresthesias, anorexia, gastrointestinal disturbances, headaches, altered taste and smell, sodium and potassium depletion, a predisposition to form renal calculi, and rarely bone marrow suppression. These side effects are possible with the topical CAIs but have a much lower incidence. With dorzolamide and brinzolamide the most common side effect is altered taste sensation.

Miotics

◆ Mechanism

Also called parasympathomimetic or cholinergic-stimulating agents, this class enhances cholinergic signal to the anterior chamber by either direct acetylcholine receptor activation or inhibition of acetylcholinesterase activity. This increased cholinergic activity causes a state of miosis that lowers IOP by enhancing aqueous humor outflow through the trabecular meshwork. A pilocarpine-induced miosis has been shown to directly increase the width of the anterior chamber angle in patients with a narrow angle.

◆ Indications

Miotics are indicated for both POAG and PAC. The side-effect profile makes miotics a rarely used glaucoma agent. This class of topical medication is also used to control accommodative esotropia.

◆ Contraindications/Adverse Effects

Systemic side effects can only occur at 5 to 10 times the normal dose. Classic parasympathetic syndrome occurs, including lacrimation, salivation, perspiration, nausea, vomiting, and diarrhea, but very rarely at prescribed dosages. The ocular side effects are problematic owing to the diminished vision with pupillary constriction and headache from ciliary muscle spasm.

Sympathomimetics (Epinephrine)

◆ Mechanism

Adrenergic stimulation decreases IOP by improving aqueous outflow through both the canal of Schlemm and the uveoscleral pathway.

◆ Indication

Sympathomimetics are infrequently used in the treatment of POAG owing to their potentially serious systemic side effects. They are also not indicated for PAC because of the adverse effect of mydriasis on the anterior chamber angle.

◆ Contraindications/Adverse Effects

Epinephrine may cause cardiac arrhythmia or an increase in systemic blood pressure owing to its systemic adrenergic stimulation. Dipivefrin is an epinephrine prodrug that causes fewer systemic side effects.

Alpha$_2$ Selective Agonists

◆ Mechanism

The first drug in this class, apraclonidine, was derived from clonidine and was intended to selectively block the α_2 adrenergic receptor. Brimonidine was then released and shown to be 23 to 32 times more selective for α_2 receptors versus α_1 receptors than apraclonidine. Activation of the α_2 receptor is thought to have a dual mechanism of decreasing aqueous production and increasing uveoscleral outflow.

◆ Indications

The different concentrations available for apraclonidine have specific indications. A single-dose applicator of a 1% solution is available for suppression of the acute IOP spikes that occur after laser treatments. A 0.5% concentration is also available in a multidose bottle for glaucoma patients whose IOP is not adequately responding to maximally tolerated therapy. Chronic use of apraclonidine is limited by its adverse effects and tachyphylaxis. The higher α_2 receptor selectivity of brimonidine allows this type of pressure-lowering medication to be used on a chronic basis.

◆ Contraindications/Adverse Effects

Apraclonidine has been associated with tachyphylaxis or rapid physiological tolerance in up to 48% of patients, rendering it less useful in the chronic forms of glaucoma. The most concerning adverse effects include orthostatic hypotension and vasovagal episodes. The topical application of apraclonidine is associated with mild pupillary dilation, whitening of the conjunctiva, and elevation of the upper eyelid. The adverse effect profile of brimonidine has been minimal but may include oral dryness, headache, and fatigue/drowsiness. Brimonidine is contraindicated in infants because of the risk of severe hypotension and apnea. Both drugs may cause a local sensitivity reaction, with apraclonidine having a fairly high rate of contact dermatitis of the lids and conjunctiva.

◆ Diagnostic Agents

Ophthalmology requires the ability to see certain pathology and manipulate the eye in certain circumstances. Not all pathology is readily visible under direct slit lamp examination. The eye is a very sensitive organ and will not tolerate manipulation without appropriate anesthesia. Anesthetics are used to help with manipulation and certain dyes to visualize pathology (**Table 14.13**).

Fluorescein

Fluorescein comes in many forms, including topical drops (Fluress), topical strips, oral forms, or intravenous (IV) solution (**Fig. 14.5**). It appears as a red-orange pigment under natural light, but when seen under a blue filter, it turns a fluorescent green color. The most common use is the topical form. It can also be topically used to evaluate corneal scarring or other damage to the corneal epithelium. When the cornea is damaged, the dye is able to pass across tight junctions and stain the underlying layers. Recent publications also note that it has a diagnostic purpose in evaluating functioning of the glands in the eyelids. IV and oral fluorescein is used to evaluate retinal pathology by direct fundus photography or confocal microscopy. Fluorescein angiography allows visualization of the vasculature of the retina at different time intervals.

Fluorescein is usually administered in combination with anesthetic or by moistened strips. Slit-lamp examination provides better diagnostic viewing when strips are used because the concentration of fluorescein delivered in most drops is too high for discriminating evaluation. IV fluorescein is usually injected at a dose of 500 mg. More recent research notes that doses as low as 166 mg are effective for evaluation when using confocal scanning laser imaging. Oral fluorescein may be a possible diagnostic agent as confocal imaging progresses, but current angiography still requires the use of IV fluorescein.

Table 14.13 Miscellaneous Drugs

Drug Class	Generic (Brand)	Dose	Mechanism	Indications	Contraindications
Anesthetics	Proparacaine HCl 0.5% (Alcaine, Ocu-Caine, Ophthetic, Paracaine)	1 drop preprocedure	Sodium channel blockade	Preprocedure anesthesia	Known drug allergy, p-aminobenzoic acid (PABA) allergy
	Tetracaine HCl 0.5% (Pontocaine)	Deep anesthesia 1 drop every 5–7 min 5–7 doses			
	Benoxinate 0.4% w/ fluorescein (Fluress) Cocaine 1–10% Lidocaine				
Dyes	Sodium fluorescein		Binds to exposed corneal stroma	Applanation, evaluation of corneal damage, angiography	Known allergies to substance
	*Drops *Strips	1 drop preprocedure Moistened strip touched to eye			
	*Intravenous	500 mg	Circulates through vasculature		
	*Oral	1–2 mg			
	Indocyanine green intravenous	25 mg	Circulates through vasculature	Angiography	Known allergies to indocyanine green or iodide
	Rose bengal strips	Moistened strip touched to eye			

(Continued on page 424)

Table 14.13 (*Continued*) **Miscellaneous Drugs**

Drug Class	Generic (Brand)	Dose	Mechanism	Indications	Contraindications
Decongestants	Naphazoline HCl 0.025% / pheniramine maleate 0.3% (Visine-A, Naphcon-A, Opcon-A, Ocuhist)	1–2 drops daily to 4x per day as needed for symptoms	α adrenergic stimulation and H-1 receptor blockade	Allergic conjunctivitis	Known drug allergy, narrow angle glaucoma, recent monoamine oxidase use
	Phenylephrine HCl 0.12%		α adrenergic stimulation		
	Tetrahydrazoline HCl 0.05%		α adrenergic stimulation		
Antihistamines	Levocabastine (Livostin)	1 drop 4x per day	H-1 receptor blockade	Allergic conjunctivitis	Known allergy to drug class
	Emedastine (Emadine)				
Mast cell stabilizers	Cromolyn sodium 0.4% (Crolom)	1–2 drops 4–6x per day	Prevents mast cell degranulation	Allergic conjunctivitis Giant papillary conjunctivitis Vernal keratitis Vernal kerato-conjunctivitis	Known allergy to drug class
	Pemirolast potassium 0.1% (Alamast)	1–2 drops 4x per day			
	Lodoxamine tromethamine 0.1% (Alomide)	1–2 drops 4x per day			
Combination antihistamines and mast cell stabilizers	Azelastine HCl 0.05% (Optivar, Astelin)	1 drop 2x per day	Prevents mast cell degranulation	Allergic conjunctivitis	Known allergy to drug class
	Ketotifen fumarate 0.025% (Zaditor, Alaway)	1 drop 2x per day spaced 8–12 h apart			
	Nedocromil sodium 2% (Alocril)	1–2 drops 2x per day			
	Olopatadine HCl 0.1% (Patanol)	1–2 drops 2x per day spaced 6–8 h apart			

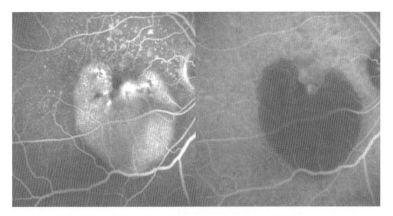

Fig. 14.5 Combined fundus fluorescein angiography and indocyanine green (ICG) angiography. It reveals a pigment epithelial detachment with pooling of dye with a notch, and the ICG is suggestive of a focal hot spot in the area of the notch. (Courtesy of Dr. Manish Nagpal)

Adverse effects are minimal for the topical forms of the drug. More effects are possible when IV fluorescein is used. Nausea, vomiting, dizziness, and a bitter taste may result during IV administration. Many patients develop cough or dry throat, and some can develop urticaria, or localized inflammation of the injection site from allergies. Anaphylactoid reactions, sickle cell crises, hemolytic anemia, seizure, myocardial infarction, and deaths are all documented in the literature, but their occurrence is rare.

Indocyanine Green

Another potential agent used to evaluate posterior compartment pathology is ICG. Much like its closely related substance, fluorescein, this dye is injected intravenously to evaluate the retina and choroid. It has a distinct advantage over fluorescein in that it can better diagnose choroidal neovascularization. This is due partly to the fact that ICG is highly plasma protein bound. Fluorescein, which usually leaks out of the capillaries, cannot define vasculature as well as ICG, which stays within the vessels. Other advantages include the fact that the fluorescent wavelength of ICG places it in the near infrared spectrum. This factor allows penetration of tissues that normally absorb the shorter wavelength fluorescence of fluorescein.

ICG is usually administered in doses of 25 mg for proper imaging. Because of advances in confocal ophthalmoscopy, adequate diagnostics can be obtained by as little as 5 mg of ICG. Adverse reactions are rare but can include nausea, vomiting, and general discomfort. Anaphylaxis has been reported in certain cases. ICG should not be used in individuals with known allergy to the substance or allergies to iodide because many preparations of ICG contain iodide. In individuals with allergies to fluorescein, use of ICG may avoid serious reactions.

Agents Used in the Diagnosis and Management of Neuro-ophthalmological Conditions

Most pupillary disorders of the sympathetic or parasympathetic nervous system are pharmacologically diagnosed by using specific ophthalmic drops (**Table 14.14**).

◆ Medications and Therapeutics for Dry Eye

An estimated 7.1 million people in the United States over the age of 40 are afflicted with keratoconjunctivitis sicca (KCS, also known as dry eye) (**Fig. 14.6**). Dry eye is particularly prevalent in women aged 50 years and older, but in patients aged 75 and older, this prevalence is diminished. **Table 14.15** provides a listing of the types of targeted and palliative treatments available.

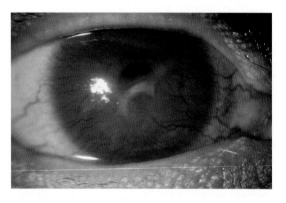

Fig. 14.6 Severe dry-eye syndrome with corneal neovascularization.

Table 14.14 Neuro-ophthalmic Agents

Ophthalmic Condition	Drug Name	Route of Administration	Mechanism of Action	Dosage
Blepharospasm	Botulinum toxin A (Botox, Allergan)	Subcutaneous	Acts presynaptically by inhibiting release of acetylcholine at the neuromuscular junction	Total periorbital treatment dose 100 units (50 units per eye)
Hemifacial spasm	Botulinum toxin B (Myobloc, Elan)	Subcutaneous	Indicated for those resistant to Botox A	750–5000 units (up to 2500 units per side)
Horner syndrome	Cocaine 4% or 10%	Topical	Prevents reuptake of norepinephrine released by postganglionic synaptic endings; used to confirm the presence of Horner syndrome	1 drop OU if no mydriasis in 1 hour then instill a second drop
Horner syndrome	Hydroxyamphetamine 1%	Topical	Releases norepinephrine from the sympathetic vesicles at synaptic endings; differentiates between preganglionic and postganglionic lesions; partial or no dilation c/w postganglionic third order lesion; dilation of involved pupil c/w preganglionic first- or second-order lesion	1 drop OU
Horner syndrome	Apraclonidine 0.5% or 1%	Topical	Weak direct action on α^1 receptors; actively dilates the affected pupil but not the normal pupil; results in reversal of the anisocoria	1 drop OU
Adie tonic pupil	Pilocarpine 1/8%	Topical	Constriction of the involved pupil due to cholinergic supersensitivity	1 drop OU
Tonic pupil	Pilocarpine 1%	Topical	Failure of the dilated pupil to constrict due to pharmacological blockade	1 drop OU

Abbreviations: OU, oculi uterque (both eyes).

Table 14.15   Therapeutic Options for Dry Eye Syndrome*

Product	Brand Name	How Supplied	Dosing
I. Targeted therapies			
Antibiotics:			
Topical:			
Bacitracin/ploymyxin	Polysporin[7]	5 mL bottle	1–2 drops 2x daily
Systemic:			
Doxycycline	Vibra-Tabs[8]	100 mg tablets	100 mg 2x daily
Immunomodulators:			
Cyclosporine A	Restasis[2]	Unit dose vials (0.4 mL)	1 drop 2x daily
Mucolytic agents:			
N-acetylcysteine	Mucomyst[10]	10–20% drops, 5 ml bottle	1–2 drops up to 4x daily
Corticosteroid & antibiotic mixtures:			
Loteprednol etabonate (0.5%) and tobramycin (0.3%)	Zylet[7]	2.5, 5, and 10 mL bottles	1–2 drops 4–6 hours
II. Palliative therapies			
Corticosteroids:			
Loteprednol etabonate (0.5%)	Lotemax[7]	5 & 10 mL dropper bottle	1–2 drops 4x daily
(0.2%)	Alrex[7]		
Prednisolone acetate (0.1%)	Pred Forte[2] Omnipred[1]	5 & 10 mL dropper bottle	2 drops 4x daily
Fluorometholone (0.25%)	FML Forte[2]	5, 10 & 15 mL dropper bottle, ointment	1 drop 2–4x daily, ½ inch into cul de sac 1–3x daily
Rimexolone (1%)	Vexol[1]	5 & 10 mL dropper bottle	
Secretagogues:			
Pilocarpine	Salagen[11]	5 mg tablets	1 daily
Therapeutic plug:			
Hydroxypropyl cellulose	Lacrisert[7]	5 mg water-soluble rod	1–2 rods per eye daily
Artificial tears:			
Low viscosity—	OPTIVE[2]	5 mL dropper or unit dose	1–2 drops as needed
	Refresh Plus[2]	Unit dose	1–2 drops as needed
	Refresh Tears[2]	Unit and Multi-dose	1–2 drops as needed
Hypoosmotic—	TheraTears[3]	Unit and multi-dose	1–2 drops as needed

Table 14.15   *(continued)*

Product	Brand Name	How Supplied	Dosing
Moderate viscosity—	Refresh Dry Eye Therapy[2]	Unit dose	1–2 drops as needed
	Tear Naturale Forte[1]	5 mL dropper bottle	1–2 drops as needed
	GenTeal[6]	Unit dose, preservative free	1–2 drops as needed
	Bion Tears[5]	Unit dose, preservative free	1–2 drops as needed
	Ocucoat[7]	Unit dose, preservative free	1–2 drops as needed
High viscosity— (best for nocturnal application)	Systane Ultra[1]	10 mL dropper bottle	1–2 drops as needed
	Refresh Celluvisc[2]	Unit dose	1–2 drops as needed
	Refresh Liquigel[2]	Unit dose	1–2 drops as needed
	Blink Tears[5]	15 mL dropper bottle	1–2 drops as needed
Gel formulations— (best for nocturanal application)	GenTeal Gel[6]	Tube delivery system	¼ inch into cul de sac
	Tears Again[5]	Tube delivery system	¼ inch into cul de sac
Lubricating ointments— (best for nocturnal application)	Refresh P.M.[2]	Tube	¼ inch into cul de sac
	Tears Naturale PM[1]	Tube	¼ inch into cul de sac
	Advanced Eye Relief[2]	Tube	¼ inch into cul de sac
	Systane Nighttime[1]	Tube	¼ inch into cul de sac

[1]Alcon Laboratories, Inc., Fort Worth, TX USA; [2]Allergan, Inc., Irvine, CA USA; [3]Advanced Vision Research, Inc., Woburn, MA USA; [4]Abbott Medical Optics, Abbott Park, IL USA; [5]Cynacon/OcuSoft, Inc., Richmond, TX USA; [6]Novartis Pharmaceuticals, St. Louis, MO USA; [7]Bausch and Lomb, Inc., Rochester, NY USA; [8]Pfizer Labs, Inc., New York, NY USA; [9]Aton Pharmaceuticals, Inc., Lawrenceville, NJ USA; [10]Mead-Johnson Laboratories, Evansville, ID USA; and [11]MGI PHARMA, Inc., Bloomington, MN USA.

Acknowledgments
This work was made possible, in part, by NEI-EY-006311 (JMH), Research to Prevent Blindness Senior Scientific Investigator Award (JMH), EY02672 (HEK) and LSU Eye Center Core Grant EY02377. The Department of Ophthalmology has an unrestricted grant from Research to Prevent Blindness, New York, NY and funds from the Louisiana Eye Foundation, New Orleans.

15 Ocular Manifestations of Systemic Disease

Soosan Jacob and Amar Agarwal

◆ Diabetes Mellitus

Diabetes mellitus (DM) is a chronic disorder characterized by persistent hyperglycemia presenting with varied manifestations and consequently resulting in microvascular and macrovascular complications. Risk factors for diabetic retinopathy include duration of DM, control of blood glucose, puberty and type of DM, nephropathy, hypertension, pregnancy, and genetic factors (**Fig. 15.1**).

◆ Presentation

- *Nonproliferative diabetic retinopathy*: This is the earliest form characterized by microaneurysms, dot and blot hemorrhages, cotton-wool spots, hard exudates, venous loops, venous beading, and intraretinal microvascular abnormality.
- *Proliferative diabetic retinopathy*: Characterized by the proliferation of abnormal new vessels either on the optic disk or elsewhere on the surface of retina.
- *Diabetic macular edema*: Types include focal, diffuse, ischemic, and mixed.
- *Posterior subcapsular cataracts*: Transient shift in refraction occurs due to lens swelling due to osmotic gradient formed by sorbitol.
- *Glaucoma*: There is increased risk of open-angle and neovascular glaucoma.
- *Corneal neuropathic changes*: It can present with decreased corneal sensations and epitheliopathy.
- *Cranial-nerve palsies*: Pupil-sparing third, fourth, and sixth cranial nerves can be involved. Diabetic papillitis, mucormycosis, and orbital cellulitis are also common.

◆ Management

Management includes systemic control of DM, correction of anemia, and maintenance of blood pressure <130/80 mm Hg, fasting blood sugar → 90 to 130 mg%, post-prandial blood sugar → 180 mg%, triglycerides <150 mg%, low-density lipoprotein (LDL) <100 mg%, high-density lipoprotein (HDL) >40 mg%, and albuminuria <30 µg/mg.

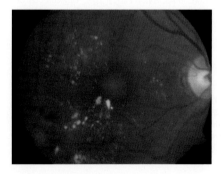

Fig. 15.1 Diabetic retinopathy.

Panretinal photocoagulation, focal and grid laser photocoagulation, pars plana vitreous surgery, and pharmacotherapy with aldose reductase inhibitors, protein kinase C-β inhibitors and intravitreal antivascular endothelial growth factor (VEGF) agents (bevacizumab, ranibizumab, etc.) are effective modalities of treatment.

◆ Acquired Immunodeficiency Syndrome

Acquired immunodeficiency syndrome (AIDS) is a potentially fatal multisystem syndrome caused by human immunodeficiency virus (HIV), characterized by profound disruption of the immune system and a propensity for various opportunistic infections and neoplasms.

◆ Presentation

- ◆ *Eyelids*: Kaposi sarcoma, herpes zoster ophthalmicus, multiple molluscum lesions
- ◆ *Orbit*: B-cell lymphoma
- ◆ *Conjunctiva*: Kaposi sarcoma, squamous cell carcinoma
- ◆ *Cornea*: Keratitis due to microsporidium, herpes simplex, herpes zoster
- ◆ *Posterior segment*: HIV retinopathy, cytomegalovirus (CMV) retinitis, toxoplasmosis, *Candida* retinitis, progressive outer retinal necrosis, pneumocystis carinii pneumonia retinopathy, *Histoplasma capsulatum*, cryptococcal infection
- ◆ *Neuro-ophthalmic*: Cranial-nerve palsies, pupillary abnormalities, optic neuritis, papilledema, and visual-field defects

◆ Management

Diagnosis is confirmed with enzyme-linked immunosorbent assay (ELISA) and Western blot test. Monitoring is done by complete blood count (CBC), CD4 count, and tests for secondary infections. Highly active antiretroviral therapy (HAART) is the recommended treatment, which involves two nucleoside reverse transcriptase inhibitors with either a nonnucleoside reverse transcriptase inhibitor or one or two protease inhibitors.

- ◆ *Nucleoside reverse transcriptase inhibitors*: zidovudine, lamivudine, and zalcitabine
- ◆ *Protease inhibitors*: Amprenavir, indinavir
- ◆ *Nonnucleoside reverse transcriptase inhibitors*: efavirenz

◆ Varicella Zoster Virus

Varicella zoster virus (VZV) is one of the herpesviruses known to infect humans. It causes chickenpox in children and both shingles and postherpetic neuralgia in adults. It is spread by airborne droplets as well as infected secretions.

◆ Presentation

After the primary infection resulting in chickenpox, the virus remains dormant within the body in the trigeminal and dorsal root ganglia and may become reactivated to produce herpes zoster. The risk of zoster increases with age and immunosuppression. Systemic involvement may cause serious complications.
Ocular involvement:

◆ Acute conjunctivitis with or without secondary bacterial infection
◆ Pseudodendrites and corneal ulcers
◆ Stromal keratitis
◆ Uveitis, retinitis, optic neuritis, ophthalmoplegia

◆ Management

Management is in coordination with the neurologist, infectious disease specialist, and dermatologist. Treatment is based on the severity, age, and immune state. Antiviral medications are thought to decrease the duration of symptoms and the likelihood of postherpetic neuralgia when started within 2 days of the onset of rash. Medications available include acyclovir, valacyclovir, penciclovir, and famciclovir.

◆ Rheumatoid Arthritis

Rheumatoid arthritis (RA) is an autoimmune systemic disease characterized by asymmetrical, destructive, deforming, inflammatory polyarthropathy, in association with a spectrum of extraarticular manifestations. Association of HLA-DW4/DR4 occurs in white persons.

◆ Presentation

Women are more frequently affected than men (3:1). RA is commonly seen in the fourth decade. Fever, malaise, weight loss, morning stiffness, joint pain and inflammation, and limitation of movements are the main complaints. Ulnar deviation and swan neck deformity, bursal effusion, Baker cyst and hallux valgus are seen. Extraocular findings include superficial rheumatoid nodule, pericarditis and pleural effusion, Caplan syndrome, and Felty syndrome.
Ophthalmic manifestations include keratoconjunctivitis sicca, scleritis, peripheral ulcerative keratitis, and acquired superior oblique tendon sheath syndrome.

◆ Management

Laboratory investigations include rheumatic factor (RF), antinuclear antibodies (ANA), CBC, and rheumatology consultation. Nonsteroidal antiinflammatory drugs (NSAIDs), gold salts, D-pencillamine, hydroxychloroquine, sulphasalazine, steroids, and cytotoxic agents are the drugs used.

◆ Systemic Lupus Erythematosis

Systemic lupus erythematosus (SLE) is an autoimmune, non–organ-specific connective tissue disease characterized by numerous antibodies and circulating immune complexes, which mediate widespread vasculitis and tissue damage.

◆ Presentation

◆ Predominantly affects young women (9:1), frequently in the third or fourth decade. Common presenting symptoms include fever, fatigue, and weight loss.
◆ Ophthalmic features include madarosis, keratoconjunctivitis sicca, peripheral ulcerative keratitis, scleritis, retinal vasculitis, and optic neuropathy.
◆ Extraocular manifestations include the following:
  ◆ *Mucocutaneous*: Butterfly facial rash, discoid rash, vasculitis, alopecia, oral ulceration, Raynaud phenomenon
  ◆ *Musculoskeletal*: Arthritis, myositis, tendonitis
  ◆ *Renal*: Glomerulonephritis
  ◆ *Cardiovascular*: Pericarditis, endocarditis, myocarditis, arterial and venous occlusions.
  ◆ *Pulmonary*: Pleurisy, atelectasis
  ◆ *Hematopoietic*: Anemia, thrombocytopenia, lymphopenia, leucopenia
  ◆ *Reticuloendothelial*: Splenomegaly, lymphadenopathy
  ◆ *Neurological*: Polyneuritis, cranial-nerve palsies, spinal cord lesions, epilepsy

◆ Management

Laboratory investigations include CBC, ANA, double stranded/single stranded (DS/SS) DNA, SSA/SSB (Sjögren syndrome), erythrocyte sedimentation rate (ESR), antiphospholipid antibody, lupus anticoagulant, and a rheumatologist's opinion. Therapies include antimalarials, NSAIDs, steroids, and cytotoxic agents.

◆ Sjögren Syndrome

Sjögren syndrome (SS) is characterized by autoimmune inflammation and destruction of lacrimal and salivary glands.

◆ *Primary SS*: When it exists in isolation
◆ *Secondary SS*: When it is associated with other disease such as RA and SLE

◆ Presentation

Primary SS affects women more commonly than men. It presents in adult life with grittiness of the eyes and dryness of the mouth. Enlargement of the salivary glands with diminished salivary flow rate and a dry fissured tongue, dry nasal passages, diminished vaginal secretions, Raynaud phenomenon, and cutaneous vasculitis are the features of the disorder.
  The main ophthalmic features include keratoconjunctivitis sicca and Adie pupil.

Management

Laboratory tests include CBC, rheumatoid factor, ANA, SSA/SSB, cryoglobulins, circulating immune complexes, gammaglobulins, and antithyroid antibodies. Diagnosis can be confirmed by salivary gland biopsy. Important therapies include systemic steroids and cytotoxic agents.

◆ Lyme Disease

Lyme disease is an infection caused by a spirochete, *Borrelia burgdorferi*, transmitted through the bite of a deer tick, *Ixodes dammini*. It is most commonly reported from the northeastern United States.

Presentation

Following are the manifestations of Lyme disease.

- ◆ Early stage
  - ◆ Presents several days after the bite
  - ◆ Erythema chronicum migrans
  - ◆ Constitutional symptoms, lymphadenopathy
  - ◆ Neurological and cardiac complications may follow within 3 to 4 weeks of the initial manifestation.
- ◆ Late stage
  - ◆ Chronic arthritis of the large joints
  - ◆ Polyneuropathy, chronic acrodermatitis
- ◆ Ophthalmic manifestations include the following:
  - ◆ Photophobia, pain, periocular edema, conjunctivitis
  - ◆ Keratitis, anterior uveitis, intermediate uveitis, optic neuritis, neuroretinitis, ocular motor nerve palsies
  - ◆ Peripheral multifocal choroiditis, retinal periphlebitis

Management

Check for a history of tick bite, exposure, and the characteristic rash. Perform a thorough dermatological, neurological, and ocular examination. Immunofluorescence and ELISA must be performed. Western blot is confirmatory. Therapies include oral doxycycline and intravenous antibiotics.

◆ Leprosy

Leprosy is a chronic granulomatous infection caused by an intracellular acid-fast bacillus, *Mycobacterium leprae*.

Presentation

- ◆ Lepromatous leprosy is a generalized, multisystem infection.
  - ◆ *Skin*: When it exists in isolation
  - ◆ *Nose*: When it is associated with other disease such as RA and SLE

◆ *Neurological*: Sensory neuropathy, autonomic neuropathy, and motor neuropathy
◆ Tuberculoid leprosy is restricted to the skin and peripheral nerves.
  ◆ *Skin*: Annular, anesthetic, hypopigmented lesions with raised edges
  ◆ *Nerves*: Thickening of cutaneous sensory nerves
◆ Ophthalmic features include the following:
  ◆ Madarosis, lagophthalmos due to seventh-nerve palsy, neurotropic keratitis due to trigeminal nerve involvement
  ◆ Anterior uveitis (granulomatous)

◆ Management

Dapsone is the drug of choice. Rifampicin and clofazimine contributes in multidrug therapy. Clofazimine is no longer available through most U.S. pharmacies. Requests for clofazimine to treat leprosy should be directed to the National Hansen's Disease program (a division of the U.S. Dept. of Health and Human Services), which holds the IND for this indication. It can thus be obtained for use in leprosy.

◆ Leukemia

Leukemias are a group of neoplastic disorders characterized by abnormal proliferation of white blood cells. Ocular involvement is more commonly seen in the acute than in the chronic form.

◆ Presentation

Acute leukemia presents with constitutional symptoms, including fever, lymphadenopathy, hepatosplenomegaly, epistaxis, and easy bruisability. Central nervous system (CNS) involvement and secondary infections are the main concern (**Fig. 15.2**). Ocular manifestations include the following:

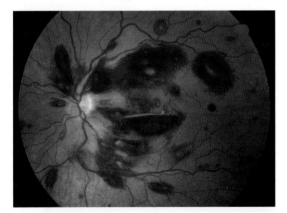

Fig. 15.2 Color fundus photograph showing superficial and deep retinal hemorrhages, and a preretinal boat-shaped hemorrhage associated with leukemia. (Courtesy of Stephen W. Wong, MD, Philadelphia, PA)

- Retinopathy, including flame-shaped hemorrhages, Roth spots, cotton-wool spots, peripheral retinal neovascularization leukemic pigment epitheliopathy, characterized by a leopard spot fundus
- Orbital involvement
- Iris thickening, iritis, and pseudohypopyon
- Subconjunctival hemorrhage, hyphema
- Optic neuropathy

Management

Bone marrow aspiration, biopsy with immunocytogenic markers, computed tomographic (CT) scan, and lumbar puncture are required for confirming the diagnosis and extent of the disease. Systemic chemotherapy, general supportive measures, and ocular radiotherapy are the mainstays of the treatment.

Lymphoma

Lymphoma is a type of solid hematological neoplasm originating from the lymphocytes. Primary intraocular and central nervous system lymphoma is a highly malignant, diffuse, large B-cell lymphoma (**Figs. 15.3** and **15.4**).

Presentation

Intraocular lymphomas generally affect elderly patients and are unilateral (20%) or bilateral (80%). Two types are recognized: vitreoretinal (not associated with systemic involvement) and uveal (associated with systemic involvement).

- Ocular features
    - Chronic anterior uveitis
    - Intermediate uveitis

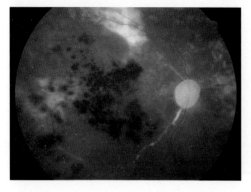

Fig. 15.3 Color fundus photograph of a patient with intraocular lymphoma showing hemorrhagic retinal vasculitis. (Courtesy of Debra A. Goldstein, MD, Chicago, IL)

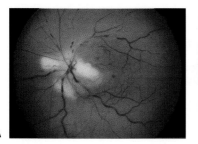 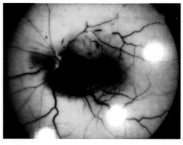

A   B

Fig. 15.4 **(A)** Color and **(B)** red-free fundus photographs of a patient with central nervous system lymphoma that resulted in central retinal artery occlusion secondary to optic nerve compression. (Courtesy of Lawrence J. Ulanski, MD, Chicago, IL)

    ◆ Posterior segment
    ◆ Multifocal, large, yellowish, subretinal pigment epithelium (RPE) infiltrates.
    ◆ Diffuse retinal infiltrates, vascular sheathing, and occlusion
◆ CNS features
    ◆ Solitary or multiple intracranial nodules
    ◆ Diffuse meningeal or periventricular lesions
    ◆ Localized intradural spinal masses

◆ **Management**

Diagnosis of ocular lymphoma is confirmed with aqueous and vitreous biopsy and cytology. CT, magnetic resonance imaging (MRI), and lumbar puncture help in ascertaining the diagnosis of CNS lymphoma. Lymphoma is treated with high-dose external beam radiotherapy to the eyes, whole-brain radiotherapy, systemic or intrathecal chemotherapy, and intrathecal methotrexate.

◆ Pregnancy

Pregnancy is associated with maternal hormonal, metabolic, hematological, cardiovascular, and immunologic alterations that can affect the ocular tissues.

◆ **Presentation**

◆ Retinal and choroidal disorders arising in pregnancy
◆ Preeclampsia and eclampsia
◆ Retinopathy—focal or generalized retinal arteriolar narrowing
◆ Choroidopathy—serous retinal detachments or yellow RPE lesions
◆ Cortical blindness
◆ Retinal arterial and venous occlusions
◆ Central serous chorioretinopathy
◆ Disseminated intravascular coagulopathy (DIC)
◆ Thrombotic thrombocytopenic purpura (TTP)

- Amniotic fluid embolism
- Uveal melanoma
- Worsened preexisting conditions
- Diabetic retinopathy (progression can be diminished by better metabolic control before pregnancy)
- Diabetic macular edema (pregnant women with diabetic macular edema should not be treated during pregnancy because of the high rate of spontaneous improvement postpartum)

◆ Management

Treatment is aimed at the pathological state and is done in coordination with the patient's obstetrician. A close watch must be kept on the retinopathies because spontaneous regression can occur with time. Proliferative diabetic retinopathy may be required to be treated to prevent vitreous hemorrhage during labor.

◆ Albinism

Albinism is a genetically determined heterogeneous group of disorders involving hypopigmentation of the eyes or skin due to a deficiency of tyrosinase, which mediates the conversion of tyrosine to melanin (**Fig. 15.5**).

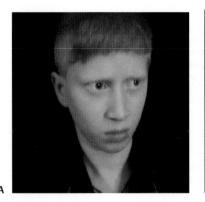
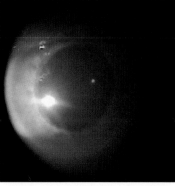

A   B

Fig. 15.5 **(A)** Albinotic patient. **(B)** Transillumination seen through the iris in the same patient.

◆ Presentation

Oculocutaneous Albinism

- ◆ *Tyrosinase-negative*: These albinos are incapable of synthesizing melanin and have blond hair and very pale skin.
  - ◆ Iris is diaphanous and translucent, giving rise to a "pink-eyed" appearance.
  - ◆ Fundus
    - ◆ Lack of pigment with conspicuously large choroidal vessels
    - ◆ Hypoplasia of vessels forming the perimacular arcades
    - ◆ Foveal and optic nerve hypoplasia may be present.
    - ◆ Refractive errors are common.
    - ◆ Nystagmus
    - ◆ The chiasm has a decreased number of uncrossed nerved fibers.

- ◆ *Tyrosinase-positive*: These albinos can synthesize variable amounts of melanin and vary in complexion from very fair to almost normal.
  - ◆ Iris may be blue or dark brown.
  - ◆ Fundus shows variables hypopigmentation.
  - ◆ Visual acuity is usually impaired owing to foveal hypoplasia.

- ◆ *Associated syndromes*: Chédiak-Higashi and Hermansky-Pudlak syndromes can be associated with oculocutaneous albinism.
  - ◆ Chédiak-Higashi syndrome is associated with white cell abnormalities resulting in pyogenic infections, lymphadenopathy, and death.
  - ◆ Hermansky-Pudlak syndrome is a lysosomal storage disease of the reticuloendothelial system characterized by easy bruising due to platelet dysfunction.

Ocular Albinism
The eyes are predominantly affected, with less evident skin and hair involvement. Inheritance is XL or less commonly AR. Female carriers are asymptomatic and have normal vision, although they may show partial iris translucency, macular stippling, and scattered areas of depigmentation and granularity in the midperiphery. Affected males manifest hypopigmented iris and fundus.

◆ Management

Tyrosinase test, electroretinography, hematological tests are helpful in the diagnosis. Dark glasses, low vision aids, genetic counseling are helpful.

◆ Marfan Syndrome

Marfan syndrome is a widespread disorder of connective tissues associated with mutation of the fibrillin gene or chromosome 15q. It is the most common cause of heritable ectopia lentis. Marfan syndrome is autosomal dominant, and the prevalence is 5/100,000 (**Fig. 15.6**).

◆ Presentation

◆ Ophthalmic features
  ◆ Ectopia lentis, hypoplasia of dilator pupillae, angle anomaly, myopia, and retinal detachment
  ◆ Lens dislocation occurs in ~80% of patients with Marfan syndrome and is usually bilateral, symmetrical, and superotemporal.
  ◆ Microspherophakia, keratoconus, and cornea plana
◆ Musculoskeletal features
  ◆ Tall, thin stature, scoliosis, increased arm span
  ◆ Arachnodactyly, mild joint hypermobility
  ◆ Narrow and high-arched palate
◆ Cardiovascular features
  ◆ Dilatation of the ascending aorta leading to aortic incompetence and heart failure
  ◆ Mitral valve disease and aortic dissection
◆ Skin
  ◆ Striae, fragility, and easy bruising

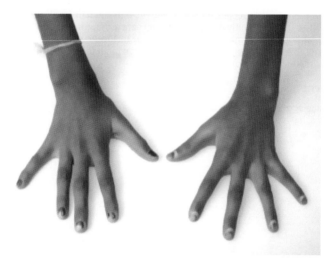

Fig. 15.6 Long, thin, and slender fingers in a patient with Marfan syndrome.

◆ **Management**

Evaluation by a cardiologist is often necessary. Rule out other causes of lens sub-luxation. The subluxation is treated according to the grade and visual symptoms.

◆ Homocystinuria

Homocystinuria is caused by deficiency of cystathionine β-synthetase leading to accumulation of homocystine and methionine. It is the second most common cause of ectopia lentis.

◆ **Presentation**

◆ Ophthalmic features
  ◆ Ectopia lentis, which is usually bilateral, symmetrical, inferonasal, and pres-ent in nearly 90% of patients. Deficient zonular integrity secondary to the enzymatic defect has been implicated as the primary cause of lens displace-ment (**Fig. 15.7**).
  ◆ Myopia, retinal detachment, retinal vein occlusions, retinal artery occlu-sions
◆ Other features
  ◆ Fair skin with coarse hair, osteoporosis, mental retardation, seizure disorder, marfanoid habitus, and poor circulation
  ◆ Thromboembolic events constitute the major threat to survival, especially following general anesthesia.
  ◆ Sodium nitroprusside test and urine chromatography help in confirming the diagnosis.

◆ **Management**

IQ testing and special needs programs and schooling may be required. Limit me-thionine intake and increase cysteine intake. Oral pyridoxine reduces homocystine and methionine levels. Rule out other causes of subluxation and treat it if the pa-tient is symptomatic.

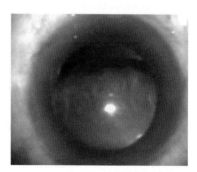

Fig. 15.7 Inferior subluxation seen in a patient with homocystinuria.

◆ Weill-Marchesani Syndrome

Weill-Marchesani syndrome is a rare autosomal, recessive, systemic, connective tissue disorder, characterized by short stature, brachydactyly, and stiff joints. Penetrance is variable and consanguinity is often present.

◆ Presentation

- ◆ Ocular features
    - ◆ Ectopia lentis, bilateral and inferior, occurs in ~50% of cases during the teen years or early twenties.
    - ◆ Microspherophakia is the most prominent feature of this syndrome.
    - ◆ Secondary angle-closure glaucoma due to pupillary block
    - ◆ Lenticular myopia, asymmetrical axial lengths, presenile vitreous liquefaction
- ◆ Other features
    - ◆ Short stature, brachycephaly, limited joint mobility, well-developed muscular appearance, and normal intelligence

◆ Management

Radiography of the metacarpals is important. Treat angle-closure glaucoma with mydriatics and laser iridotomy. The fellow eye must be kept on miotics to prevent a similar occurrence. Rule out other causes of lens subluxation and treat it if the patient is symptomatic.

◆ Pseudoxanthoma Elasticum

Pseudoxanthoma elasticum (PXE) is a rare genetic disorder characterized by progressive calcification and fragmentation of elastic fibers in the skin, retina, and cardiovascular system, which is referred to as *elastorrhexia*.

◆ Presentation

- ◆ Ocular features
    - ◆ Angioid streaks of the retina, which are slate gray to reddish brown curvilinear bands radiating from the optic disk. They result from calcification of the elastic fibers in the Bruch membrane of the retina. They are present in 85% of patients with PXE.
    - ◆ Fibrovascular ingrowth in the retina may lead to retinal hemorrhage.
    - ◆ Development of subretinal neovascular membrane can cause loss of central vision.
    - ◆ Yellowish speckled mottling described as peau'd'orange in seen in the temporal quadrant of the retina.
- ◆ Cutaneous findings
    - ◆ Plaques are seen on the lateral part of the neck and involve the antecubital fossa.
- ◆ Cardiovascular findings
    - ◆ Hypertension, coronary infarction, mitral valve prolapse
- ◆ Other findings
    - ◆ Gastrointestinal bleeding, peripheral vascular diseases

◆ Management

Skin biopsy is diagnostic. Fundus fluorescein angiography (FFA) and optical coherence tomography (OCT) help in determining underlying choroidal neovascular membrane if the patient complains of metamorphopsia. Patients should avoid heavy lifting, straining, and head trauma. Treatment of the choroidal neovascular membrane either with laser photocoagulation or with intravitreal anti-VEGF injection is recommended.

◆ Phakomatoses

Neurofibromatosis (von Recklinghausen Disease)

Neurofibromatosis 1 (NF-1) is by far more common, associated with skin, nervous system, and bone and joint manifestations. Patients with NF-2 have few dermatological findings, but they have a high incidence of meningiomas and acoustic neuromas. Prevalence is estimated to be ~1/3000 (**Fig. 15.8**).

◆ Presentation

◆ *Cutaneous involvement*: Hyperpigmentation, hypomelanotic macules, cutaneous neurofibromas
◆ *CNS involvement*: Simple megalencephaly, hydrocephalus, vascular occlusions, dural ectasia, absence of the sphenoid wing, lambdoidal suture defect, seizures, learning disabilities, emotional/behavioral disturbances, gliomas, and meningiomas
◆ *Skeletal involvement*: Progressive kyphoscoliosis, plexiform neurofibromas, lytic metaphyseal, diaphyseal defects, and short stature
◆ *Visceral involvement*: Neurofibromas of the gastrointestinal tract and pheochromocytomas
◆ *Ophthalmic involvement*: Lisch nodules, multiple nodules, nevi, plexiform neurofibromas of the eyelid, congenital glaucoma, prominent corneal nerves, hamartomas of the choroid, astrocytic hamartomas (white tumors involving the optic nerve), combined hamartomas, retinal capillary hemangiomas. Absence of the greater wing of the sphenoid bone may lead to pulsatile proptosis, choroidal melanomas, and optic nerve gliomas

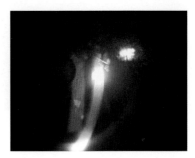

Fig. 15.8   Lisch nodules.

◆ **Management**

Skin biopsy is diagnostic. Radiographs of the metaphyseal joints and neuroimaging are done to rule out associated lesions.

Tuberous Sclerosis (Bourneville Disease)

Tuberous sclerosis is an autosomal dominant disease with incomplete penetrance. It is a rare, multisystem disorder with hamartomas in the brain and on other vital organs such as the kidneys, heart, eyes, lungs, and skin (**Fig. 15.9**).

◆ **Presentation**

The cutaneous features include adenoma sebaceum (angiofibroma, which appears on the nose and cheeks in a butterfly distribution), ungula or subungual fibromas, hypomelanic macules called ashleaf spots, café-au-lait spots, lumbosacral shagreen patches, and forehead plaques. Other features include CNS involvement in the form of subependymal nodules and cortical/subcortical tubers, learning difficulties, seizures, renal angiomyolipomata, cardiac rhabdomyoma, and pulmonary fibrosis.
   Ocular involvement includes the following:

◆ Retinal astrocytic hamartomas, which appear as a grayish or yellowish white lesion, 1 to 2 disk diameters on the retina. These can calcify and may be seen on a CT scan.
◆ Giant drusen of the optic nerve head
◆ Angiofibromas of the eyelids, colobomas, and papilledema may be seen.

◆ **Management**

A multidisciplinary team approach is required with periodic monitoring for internal tumors. Prognosis is generally poor, with death by the second or third decade.

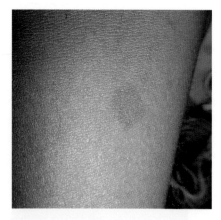

Fig. 15.9   Bourneville disease spot in a patient with suspected tuberous sclerosis.

Sturge-Weber Syndrome (Encephalofacial Cavernous Hemangiomatosis)

This neurocutaneous disorder comprises angiomas involving the leptomeninges (leptomeningeal angiomas) and skin of the face, typically in the ophthalmic (V1) and maxillary (V2) distributions of the trigeminal nerve (nevus flammeus or port-wine stain). It has no definite inheritance pattern.

◆ Presentation

Classification uses the Roach scale:

◆ *Type I*: Both facial and leptomeningeal angiomas; may have glaucoma
◆ *Type II*: Facial angioma alone (no CNS involvement); may have glaucoma
◆ *Type III*: Isolated leptomeningeal angiomas; usually no glaucoma

Cranial hemangiomas, cerebral calcification, mental retardation, and seizures may also be seen.

Ocular involvement may consist of glaucoma in 30 to 71%, which may develop early or in adulthood. Conjunctival or episcleral hemangiomas, heterochromia of the iris, and choroidal hemangiomas may also be seen. Tomato-catsup color of the fundus may be seen ipsilateral to the nevus flammeus. Choroidal hemangiomas may lead to RPE degeneration, fibrous metaplasia, cystic retinal degeneration, and retinal detachment. Retinal vascular tortuosity, iris heterochromia, optic disk coloboma, and cataracts may also be seen in these patients.

◆ Management

Systemic evaluation should be done by an internist. Treatment includes yearly examinations, looking for optic nerve damage (with measurement of intraocular pressure and visual fields) and corneal diameter and refractive changes in children. Choroidal lesions may be treated when indicated with photocoagulation, diathermy, cryotherapy, and local irradiation.

Von Hippel-Lindau Syndrome (Retinocerebellar Capillary Hemangiomatosis)

Von Hippel-Lindau Syndrome is a benign capillary hamartoma with autosomal dominant inheritance with variable penetrance.

◆ Presentation

Hemangioblastomas in the cerebellum and other organs of the body along with cysts of the pancreas and kidneys, pheochromocytoma, and hypernephroma may be seen. Ocular involvement includes the following:
◆ Retinal capillary hemangiomas, 1 to 3 disk diameters in size and supplied by a feeder artery, may be seen.
◆ Choroidal mass (tumor/metastasis)
◆ Retinal telangiectasis
◆ Retinal macroaneurysms
◆ Leakage from these vessels and hemangiomas may lead to retinal exudates, fibroglial bands, traction retinal detachment, and vitreous hemorrhage.

◆ Management

Vanillylmandelic acid levels in urine and imaging studies are required with periodic evaluation.

Wyburn-Mason Syndrome (Racemose Hemangiomatosis)

Arteriovenous malformations (AVMs) are seen in the CNS and the retina.

◆ Presentation

Neurological symptoms may be seen depending on the location and severity.

Classification of Retinal Arteriovenous Anastomoses (Archer et al)
◆ *Group I*: Small arteriole-venule anastomoses, which may be subtle and difficult to detect clinically. These vessels are usually isolated to a sector or quadrant of the retina, and they often involve the macula.
◆ *Group II*: Represents direct artery-to-vein communication without intervening capillary or arteriolar elements. This group may represent an exaggerated form of the abnormalities included in group I, and it is likewise geographically segmented within the fundus.
◆ *Group III*: Includes malformations characterized by markedly convoluted, dilated, and tortuous retinal vessels extending throughout the entire fundus, making it virtually impossible to differentiate between arterial components and venous components. These eyes are usually severely vision impaired, which generally leads to earlier diagnosis in childhood. Patients in this group are at higher risk for systemic vascular involvement.

◆ Management

Refer for neurological evaluation, and perform routine, periodic ophthalmic examinations.

Ataxia-Telangiectasia (Louis-Bar Syndrome)

◆ Presentation

This is an autosomal recessive disorder with multisystem involvement in the form of progressive neurological impairment, cerebellar ataxia, variable immunodeficiency with susceptibility to sinopulmonary infections, impaired organ maturation, x-ray hypersensitivity, ocular and cutaneous telangiectasia, and a predisposition to malignancy.

Bulbar conjunctival telangiectasias along with oculomotor signs are diagnostically important. Saccadic imbalance may also be seen along with squint and nystagmus.

◆ Management

Laboratory studies for detecting humoral or cellular immunologic defects, imaging studies, electro-oculography, and ocular evaluation are required. The patient should be referred to an internist for treatment of infections.

16 Contact Lenses
Kenneth M. Daniels

◆ Corneal Edema

Corneal edema is the leakage of fluid into the cornea due to a change in the endothelial pump mechanism leading to fluid influx into the stromal layer. Corneal stroma, made of hydrophilic glycosamine glycans and glycoproteins (GAGS) can absorb a tremendous amount of water. Fluid leakage due to defects in the endothelium more so than the epithelium leads to fluid intumescence with subsequent disruption to the regularity of the collagen fibrils seen as either striae, folds, or central corneal clouding (**Fig. 16.1**).

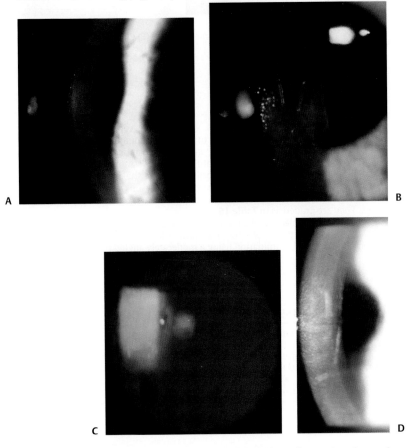

Fig. 16.1 **(A)** Central corneal striae. **(B)** Corneal folds. **(C)** Retroillumination of corneal folds. **(D)** Parrellapiped image of folds. (*Continued on page 448*)

447

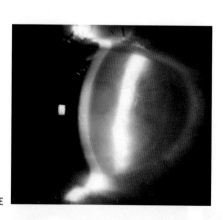
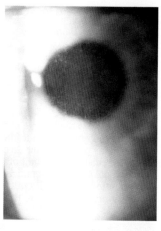

E

F

Fig. 16.1 (*Continued*) **(E)** 4+ (severe) corneal edema. **(F)** Clinically significant corneal edema.

◆ **Presentation**

Striae are recognized as fine, meshlike, grayish white vertical lines that do not interconnect. They may appear similar to white branching neural fibrils. Contact lens–induced hypoxia leads to a change in the homeostatic balance of the cornea and the deturgence or uptake of fluid into the corneal stroma. The subtle increase in fluid induces swelling of collagen fibrils leading to the appearance of the fine, meshlike character of striae. The striae with contact lens corneal edema tend to appear slightly more oblique than the Vogt vertical striae associated with keratoconus. They are graded as in **Table 16.1**.

Folds are seen as black, vertical criss-crossing creases that represent a buckling of the cornea at the posterior stroma–Descemet layer. Both findings are best observed in direct focal illumination using a moderately angled parallelepiped.

Table 16.1   Grading Corneal Striae

Grade	Finding
Grade 0	No striae
Grade 1	One to two faint lines
Grade 2	Two to six lines
Grade 3	Greater than six lines without folds

Table 16.2   Corneal Edema Levels

Corneal Swelling	Signs	Relationships	Level
< 2%	Undetectable edema	Unknown	Benign
2 to 5%	Early stages of striae	Implies chronic hypoxia	Safe
> 5%	Vertical striae observed	Chronic hypoxia	Caution
> 8%	Posterior folds and striae	Acute edema	Danger
> 20%	Loss of corneal transparency, folds, striae	Pathological	Pathological

Central corneal clouding or haze occurs at the corneal apex as a whitened region throughout the stromal depth, which will bulge. The central cornea will exhibit severe epithelial thinning with subsequent reduction in vision and lens intolerance. Central corneal clouding is best visualized with sclerotic scatter and/or moderate angle parallelepiped (**Table 16.2**).

In the initial stages, patients will generally have no symptoms other than a minor to moderate level of lens awareness, glare sensitivity, and halos. Visual acuity will be slightly to moderately reduced and possibly notable keratometric–topographic distortion will be present. Pachymetry will be showing a mild to moderate increase from baseline. As the corneal edema progresses, there will be a marked visual distortion appreciated by the patient as well as noticeable cloudiness or haze to vision. If the patients enter the severe state, then there will a much defined decrease in vision and increased ocular discomfort accompanied by a variable level of "red eye" and ocular congestion. This may actually mimic a form of iridocyclitis. If epithelial breaks subsequently occur, there is a higher potential for opportunistic infection.

◆ Differential Diagnosis

Tight lens syndrome, corneal warpage, corneal ulcer, other causes of contact lens–related discomfort, and redness. Rule out other corneal degenerations and dystrophies such as keratoconus, pellucid, posterior polymorphous dystrophy, or Fuchs endothelial dystrophy, as well as postoperative edema, acutely elevated intraocular pressure (IOP), or iridocyclitis.

◆ Management

Discontinue wearing lenses until resolution. Clinical aftercare and patient education need to be more aggressive to monitor for more advanced signs of edema and possible corneal irregularities via biomicroscopy, pachymetry, topography, endothelial cell count, and refraction. Endothelial cell count will be necessary only if one suspects endothelial cell disease or loss. Pachymetry of the normal corneal thickness measures ~0.55 mm centrally, progressing in natural thickness to ~0.8 mm in the corneal periphery. Resultant corneal edema associated with various disease states will be suspect with the central corneal thickness above 0.6 mm. Serial measures will assist in the determination of treatment success.

If the corneal edema is less than 5% (caution), the patient requires a refit to high water content hydrogel or silicone hydrogel material. High water content materials that maintain proper hydration are critical, and therefore a group 2 nonionic, high water material is suggested. A refit to a high diffusion coefficient rigid gas permeable lens is also highly advisable. Both gas permeable and soft lens modalities should be strictly prescribed for a daily wear schedule; extended wear should be forbidden. If the edema is greater than 5%, but less than 8% (moderate to dangerous), the same contact lens refit approach is pursued with the intent of introducing medicinal intervention based on subjective findings, such as reduced visual acuity, clinically significant corneal haze, and pachymetry.

Finally, if the edema is 9% or more (pathological), lenses need to be discontinued with the administration of either or both hypertonics and steroids to draw corneal fluids anteriorly out of the stroma. At this stage, corneal irregularities such as microcystic eruptions, a decrease in epithelial thickness, and an increase in stromal thickness will be noted. Lenses should not be refit until microcysts partially resolve and the edema is reduced. When refit, the patient should limit the hours of wear and be restricted to daily wear high dK water content lenses.

Hyperosmotic agents such as sodium chloride 2 to 5% drops or ointment are the first nonmedicinal treatment. Steroid agents such as prednisolone 1% with a taper to fluorometholone or loteprednol 1% will be of assistance in a more rapid reduction of appreciable corneal haze from edema. Caution should be taken if there is bacterial or viral co-disease or if the patient may be a steroid responder. Also, owing to the superficial corneal treatment, a steroid of a phosphate agent, lower corneal–anterior chamber penetration is more appropriate than an acetate preparation. In general, based on the level of corneal edema, treatment results may be seen within 24 to 48 hours of lens discontinuance alone, but resolution in relation to severity will take place over 2 days to 2 weeks. As a note, if the corneal edema is related to a disease state, such as pseudophakic bullous keratopathy, a bandage contact lens should be considered for pain control as well as allowing the dosing of steroid as necessary.

◆ Contact Lens–Induced Papillary Conjunctivitis or Giant Papillary Conjunctivitis

Contact lens–induced papillary conjunctivitis (CLPC) was first described as a "contact-related spring catarrh" or vernal keratoconjunctivitis (VKC). Later, giant papillary conjunctivitis (GPC) received its name from Allansmith et al, who described the palpebral conjunctival lid formations as an elevation with a central core vascularization, unlike a follicle, which is a fluid-filled cyst formation.

◆ Presentation

CLPC is a chronic inflammatory response isolated to the superior lid in relation to either mechanical or antigenic response, found more so with longer-duration-wear hydrogel lenses than with gas-permeable lenses. (With longer duration wear hydrogel lenses [continuous, 14 to 30 days] > extended [3–7 days] > flexible [1–3 days] > daily wear [1 day] > single use or daily disposable lenses.) It is described as a cutaneous basophilic hypersensitivity to surface proteins. It is considered that the combination of the irritative mechanics induced by surface deposits as well as the antigenic response of the denatured surface proteins within the deposits lead to the inflammatory response and the development of the papillae. Mechanical irritation of the conjunctiva not only occurs with contact lenses but can also occur in isolated areas associated with sutures. Also, the introduction of silicone hydrogel contact lens materials, and the related continuous wear, has given a rebirth to an increasing incidence of CLPC. This is related to a higher modulus of elasticity (1.1 to 1.2 megapascals) making the lens stiffer than hydrogel lenses. The rigidity of the material encourages mechanical irritation by rubbing against the superior palpebral conjunctiva, producing a local response.

Papillae are morphologically different from follicles and less severe compared with an acute, hypersensitive follicular or cobblestone appearance of a vernal conjunctivitis. GPC or CLPC is best observed using a white, diffuse light on low magnification. Papillae, which are space-occupying elevations, will tend to grab the lens upon the blink and hold it in a slightly superior, decentered position while impeding the downward translation of the lens. Because of the constant irritation of the palpebral conjunctiva, a reactive mucous discharge will increase, leading to additional lens surface depositing.

The palpebral conjunctiva can be described as smooth or satin, uniform or nonuniform. Under low magnification, with or without NaFl staining, a variable level of hyperemia will appear with an increasing degree of edema. The papillae will be of varying sizes, from 0.5 mm and greater. With the instillation of NaFl, distinct crevices can be visualized between each papillae, which will assist in the delineation of the severity of the papillary reaction.

In the earliest stages the patient is generally asymptomatic yet complains of frequent depositing of lenses and variable vision. As the condition progresses, the patient starts to find that cleaning the lenses becomes somewhat futile, and there is a slight to more purulent mucous discharge. This may or may not be symmetric to both eyes and is often bilateral, asymmetric in presentation. As the discharge and the vision depreciate, so does the patient's lens-wearing time. The patient will also find that the lens tends to decenter significantly and may even complain of a greater lens awareness. Most often the patient will present with a self-diagnosis of a "common conjunctivitis or red eye" and may have self-treated with over-the-counter vasoconstrictive agents or been treated by the primary care physician for a "garden variety" bacterial conjunctivitis without response to antibiotics. There may be some tenderness to tactile manipulation of the lid but no significant pain, nor do systemic symptoms suggest bacterial or viral conjunctivitis.

CLPC can be staged into four levels of severity. Stage 1 demonstrates no anatomical signs, and only minor symptoms of mucous discharge and itching. Stage 2 exhibits papillary enlargement to 0.5 mm but less than 1 mm, mucous strains, hyperemia, and an increase in lens deposits. The patient will describe itchiness, discharge, lens awareness, and blurred acuity. Stage 3 shows papillae greater than 1 mm, increased mucus, lens awareness, hyperemia, edema, and lens decentration superiorly. The patient will describe moderate to severe symptoms with decreased wear time, frequent lens depositing, and increased lens movement and blur. Stage 4 demonstrates papillae larger than 1 mm, which have a mushroom shape accompanied by severe symptoms and signs (**Fig. 16.2**).

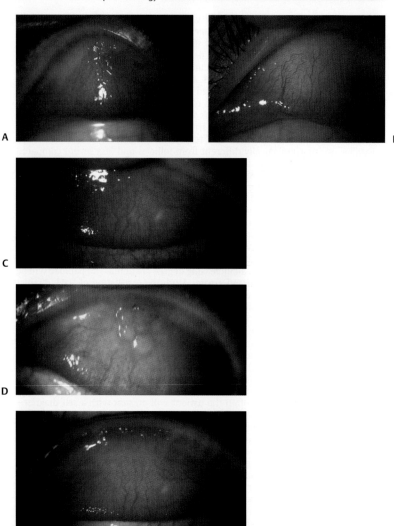

Fig. 16.2 **(A)** Papillary formation right eye (ocular dextrose, OD). **(B)** Nonpapillary satin left eye (ocular sinistras, OS). **(C)** Grade 1 contact lens–induced papillary conjunctivitis (CLPC) marginal papillary formation with hyperemia Pre-Tx OD. **(D)** Grade 3 CLPC with isolated giant papillary formation with hyperemia Pre-Tx OS. **(E)** Grade 1 CLPC with hyperemia post-Tx OD 2 weeks: significant decrease in hyperemia and early papillary formation.

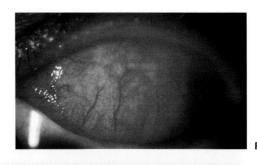

F

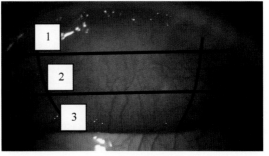

G

Fig. 16.2 *(Continued)* **(F)** Grade 3 CLPC with hyperemia post-Tx OS 2 weeks: significant decrease in hyperemia and early papillary formation. **(G)** Zonal diagram of the superior everted lid.

◆ Differential Diagnosis

Involves identifying the underlying culprit of mechanics, protein denaturation, antigenic-related response, or environmental influences giving rise to similar findings and symptoms exacerbated by the use of contact lenses, yet they are not the cause. By history alone, the etiology and differential can be made. If there is hydrogel contact lens wear, extended more than daily; if there is a history of cataract or corneal procedures with sutures; or if the patient has a significant history of seasonal or vernal allergy, the history is the true story. Treatment will thus follow the scenario of the history.

CLPC may also present with similar symptoms typical of a variety of conjunctivitis, including bacterial, viral, vernal, atopic, or mechanically induced by sutures postoperatively. The hallmark differential of CLPC is a more rapid onset with increased mucous discharge and the inability to properly maintain the contact lens on the eye, usually exhibited by excessive lens movement due to the mechanical influence of the enlarged pappilae. Follicles of variable size are seen in a hyperemic conjunctiva, inferior more so than superior (unlike CLPC seen in the superior palpebral conjunctiva) with translucent, avascular fluid–lymphoid accumulation and are accompanied by systemic findings as in pharyngoconjunctival fever (PCF) or epidemic keratoconjunctivitis (EKC), as well as ruling out chlamydial disease. The Academy of Ophthalmology has presented an excellent differential format for conjunctivitis as seen in **Table 16.3**.

Table 16.3   Typical Clinical Signs of Conjunctivitis

Typical Clinical Signs of Conjunctivitis	
Type of Conjunctivitis	**Clinical Signs**
Allergic/immunologic	
Seasonal allergic	Bilateral; conjunctival injection, chemosis, watery discharge, mild mucous discharge
Vernal	Bilateral; giant papillary hypertrophy of superior tarsal conjunctiva, bulbar conjunctival injection, conjunctival scarring, watery and mucoid discharge, limbal Trantas dots, limbal "papillae," corneal epithelial erosions, corneal neovascularization and scarring, corneal vernal plaque/shield ulcer
Atopic	Bilateral; eczematoid blepharitis; eyelid thickening, scarring; lash loss; papillary hypertrophy of superior and inferior tarsal conjunctiva; conjunctival scarring; watery or mucoid discharge; boggy edema; corneal neovascularization, ulcers, and scarring; punctate epithelial keratitis; keratoconus; subcapsular cataract
Giant papillary	Laterality associated with contact lens wear pattern; papillary hypertrophy of superior tarsal conjunctiva, mucoid discharge; in severe cases: lid swelling, ptosis
Mechanical/irritative	
Superior limbic keratoconjunctivitis (SLK)	Bilateral superior bulbar injection, laxity, edema, and keratinization; superior corneal punctate epitheliopathy and filaments
Contact lens-related SLK	Injection of superior bulbar conjunctiva, epithelial thickening of limbus with neovascularization and/or extension of conjunctival epithelium onto superior cornea; papillary hypertrophy of tarsal conjunctivitis is variable
Floppy eyelid syndrome	Upper eyelid edema; upper eyelid easily everted, sometimes by simple elevation or lifting of lid; diffuse papillary reaction of superior tarsal conjunctiva; punctate epithelial keratopathy; pannus; bilateral often asymmetric
Pediculosis palpebrarum (*Pthirus pubis*)	Unilateral or bilateral follicular conjunctivitis; adult lice at the base of the eyelashes, nits (eggs) adherent to the eyelash shafts, blood-tinged debris on the eyelashes and eyelids
Medication-induced keratoconjunctivitis	Laterality based on drug use; conjunctival injection, inferior fornix conjunctival follicles; distinctive signs: contact dermatitis of eyelids with erythema, scaling in some cases

Table 16.3 (*Continued*) **Typical Clinical Signs of Conjunctivitis**

Typical Clinical Signs of Conjunctivitis	
Type of Conjunctivitis	**Clinical Signs**
Viral	
Adenoviral	Abrupt onset; unilateral or bilateral; varies in severity; bulbar conjunctival injection, watery discharge, follicular reaction of inferior tarsal conjunctiva, chemosis
	Distinctive signs: preauricular lymphadenopathy, petechial and subconjunctival hemorrhage, corneal epithelial defect, multifocal epithelial punctate keratitis evolving to anterior stromal keratitis, membrane/pseudomembrane formation, eyelid ecchymosis
Herpes simplex virus	Unilateral: bulbar conjunctival injection, watery discharge, mild follicular reaction of conjunctiva; may have palpable preauricular node
	Distinctive signs: vesicular rash or ulceration of eyelids, pleomorphic or dendritic epithelial keratitis of cornea or conjunctiva
Molluscum contagiosum	Typically unilateral but can be bilateral: mild to severe follicular reaction, punctate epithelial keratitis; may have corneal pannus, especially if longstanding
	Distinctive signs: single or multiple shiny, dome-shaped umbilicated lesion(s) of the eyelid skin or margin
Bacterial	
Nongonococcal	Unilateral: bulbar conjunctival injection, purulent or mucopurulent discharge
Gonococcal	Unilateral or bilateral: marked eyelid edema, marked bulbar conjunctival injection, marked purulent discharge, preauricular lymphadenopathy
	Important sign to detect: corneal infiltrate
Chlamydial	Unilateral or bilateral
Neonate/infant	Eyelid edema, bulbar conjunctival injection, discharge may be purulent or mucopurulent, no follicles
Adult	Bulbar conjunctival injection, follicular reaction of tarsal conjunctiva, mucoid discharge, corneal pannus, punctate epithelial keratitis, preauricular lymphadenopathy
Immune-mediated	Distinctive sign: bulbar conjunctival follicles
Ocular cicatricial pemphigoid	Bilateral: bulbar conjunctival injection, papillary conjunctivitis, conjunctival subepithelial fibrosis and keratinization, conjunctival scarring beginning in the fornices, punctal stenosis and keratinization, progressive conjunctival shrinkage, symblepharon, entropion, trichiasis, corneal ulcers, neovascularization, and scarring

(continued on page 456)

Table 16.3   (*Continued*)   Typical Clinical Signs of Conjunctivitis

<table>
<tr><th colspan="2">Typical Clinical Signs of Conjunctivitis</th></tr>
<tr><th>Type of Conjunctivitis</th><th>Clinical Signs</th></tr>
<tr><td>graft-versus-host disease</td><td>Bilateral; conjunctival injection, chemosis, pseudomembranous conjunctivitis, keratoconjunctivitis sicca, superior limbic keratoconjunctivitis, cicatricial eyelid disease, episcleritis, corneal epithelial sloughing, limbal stem cell failure, calcareous corneal degeneration; rare intraocular involvement</td></tr>
<tr><td>**Neoplastic**
Sebaceous gland carcinoma</td><td>Unilateral: intense bulbar conjunctival injection, conjunctival scarring; corneal epithelial invasion may occur
Eyelids may exhibit a hard nodular, nonmobile mass of the tarsal plate with yellowish discoloration; may appear as a subconjunctival, multilobulated yellow mass, may resemble a chalazion</td></tr>
</table>

Note: Typical clinical signs may not be present in all cases. Distinctive signs are most useful in making a clinical diagnosis, but may occur uncommonly. In all entities, laterality may vary and may be asymmetrical.

Source: Matoba AY. Preferred Practice Patterns, Conjunctivitis. San Francisco: American Academy of Ophthalmology; 2003. Available at: http://www.aao.org/aao/education/library/ppp/upload/Conjunctivitis_.pdf. (Accessed 12–08–2008). Reprinted with permission.

◆ Management

As with any potential antigenic–allergic response, one must first remove the initiating stimulus. The simple removal and discontinuance of the lens are the easiest treatment, but for some patients the most traumatic. Therefore a combination therapy is suggested based on the level of disease. It is important to note that the use of vasoconstrictive agents, antibiotics, and/or antivirals that have been started prior to presentation can be safely discontinued. However, if there is concern about bacterial coinfection, maintain the appropriate level of antibiotics such as fourth-generation fluoroquinolone when involving contact lens.

The most expedient treatment is the simple discontinuation of wearing contact lenses and converting to eyeglass wear until the condition improves. However, in many cases, the patient may not have eyeglasses or may not be tolerant of the alternative. Therefore, the use of soft daily disposable lenses with a high moisture content in conjunction with a steroidal antiinflammatory serves as the best overall therapy.

Stage 1 CLPC requires minimal intervention, such as refitting the patient with a frequent replacement or disposable lens. In this situation, the simple conversion to a "daily disposable–single use lens" is the most appropriate. Another option would be to continue conventional, disposable, or frequent replacement lenses but change the care product to a peroxide-based system and possibly add an enzymatic cleaning solution.

In an unpublished study by K. Daniels, daily disposable lenses demonstrated a more rapid resolution of patient symptoms with grade 2 to 4 CLPC without the use of medicinals followed by 1-week and 2-week disposable lenses, respectively. This suggests that the simple use of daily disposable–single use lenses might be the most appropriate single or adjuvant treatment for CLPC.

Stage 2 CLPC requires lens replacement, frequent irrigation with lubricating drops to rid mucus, lid hygiene to avoid lid wipers epitheliopathy, and possibly a prescription for a mast cell stabilizer such as such as Iodoxamide (Alomide, Allergan, Irvine, CA), cromolyn (Crolom, Bausch & Lomb, Rochester, NY) (Opticrom, Allergan, Irvine, CA), nedocromil (Alocril, Allergan), pemirolast (Alamast, Vistakon Pharmaceuticals, Jacksonville, FL), or olopatadine (Pataday or Patanol, Alcon Laboratories, Fort Worth, TX) for short-term to chronic therapy.

Stage 3 CLPC requires a discontinuation of lenses for a short time while prescribing a mast cell stabilizer or low-concentration steroid such as prednisolone 1%. Lenses can be refit to daily disposable or short-term frequent replacement lenses with peroxide care products until resolution of the papillae to a whitened cap called *hypertrophy*.

Stage 4 CLPC requires complete discontinuation of lenses and more aggressive steroid intervention until resolution. Upon resolution, frequent replacement or disposable lenses should be fitted using a peroxide-based product system.

In general, when utilizing steroids for treatment, it is highly suggested to adjuvantly treat the patient with single-use daily disposable lenses, which will satisfy the patient's needs while allowing for a bandage lens–drug delivery efficiency. The steroid (prednisolone 1%) should be aggressively dosed for the first 1 to 2 weeks at four times a day and then taper slowly over the next 2 to 3 weeks. As one tapers the prednisolone down to twice a day, start the addition of a soft steroid such as loteprednol either 1% or 0.2% for 1 to 2 weeks or until resolution of clinical findings. Long-term maintenance is most appropriate with shorter-term, frequently replaced hydrogel lenses of 2 to 4 weeks of nonionic, high-water-content materials and peroxide cleaning or a conversion to gas permeable high Dk–plasma-treated designs.

Also consider the long-term use of antihistamine–mast cell stabilizer for long-term maintenance. Additionally, if one was to be conservative with long-term medicinals, consider twice-a-day to three-times-a-day use of physiologically based wetting drops such as vitamin A drops (ViVa, Corneal Sciences, Gaithersburg, MD) or electrolyte-balanced formulas such as Thera–Tears (Advanced Vision Research, Boston, MA) or Soothe (Bausch & Lomb, Rochester, NY; Almira Sciences, Atlanta, GA). There is also suggestion that cyclosporine drops (Restasis, Allergan, Irvine, CA) may also be helpful in a twice-a-day dosage for long-term control of ocular inflammatory response as well as being a vehicle carrier helpful in maintaining a healthy ocular mucin surface to avoid mechanical irritation from the lens material.

◆ Vascularization

Vascularization is considered to be the general formation and extension of capillaries that had not previously existed within the avascular cornea. Neovascularization is the formation of new vessels as an extension or shunts to preexisting vascularized areas of the avascular cornea. To differentiate further is to classify forms of redness and vascularization by location. Limbal engorgement or hyperemia is the distension of limbal blood vessels in the absence of new vessel growth. Vessel ingrowth or penetration is not neovascularization, but simply an extension of a vessel inward toward the central cornea. Pannus, which is highly vascularized, is extension of conjunctival tissue overlapping the clear avascular cornea seen as an anatomical variance or induced by trauma to the eye.

Chronic hypoxia is the underlying condition that initiates the vascularization response. Hypoxia causes lactate acidosis, which decreases the integrity of the epithelium and stromal softening. This yields an opportunity for vessel ingrowth. Due to hypoxia, an early phase of vascularization occurs inducing a release of inflammatory mediators. This stimulates additional vessel growth called an *angiogenic response*. Tight lenses, limbal compression, and/or trauma may also stimulate a vascular response, which will increase the release of inflammatory and vasostimulatory mediators. There are several possibilities that encourage vascularization under hypoxic conditions: (1) vasostimulation and inflammation, (2) tight lens syndrome, (3) limbal-plexal compression, (4) solution sensitivity, and (5) vasogenic response to trauma (**Fig. 16.3**). The main causes of vascularization associated with contact lens wear are tight lens (edge suction) central corneal edema (hypoxia), solution toxicity, mechanical abrasion, lens damage and mechanical stimulus association with irritation, surface deposition, and poorly fitting lenses.

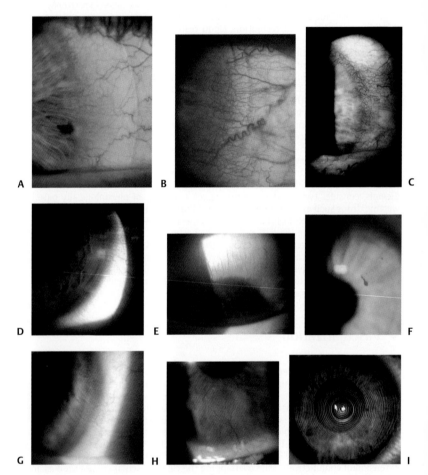

Fig. 16.3 **(A)** Limbal congestion–hyperemia. **(B)** Combination of vasodilatation (corkscrew vessels)–vasoproliferation–vasolimbal congestion. **(C)** Severe limbal vascularization congestion with early neovascularization. **(D)** Vessel penetration with early pannus. **(E)** 4+ superior limbal neovascularization leading toward the central cornea and papillary zone encroachment. **(F)** Intracorneal hemorrhage from neovascularization post-LASIK on an extended-wear contact lens wearer. **(G)** Sectoral pannus associated with overwear. **(H)** Sectoral pannus with corneal decompensation. **(I)** Sectoral pannus with corneal decompensation–placido topographic image.

◆ Presentation

Vascular responses to chronic hypoxia can vary from minor to severe based on the association with possible microbial infiltration. Some form of corneal vascularization occurs in ~34% of cases associated with hydrogel lens use versus 2% with nonlens wearers, with 98% of the vascularization occurring within the superficial stroma. The patient is otherwise asymptomatic other than noting an apparent hyperemia or limbal engorgement, which appears to the patient as a "chronic red eye" when wearing contact lenses. This is simply an engorgement of the marginal arcade capillaries. These vessels have a straight protuberance with a defined loop at the end. Hyperemic episcleral limbal vessels are differentiated from neovessels that extend forward with leaflike fronds that interdigitate.

Vascularization appears similar to a meshlike plexal growth in the midepithelium projecting toward the cornea like small, linear spikes and branches called *fronds* (similar to the veins within a leaf). There is generally no symptomatology associated with the findings. These are differentiated from normal limbal vessels that "loop" back toward the limbus. Low-grade (grade 1) vessels will tend to migrate inward to approximately 0.4 to 0.6 mm (daily wear) to 1.4 mm (extended wear). Grade 2 will be grade 1 vessels that will tend to migrate toward the pupil without passing into the pupillary zone. The most severe, grade 3, will penetrate the pupillary region. It is important to photodocument the vessels and determine the location on the limbus, depth (superficial or deep), degree of penetration, and severity defined as the depth of penetration (and the advancement of growth toward the papillary region).

◆ Differential Diagnosis

Vascularization and neovascularization are differentiated from limbal vessels that may be dilatated by trauma, infection, inflammation, tumor, conjunctival ingrowth or pterygium, or postoperative complication. Differentiation must also be made from vascularized pannus, which is the ingrowth of vessels and connective within the epithelium. The differentiation of vessel depth is important. Superficial vessels or vascularization initiates from the limbal capillary arcade, and the vessels are more tortuous and of smaller caliber than deep stromal vessels, which emerge from within the limbal midstromal region and are larger in caliber, have abrupt end bulbs, and may disrupt the regularity of the limbal cornea. Other factors that may be associated with contact lens–related vascularization are dry eyes (keratoconjunctivitis sicca) or ocular surface disease and other diseases, such as blepharitis, acne rosacea, Sjögren syndrome, and immune dysfunction, as well as interstitial keratitis, herpes keratitis, tuberculosis, measles, syphilis, and the possibility of amino acid deficiencies.

Because of the potential of non–contact lens–related concerns associated with corneal vascularization, biomicroscopic exam should include direct illumination and retroillumination, particularly of the limbal peripheral vessel arcades. In general, superficial vessels will emerge into the anterior stroma and appear as single or multiple (pannus) tortuous vessels under low magnification, yet deeper stromal vessels course through the cornea as more linear vessels that arborize. Lipid deposition appears as yellow-white opacities at the leading edge or surrounding the stromal vessels. Observation of lipid exudates surrounding an actively engorged vessel(s) should raise the concern of a possible iris-angle carcinoma requiring diligent gonioscopic examination. If there is a conjunctival growth closely juxtaposed to the limbus adjacent to the corneal vascularization, conjunctival carcinoma may be suspected.

◆ Management

The patient with limbal hyperemia or vessel engorgement tends to self-treat with over-the-counter vasoconstrictive agents. These patients will finally present stating that even with these agents their lenses feel dry and their eyes are red. In this situation, simply and forcefully tell the patient to discontinue drops that "get the red out." These drops tend to yield rebound congestion as well as a mild mydriasis and slowing of accommodation due to the sympathomimetic effects. In this situation, it is best to discontinue the lenses for a short period—2 to 3 days—and prescribe a soft steroid to rid any low-level inflammatory components.

In conjunction, implement physiologically based wetting drops such as vitamin A (ViVA, Corneal Sciences, Gaithersburg, MD), Thera-Tears (Advanced Vision Research, Boston, MA), Bion Tears (Alcon Laboratories, Fort Worth, TX), or Soothe (Bausch & Lomb, Rochester, NY, Almira Sciences, Atlanta, GA). In addition to topical supplementation, consider the use of omega 3-6 combinations for their inherent antiinflammatory and mucin complementary abilities. Also, one should consider agents such as Systane (Alcon Laboratories, Fort Worth, TX) or Endura (Allergan, Irvine, TX) for topical surface treatment.

After the discontinuance of the contact lens use and after vessel regression, there will be ghost vessels or channels that develop. These must be well documented to differentiate then from ghost vessels that may be associated with an interstitial keratitis.

Once the limbal hyperemia is tended to, a refit to contact lenses should be completed with the philosophy of high wetability, moderate modulus, and high oxygen permeability. The patient can be refit to nonionic, high-water-content hydrogel, silicone hydrogel of a lower modulus. If the modulus is high, there tends to be stiffness to the lens that can induce conjunctival irritation and repeat of conjunctival hyperemia. In addition, one should consider a high diffusion coefficient of a rigid gas permeable lens with sufficient axial edge clearance to enhance the fluid–tear channel and avoid corneal and limbal edge influences. These lenses should also incorporate an appropriate plasma treatment for wetability. Care products and lens schedules should be revisited, and patient education needs to be comprehensive.

In the event of more pronounced and progressive vascularization, such as neovascularization, one must be concerned about the fragility of these vessels.

It is not uncommon to observe an intracorneal hemorrhage as a direct sequela of neovascularization. If a hemorrhage occurs, it will appear as a "red spot on the cornea" similar to a "petechial conjunctival hemorrhage" located at the proximal end of a vascular frond. These hemorrhages should be photographed and monitored for spread. The patient should refrain from any agent that has an anticoagulant effect such as aspirin, Plavix, warfarin, as well as neutraceuticals that have an antithrombotic character. Additionally, these need to be well documented as well as the neovascularization in the event the patient decides to pursue intracorneal refractive surgical procedures in which intraoperative corneal hemorrhage could be significant.

Essentially, the treatment for any vascular response within the cornea from contact lenses is the same, and the variance is the underlying cause and intervention. Once the patient has been properly refit, education and monitoring are the keys to avoidance of recurrence. Additionally, as part of the treatment guideline, one must clinically monitor for issues that may induce ocular irritation and vascularization other than contact lenses, such as acne rosacea, systemic medications, and conditions that include connective tissue disorders, autoimmune and inflammatory disease, immunocompromised disorders, vascular stimulatory disease such as kidney problems and diabetes, keratoconjunctivitis sicca, and associated hormonally related disorders of the eye, as well as environmental irritants, use of diuretics (medicinal or as beverage–alcohol and caffeine), and smoking.

◆ Subepithelial Infiltrates

Subepithelial infiltrates (SEIs) are an inflammatory reaction secondary to chronic hypoxia or an acute reaction that threatens the avascular cornea and anterior segment. This acute reaction induces an inflammatory reaction that encourages an aggregation or accumulation of cellular components, such as polymorphonuclear cells, to migrate through the avascular corneato and settle within the subepithelium adjacent to Bowman's layer or basement membrane. This occurs in ~2% of lens wearers regardless of wear and replacement schedule. The etiology of SEI, when associated with contact lenses, is chronic hypoxia, prolonged edema, an immune response, solution toxemia, mechanical irritation–foreign debris, or a local infection or the exotoxins from bacterium resident in the ocular flora. They are thought to represent a delayed hypersensitivity immune response to viral antigens in the corneal stroma.

Corneal infiltrates are aggregates of gray or white migrating inflammatory cells arising from normally transparent corneal tissue. The inflammatory response stimulates the migration from the limbal vasculature or from the tears as a response to tissue damage or a secondary chemotactic reaction associated with an environmental antigenic activity or toxins, contact lens solutions, or from microbial organisms themselves. Infiltrates are defined as polymorphonuclear leukocytes (neutrophils) but may also contain lymphocytes and macrophages. In contact lens wear, infiltrates are most often sterile (noninfectious) but can also be infectious (**Fig. 16.4**).

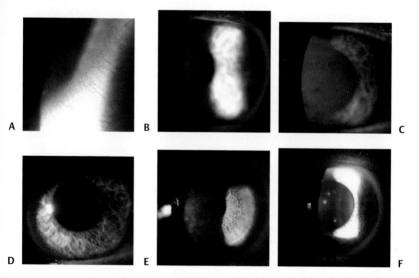

Fig. 16.4 **(A)** Subepithelial infiltrate with limbitis secondary to contact lens wear. **(B)** Subepithelial infiltrate (SEI) secondary to extended-wear contact lenses pretreatment. **(C)** Epithelial compromise with migration of SEI forward through epithelium. **(D)** Subepithelial Infiltrate secondary to extended-wear contact lenses posttreatment with steroid. **(E)** Adenovirus with infiltrates. **(F)** Viral Infiltrates with secondary scarring. (*Continued on page 462*)

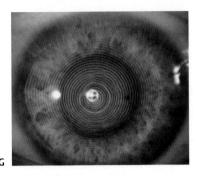

Fig. 16.4 (*Continued*) **(G)** Viral infiltrates with secondary scarring topography.

G

◆ Presentation

There is an initial and pronounced limbal–vascular response in the area of the ocular insult. Subsequently there is a release of mediators from the limbal plexus. The cellular or humoral components will migrate into and through the corneal tissue leading to the accumulation of cells that will appear as discrete white-gray subepithelial pockets or opacities. SEIs are seen as hazy gray, circumscribed infiltrates, at an intra- or subepithelium (at the surface of Bowman's layer without infiltration into the stroma; therefore, no scarring) or with anterior stromal level with infiltration, thus with a potential for scarring. They will be predominantly unilateral and concentrated focally or diffuse with a preference to the limbal and paracentral areas of the cornea. Adjacent to the SEI may be an area of localized conjunctival injection at the limbal juncture of mild to moderate severity. If there is significant corneal vascularization of any form, there will be the potential for a higher incidence of subepithelial infiltrates. As SEI migrates forward, there may be a subtle epithelial compromise or break that will stain.

The patient may have subtle symptoms ranging from mild to moderate. With inflammation of any form there will be an associated hyperemia localized to the area of occurrence, localized edema, and a variable degree of discomfort. The patient may also experience a mild to moderate level of lacrimation and photophobia and a decrease in visual acuity based on the location of the infiltrates, irritation, and/or foreign body sensation.

◆ Differential Diagnosis

If there is another anterior chamber reaction, one must differentiate between an infiltrative keratitis associated with several other anterior segment pathologies. These may also have a systemic relationship that needs to be looked for. These include episcleritis, marginal ulcer, iritis, adenovirus or EKC, or keratoconjunctivitis. Additionally, quiet noninflammatory opacities may be in actuality a subtle asymptomatic infiltrate or a simple scar. History in this case will assist in the differential. If there is significant corneal vascularization of any form, there will be the potential for a higher incidence of subepithelial infiltrates.

NaFl will be an important differential in distinguishing between a scar, ulcer, or SEI. Scars and SEI will not stain, but ulceration with an epithelial defect will. This will allow a differential between SEI and microbial epithelial defects. Upon treatment, the infiltrates may migrate forward and disrupt the epithelial surface, causing a topographic irregularity and possibly a negative staining superficial punctate keratopathy. To ensure no epithelial compromise and to rule out an early stage of masquerader such as a herpetic lesion (dendritic) *Pseudomonas*, *Acanthamoeba*, or *Fusarium*, the use of rose bengal or lissamine green will stain early bulbs of a dendritic lesion and detail devitalization of tissue much more readily than sodium fluorescein.

If the SEI is associated with an adenovirus, there will be systemic and constitutional findings such as fever, malaise, lethargy, myopathy (muscle weakness), periauricular lymphadenopathy, and/or the presence of a follicular conjunctivitis. If the SEI is associated with a keratoconjunctivitis, the clinician should consider the possibility of a transmittable disease. An example would be a chlamydial infection if there is a severe follicular conjunctivitis and history of urogenital infection. The patient should be referred to an internist, particularly in pediatric cases.

Anterior segment findings associated with SEI may also be found with an episcleritis, which may have a relationship to a connective or collagen tissue disorder (rheumatoid). Inflammatory conditions, such as a rheumatologic disorder, inflammatory bowel disease, or sacroidosis may have an associated iritis, which presents with an acute red eye, discomfort or pain, miosis, decrease in IOP, and a decrease in acuity. Even though corneal subepithelial infiltrates are considered a representation of a low-grade immune response to bacterial exotoxins, subepithelial infiltrates can complement other vasostimulatory responses as seen with corneal vascularization, atopic or viral disease, as well as postsurgical causes such as postLASIK.

Scars and ulcers can easily masquerade as an infiltrate because of their similar appearance of hazy, gray opaqueing, nontranslucent cornea, and location at the subepithelial anterior stromal level. Patients with corneal scars will have a positive history and will not respond to any therapy. Also, marginal ulcers can be mistaken for infiltrates barring the history. Ulcers will have a more rapid onset and noticeable injection and decreased comfort. Ulcers will tend to be located centrally. Infiltrates may be diffuse and central; however, more typically they are limbal. SEIs will appear less dense than marginal ulcerations and demonstrate a lesser anterior chamber and conjunctival reaction. For a differential of ulcers versus infiltrate see **Table 16.4**.

◆ Management

In the most basic treatment format it would be appropriate to discontinue contact lens use until resolution. Lens wear should not be resumed until all signs and symptoms are completely resolved. Medication is usually unnecessary in most cases of infiltrative keratitis (IK), with palliative use of preservative-free ocular lubricants. The use of a hyperosmotic agent is prescribed, such as NaCl 5% prescribed four times a day is more than sufficient if vision is not affected and there is a limited vascular response. If there is a greater vascular response and vision is decreased a more aggressive approach with a steroid such as prednisolone 1% four times a day for 1 week with a slow taper to a soft steroid (loteprednol 1%) is highly recommended. Prophylactic use of antibiotics to prevent secondary infection or antibiotic/steroid combination drops to mitigate the inflammatory response is sometimes beneficial. Such topicals would include tobramycin with dexamethasone or loteprednol (Tobradex, Alcon Laboratories) or Zylet (Bausch & Lomb) four times a day for 5 to 7 days and slow taper. Caution once again for steroid response and a corneal toxic keratopathy to tobramycin.

Because many cases of recurrent IK are secondary to exotoxins released by lid margin bacteria (*Staphylococcus* and *Streptococcus*), it is wise to recommend lid hygiene in these cases and to limit lens wear to daily wear complemented by a

Table 16.4   Differential of Ulcers versus Infiltrate

Ulcer	Infiltrate
Epidemiology: relatively rare	Epidemiology: relatively common; usually the result of hypoxia
Represents active bacterial infection	Represents migration of inflammatory white blood cells from the limbal vasculature and precorneal tear film
Generally causes significant pain	Pain is mild to moderate; rarely marked
Tends to be central rather than peripheral (*Staphylococcus*, exotoxin "peripheral ulcers" are toxic/inflammatory epithelial defects)	Tends to be peripheral because of proximity to the cellular inflammatory mechanisms released from the limbal blood vessels
Usually a solitary lesion	Can be multiple lesions
Size of the fluorescein epithelial staining defect closely mirrors the underlying stromal lesion	Size of the fluorescein epithelial staining defect is usually much smaller than the underlying stromal lesion; in any situation where there is a stromal inflammation, it is a real challenge for the overlying epithelial cells to remain physiologically intact, which explains why there can be some fluorescein staining even in these stromal inflammatory responses
There is almost invariably a cellular inflammatory response in the anterior chamber	Secondary anterior chamber reaction is rarely elicited
Pattern of bulbar conjunctival injection is usually generalized rather than sectoral	The pattern of bulbar conjunctival injection is usually sectored and proximally associated with the infiltrate; even if there is 360-degree injection, the vascular injection pattern is skewed toward the sector nearer the infiltrate, particularly if it is peripherally located
Possible tear lake debris	Tear lake is clear
Treatment options:	There are two therapeutic approaches:
◆ Aggressive use of a topical fluoroquinolone with fluoroquinolone or polysporin ointment at bedtime and daily follow-up until good control is achieved ◆ Fortified tobramycin or gentamicin (for gram-negative) and fortified cephazolin or bacitracin (for gram-positive); therapeutic cycloplegia with 5% homatropine or 0.25% scopolamine is usually wise	◆ If diagnosis is clear: Treat with antibiotic/steroid combination such as tobramycin with dexamethasone, or tobramycin with loteprednol, one drop every 2 h for 2 days, and then modify and taper according to circumstances ◆ If diagnosis is unclear: Treat with a fluoroquinolone every 1 to 2 h and follow up in 24 hours; if it is an ulcer, there may be no or minimal improvement in 24 h; if the defect is an infiltrate, it will be the same or worse the following day; at day 1 follow-up, the conservative antibiotic therapy can be continued for another day, or if your diagnostic decision is now infiltrate, then add loteprednol four times a day while continuing the antibiotic

peroxide care system. Lid treatment would include standard lid scrubs with nonirritative agents, doxycycline 20 mg, 50 mg by mouth, or up to a 100 mg for blepharitis or minocycline with lid cleansing (Cleeravue–M, Stonebridge Pharma, Duluth, GA) and/or possibly cyclosporine A drops—Restasis twice a day if there is a history of chronic rosacea.

The major concern is whether the infiltrate is actually a noninfectious sterile ulcer or contact lens–related peripheral ulcer (CLPU). If suspicious of ulcers, prescribe antibiotics only. Refrain from steroid use, culture when possible, and treat with fluoroquinolone antibiotics. In this case, the initial use of a steroid would be contraindicated until after a short course of a potent antibiotic such as moxifloxacin (Vigamox, Alcon Laboratories) or gatifloxacin (Zymar, Allergan). In the case of infiltrates, there will be no response to antibiotics. If there is an ulcer, there will be a favorable response to antibiotics, which can be followed by the introduction of steroids after the loading dose has reduced the bacterial burden. As an added comment for pain control with corneal ulceration, ample cycloplegia using homatropine 2 to 5% or a more frequent dose of cyclopentolate 1% will in many cases suffice without the need for steroid utilization. Oral analgesia for pain can be introduced using basic acetaminophen or ibuprofen or both as needed.

The prognosis of treating infiltrates is highly favorable with symptoms and findings dissipating in a short course of a few days. Infiltrates that are denser and more centralized, such as with an adenovirus, will take longer to resolve and may have a profound effect on vision requiring longer-term care and slow tapering of medications, particularly when using steroidal therapy from hard to soft steroid topicals.

◆ Contact Lens-Related Acute Red Eye

Contact lens-related red eye (CLARE) is an acute, nonspecific, nonulcerative sterile keratoconjunctivitis has inflammatory association with the adherence of debris from exogenous matter, metabolic by-products, or vestiges of bacterial debris and exotoxins that induce the recruitment of inflammatory cells. The exotoxins are from the breakdown of trapped debris or devitalized bacteria within the closed eye environment. Presumptively, the greater risk is bacterial infiltration and colonization by *Staphylococcus* and *Pseudomonas* that may lead to CLPU; there is suggestion that some patients have higher levels of gram-negative contamination.

Contact lens acute red eyes (CLAREs) have a variety of causes. CLARE could be considered an inflammatory condition associated with hypoxia, toxic effects from post-lens tear debris, mechanical irritation from a poorly fitting lens, dehydration of the lens during sleep, solution hypersensitivity or toxicity, or a reaction to bacterial toxins. Due to potential hypoxic conditions associated with lens use, cellular glucose converts to lactate. In addition, lactate diffusing into the stroma increases the osmolarity, leading to metabolic acidosis with resultant corneal edema. A decrease in normal corneal metabolism compromises corneal tissue leading to CLARE. White blood cells migrate from the limbal vasculature and form infiltrates in the peripheral cornea.

◆ **Causes of Acute Red Eye**

The contact lens relationship is via lens-induced mechanical factors or from lens deposits that lead to injury or microtrauma to the cornea. Microtrauma encourages the migration and infiltration of inflammatory cellular constituents. In the case of lens deposits, these serve as an antigenetic source that triggers an immune response leading to infiltrates. The casual relationships are either (1) tight lens syndrome, (2) tear-film deficiency/dry eye [i.e., contact lens–induced dry-eye (CLIDE)], (3) bacterial conjunctivitis, (4) inflammatory reaction to debris on the back surface debris (metabolic and/or exogenous debris stagnant between the lens and corneal surface), (5) mechanical irritation/abrasion, (6) solution toxemia/hypersensitivity, or (7) irritation to lens deposits. The incidence of corneal findings with 30-day continuous-wear silicone hydrogels has been found at an occurrence rate of 10% for CLPU and 29% for CLARE (**Fig. 16.5**).

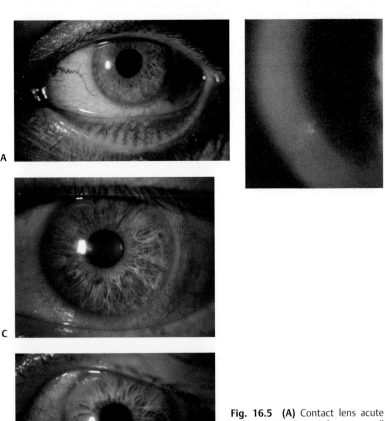

A

B

C

D

Fig. 16.5 **(A)** Contact lens acute red eye (CLARE) secondary to a small foreign body. **(B)** CLARE secondary to a small foreign body. **(C)** Sectoral CLARE—tight lens syndrome—differential diagnosis episcleritis. **(D)** CLARE secondary to solution toxemia.

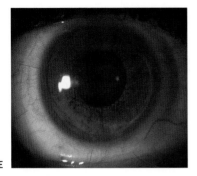
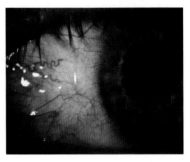

E

F

Fig. 16.5 (*Continued*) **(E)** CLARE—tight lens syndrome. **(F)** CLARE—tight lens syndrome—CLIDE.

◆ Presentation

CLARE has a generic appearance of a nondescript "red eye" directly associated with the use of contact lens extended wear more often than with daily wear. The acute reaction could be observed as a nonspecific red eye with limbal hyperemia, conjunctival injection, corneal infiltrates, and a possible corneal edema that is limbal more so than central. Upon lens removal, the patient may experience a greater level of ocular discomfort and may exhibit punctate keratopathy evidence with positive fluorescein staining associated mostly with trapped debris, a primary cause for the induced inflammatory condition.

The patient will describe a "garden variety" red eye with unilateral, sometimes bilateral, variable levels of discomfort or pain, redness, epiphoria, photophobia, and discharge described as watery to mucopurulent. The amount of vision reduction, pain, and discharge will assist in the differential diagnosis and underlying etiology. If the condition is contact lens related, a history of extended or continuous lens use will have a higher incidence than daily wear reusable more so than single-use lenses. If a contact lens patient presents with an ARE (acute red eye), it is important in the history to determine the wear modality of the lens. Continuous and extended wear schedules will demonstrate a higher incidence of CLARE than daily wear or single use lens wear schedules. It should be assumed that all contact lens wearers may have the presence of microbial keratitis and ulcer, until proven otherwise. This is important in clinical management, for many patients tend to self-treat or have been treated inappropriately for a "garden variety conjunctivitis" by a primary care physician (PCP). Because of the potential of a potentially devastating ulcer, such as *Acanthamoeba, Pseudomonas*, or *Fusarium*, it is important to stress to PCPs that if a "red eye–contact lens" patient presents to their office, they should defer treatment and seek a consult with an ophthalmologist or optometric physician.

◆ Differential Diagnosis

As stated, an acute red eye presents as a garden variety of red eye that has a distinct characteristic of rapid onset when related to contact lens, with the high potential of being ulcerative, but can also mimic or be directly related to many other forms of ocular disorders such as bacterial, viral, allergic, or chlamydial infections. If the patient is not a contact lens wearer, this is not CLARE but is more probably a bacterial conjunctivitis. The differential of the CLARE patient, due to the contact lens association, is always ulcer first until proven otherwise. Once proven otherwise, by culture or by antibiotic treatment, CLARE will remain as a red eye given the inflammatory nature. The inflammation could also be an underlying iritis in absence of an anterior chamber reaction and normal pupils. If there is a sectoral component to the CLARE, then consider a contact lens peripheral ulcer (CLPU), episcleritis, superior limbic keratitis (rule out thyroid disease), vascularized limbic keratitis, or ocular surface inflammation associated with a pingueculae or pterygium. These are anatomically obvious.

◆ Management

In many cases, the patient self-treats with over-the-counter vasoconstrictive lubricant drops without relief. In many other cases, the patient will present to a PCP for a garden variety conjunctivitis that is first treated with antibiotics. Precautionary care is required. In many instances, a nonophthalmic–nonoptometric provider may have started treatment, thereby disguising a possible etiology of CLARE. As such, the patient may have already been treated with a sulfacetamide 10% ophthalmic preparation that does not allow the condition to resolve and in fact worsens the condition if the patient has sulfa drug sensitivity. Or in other cases, the patient may have been given a variety of either aminoglycosides, fluoroquinolones, macrolide, or antiallergy medications, some having an effect or no effect at all.

In many cases the simple discontinuance of the contact lens and use of glasses for a few days is satisfactory. If the condition resolves with this mode of treatment, it suggests a simple material and wear condition issue that needs to be addressed. If the patient reintroduces, or rechallenges the use of the same material and wear schedule (i.e., extended-wear or continuous-wear modality), and the condition re-manifests, the rechallenge defines the need to readdress lens use by refitting the patient with a new material, wear schedule, and care product.

Treatment sometimes determines the differential diagnosis in the absence of corneal findings. As the caveat would suggest, "do no harm," therefore it is best to treat the eye with antibiotics, and if needed for cycloplegia, for a minimum of 24 to 48 hours prior to the introduction of a steroid to avoid a possible exacerbation of an underlying ulcerative or herpetic: viral, fungal, or protozoan entity. Aggressive antibiotic therapy should be the first course of therapy when making the assumption of ulcer, and a fluoroquinolone should be introduced. Moxifloxacin (Vigamox, Alcon Laboratories) or gatifloxacin (Zymar, Allergan) should be the first choice; however, third-generation fluoroquinolones will suffice. If there is some resolution with the antibiotic, then the CLARE was not inflammatory but infectious. If there is minimal to no response to antibiotics, then a steroid, such as prednisolone 1% four times a day, to rid the inflammatory component of CLARE can be introduced safely, after the loading dose of antibiotic reduces the bacterial load.

After the successful resolution of CLARE, the patient should be refit with a nonionic, high-water-content, deposit-resistance lens or a nonionic silicone hydrogel lens material with the restriction to daily wear use and no extended or continuous wear. Peroxide-based care products are recommended with vigorous rubbing to cleanse debris and contaminants. Also consider gas-permeable lenses that will allow for not only an appropriate high oxygen permeability but also a flatter or hyperbolic peripheral curve and edge design that facilitates sufficient tear pump and exchange.

◆ Contact Lens-Induced Dry Eye

Sometimes described as the minimal sicca syndrome, contact lens–induced dry eye forces a borderline keratoconjunctivitis sicca patient into a full manifestation of symptoms and findings associated directly with a fully manifested dry eye with the introduction of a contact lens onto the ocular surface. The lens acts as an obstacle and competitor with the natural tear film, leading to insult that will justifiably cause a reaction by the eye leading to the change in its natural tear film physiology and metabolism. This will lead to intolerance, inflammation, and a compromise of the ocular surface.

◆ Causes of Contact Lens-Induced Dry Eye

The normal tear-film environment is attacked by the introduction of a contact lens. Initially, there is a reflexive increase in tear production. However, over time tear production will "fatigue" the system, decreasing the efforts of the lacrimal system and increasing the potential for contact lens deposits, microbial infection, and corneal infiltration, corneal edema, and ultimately patient dissatisfaction and intolerance to contact lenses.

The introduction of the contact lens to the ocular surface will disrupt the homeostatic balance of the tear film, requiring a new balance to be established between the pre-lens ocular tear film and the post-lens ocular tear film–precorneal tear film. As deposits or surface film accumulates, blinking compresses the tear film and removes the lipid-contaminated, hydrophobic mucus and debris from the lens–tear surface. The integrity of the precorneal and lens tear film is directly proportional to the ability to maintain proper contact lens wettability and lens surface hydration.

If the lipid layer is poor, the evaporative process increases, leading to a greater loss of aqueous and the induction of a forward osmotic draw across the contact lens surface leading to lens dehydration and corneal desiccation. With lens dehydration, the hydrophilic lens will steepen, mechanically pulling on a weakened epithelial surface, allowing for corneal compromise visualized as central corneal epithelial desiccation and/or cell juncture splitting or separation.

Also, when the ocular surface becomes "unprotected," there is the development of neuronal hyposensitivity associated with hypoxia and the barrier effect created by the contact lens interface. As the contact lens develops a substantial dehydration it will tend to vault away from the ocular surface, leaving an exposed gap between the post-lens surface and the corneal surface. The gap however is not fluid filled and leaves the ocular surface unprotected, leading to compromise and dessication of the epithelium and aberration to neural regulation and biofeedback to the lid structure (**Fig. 16.6**).

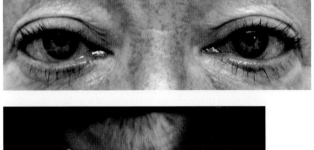

A

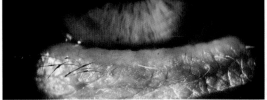

B

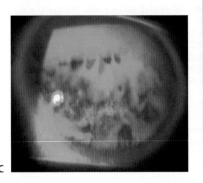

C

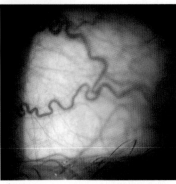

D

Fig. 16.6 **(A)** Classic appearance of contact lens acute red eye (CLIDE) in patient exhibiting circumlimbal injection, marginal erythema, conjunctival injection, and immobile lenses. **(B)** Minimal lacrimal lake as demonstrated by lissamine green. **(C)** Disrupted tear film spread with subsequent paracentral punctate keratopathy associated with CLIDE. **(D)** Lissamine green staining of the conjunctiva in a CLIDE patient.

◆ **Presentation**

The patient will present with a CLARE-type appearance that had been somewhat chronic. The eyes will be described as feeling tired, dry, and irritated and always red, particularly later in the day. It would also be noted that patients have difficult lens removal and describe a feeling of relief upon lens removal. Often the patient will proceed with vigorous eye rubbing after lens removal. In some cases of difficult lens removal, the eye feels overly sensitive and presents with an increase in injection due to the inadvertent removal of superficial epithelial tissue and neuronal exposure due to epithelial compromise during lens wear associated with lens dryness and binding. Supplementation with topical drops such as lubricants may or may not benefit the patient, leading to self-limitation of lens wear or even discontinuance.

The clinician will observe a CLARE-type red eye without infection that appears to be chronic. There maybe a mild to moderate corneal staining present due to lens vault. The lens may appear somewhat immobile, suggesting an induced tight lens syndrome or small petechial hemorrhages on the conjunctiva juxtaposed to the lens edge or on the paralimbal conjunctiva. There is neither apparent discharge nor follicular nor papillary reaction. However, in the long-term sufficient debris and lens surface dryness can induce a CLPC reaction. Tear film spreading abnormalities will be seen with the use of various diagnostic testing such as Schirmer strips, lissamine green, assessment of the tear break-up time, sodium fluorescein staining of the cornea and conjunctiva, assessment of the lacrimal lake–marginal tear volume as a variety of test.

◆ Differential Diagnosis

Contact lens–induced edema, warpage, overwear, other causes of redness and discomfort associated with contact lens use. CLIDE is directly related to other ocular conditions affecting the lacrimal–ocular surface balance including eyelid and glandular dysfunction or disease, poor blinking mechanism such as lagophthalmos, floppy lid, and/or dysfunction of the lacrimal and meibomian glands. Other associations to CLIDE and dry eye include Sjögren syndrome, autoimmune disease, rheumatoid disorders, and medications, especially antihistamines, antidepressants, and oral contraceptives.

◆ Management

The treatment for dry eye and CLIDE is to relieve the underlying problem by first identifying the portion of the tear film that is dysfunctional. Once identified, the treatment should be biased to complement the lens with minimal complexity to the patient. With the use of ocular lubricants as a supplement or stimulant, the eye becomes "subjectively comfortable," but little is known in regard to their long-term effect on the various tear film structures and corneal physiology. With respect to supplement interaction with the material and the material's interaction with the eye, the contact lens design and material are the key long-term comfort and physiological balance in the potential success of the contact lens patient.

To achieve the proper tear-film balance, the CLIDE patient must be treated as a normal dry-eye patient. Following a flow chart of treatment such as proper tear and nutritional supplementation is the first step. The selection of supplementation and/or medicinal treatment is critical. I prefer to try to define medicinal care by the determination of dry eye as a "white" or "red" dry eye. If the patient presents symptomatically and objectively as a dry eye yet has a white, noninflamed conjunctiva, the use of goblet cell–mucin enhancers in conjunction with lacrimal gland stimulus (e.g., cyclosporine) would be considered appropriate. If the patient appears with a red, inflamed dry eye, then the intervention with steroids would be deemed more appropriate. This may also be complemented with the use of nutritional supplementation of omega 3 and 6 essential oils (fish and seed oil sources), which have a natural nonsteroidal antiinflammatory effect. In addition, tear and lens rehydration is well accomplished by using antioxidant or electrolyte-balanced tear supplements. At the same time, a clinical decision must be made to refrain from contact lens use or limit it during the initial stages of therapy. Punctal occlusion should be reserved for long-term lens comfort maintenance until positive results are established with topical and oral therapies.

Material selection is critical in the treatment of the CLIDE patient. Always consider RGP lenses first for borderline dry eye patients. A deficient or unstable tear film requires high oxygen permeability and a lens with low surface reactivity that moves adequately to minimize the risk of complications. Also consider the rechallenge of hydrogel-based group 2 materials of high-water, nonionic character such as hioxifilcon and phosphatylcholine. As noted, silicone hydrogel materials may be appropriate for oxygen enhancement but are not promising when treating a defined CLIDE patient. Silicone hydrogels would be highly desirable once the CLIDE patient has been treated and the eye has resumed a feasible level of comfort and proper tear film balance.

◆ Superior Epithelial Arcuate Lesions

The separation of the corneal epithelium, occurring more so at the superior limbal margin, is known as superior epithelial accurate limbal split (SEALS), or a similar form of epithelial splitting that follows the corneal-limbal border around the cornea is known as intra-epithelial splitting (ILES). It is characterized by an observation of an arcuate staining juxtaposed to the limbus. The pattern of the full-thickness corneal epithelial separation usually occurs in the limbal cornea covered by the upper eyelid, within 2 to 3 mm of the superior limbus in the 10- and 2-o'clock region.

The main cause for this entity is considered to include mechanical irritation and dehydration of the lens surface. The etiology of SEALS and/or ILES is considered to be either a mechanical pull or stress on the epithelial junctures due to a tight lens or lens dehydration or a mechanical chafing within the paralimbal cornea. As for SEALS, superior mechanical chafing may be the result of inward pressure of the upper lid at the superior intralimbus associated with lens design, rigidity, and surface characteristics. In combination the excessive "frictional" pressure and abrasive shear force on the epithelial surface induce a separation of the epithelial cell junctures. New materials, first-generation silicone hydrogels, which possess a stiffer elastic modulus, may cause an increase in the shearing force not only on the cornea, but also may induce a similar force on the conjunctiva leading to a pseudo-impression ring called a conjunctival flap.

The concerns with SEALS or ILES are the provocation of an inflammatory and/or bacterial infiltrative response. Additionally, excessive shearing forces may lead to a degradation of limbal stem cells require for corneal repair mechanisms (**Fig. 16.7**).

◆ Presentation

Presentation is generally asymptomatic other than mild, observable injection to the eye, particularly upon lens removal. The patient may also complain of a mild to moderate lens awareness, difficult lens removal, burning, or itching sensation. The patient may describe a slightly greater lens intolerance to standard low modulus 2-hydroxyethyl methacrylate-based lenses as compared with higher modulus silicone–hydrogel combined polymers.

Upon biomicroscopic exam, the generally asymptomatic patient may present with conjunctival injection juxtaposed to the affected area. In the case of SEALS, the conjunctival injection would appear more strictly between 10 o'clock and 2 o'clock versus a 360-degree-type epithelial splitting, which would appear more as the CLARE-type eye associated with a tight lens syndrome. Subsequently, significant paralimbal staining appears in an arc about the intralimbal cornea.

Fig. 16.7 **(A)** Classic circumlimbal epithelial splitting with tear-film ir-regularity. **(B)** Classic circumlimbal superior epithelial arcuate limbal splitting (SEALS) due to a tight lens syndrome with tear-film disruption and conjunctival congestion [contact lens acute red eye (CLARE)]. **(C)** Classic SEALS due to a tight lens syndrome with tear film disruption and conjunctival congestion (CLARE).

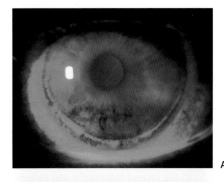

A

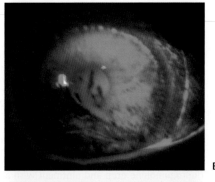

B

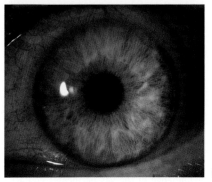

C

◆ **Differential Diagnosis**

This is simply related to the history of lens use or the lack thereof. If there is no his-tory of lens use, then one needs to evaluate the localized conjunctival response to determine the level of injection. A superior limbic keratitis (SLK) may be an indica-tor of subsequent thyroid disease. If the conjunctival response is temporal or nasal, then determine inflammatory concerns of vascularized limbic keratitis, episcleritis, phylctenulitis, pinqueculitis, pterygium, and/or early marginal degenerations. Fortunately, SEALS or ILES, are more consistent with contact lens use, extended wear more so than daily wear. If superior limbal injection occurs, particularly bilateral, consider other issues such as thyroid disorder or corneal disorder.

◆ **Management**

Simple lens discontinuance is the most appropriate, allowing the lesion to recover within a few days to several weeks. If the SEALS or split is minor, the simple discontinuance of the lens is proper based on the patient's ability to function with spectacles. As a precaution against bacterial infiltration, a short course of topical antibiotics may be beneficial. In this scenario, a simple refit to a daily disposable lens with adequate and frequent rehydration is deemed appropriate. The refit of lens should not only reevaluate the hydration ability of the lens but the lens' relation to the corneal topography and asphericity or corneal contour. Therefore, the lens design should complement the anatomy suggesting a flatter base curve or higher eccentricity value. In conjunction, short-term punctal plugs can be considered an ample adjuvant therapy to enhance epithelial healing and maintain lens and corneal hydration.

If there is a low-grade conjunctival response, a break within the epithelium could be the potential opportunity for bacterial contamination and/or inflammatory responses. As such, the level of the condition will warrant the level of therapy. Again, discontinuance is appropriate, yet the addition of a soft steroid with mild antibiotics such as tobramycin/loteprednol (Zylet, Bausch & Lomb) four times a day for 5 to 7 days with the addition of a bacitracin ointment during sleeping hours is considered prophylactically safe.

If there is a greater (mild–moderate–severe) ocular injection and significant splitting, complete discontinuance of the lens is required with a more aggressive therapy utilizing a combination steroid-antibiotic drop and ointment or a separate fluoroquinolone drop and ointment with a secondary steroid such as prednisolone acetate if the condition has associated infiltrates or may lead to an ulcerative keratopathy.

Once the condition is resolved, the patient can be refit to a lower elastic modulus lens, avoiding extended or continuous wear or be refit to a high Dk gas permeable lens.

◆ Dellen-Epithelial Hyperplasia

Dellen are focal areas of corneal thinning typically located, usually at the 3- to 9-o'clock limbus due to dehydration of the region. These formations are the active state of mechanical irritation of a sector or portion of the cornea juxtaposed to the edge of the gas permeable contact lens. They are considered a transient form of corneal degeneration that results from stromal dehydration secondary to poor wetting by the tear film seen not only with contact lens wear but also postsurgically (e.g., cataract, LASIK, strabismus). It represents a localized thinning of the corneal and scleral tissue. Epithelial hyperplasia is more related to the chronic dehydration and mechanical chafing of the gas permeable lens in a specific juxtaposed area of the cornea.

The etiology of the dellen is local dehydration. It is thought that breaks in the oil layer of the tear film prevent the proper wetting of the tissue, leading to devitalizing dehydration of the epithelial cells. Due to the lack of proper oil and aqueous

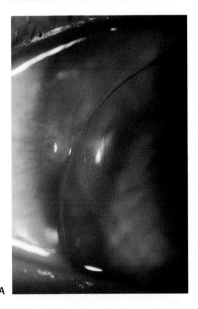 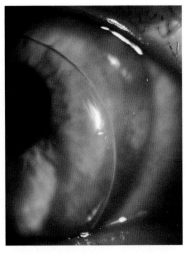

Fig. 16.8 **(A)** Corneal dellen secondary to gas permeable lens wear. **(B)** Epithelial hyperplasia secondary to gas permeable lens wear.

fluids in the location, there is a greater tendency for lens binding and mechanical chafing. Mechanical influences are induced by the eyelids, which are unable to follow the changing contour of the lens edge forcing it to lift or bore into the epithelium. If the lens edge creates a gap, then there is a subsequent lack of wetting and hydration of the corneal tissue in which mucins are not spread over the epithelium, resulting in an area of nonwetting results. Further dehydration either eventually causes corneoscleral thinning to occur, with the formation of a dellen or long-term local epithelial hyperplasia (**Fig. 16.8**).

◆ Presentation

Patients with corneal dellen may be asymptomatic but often report mild ocular discomfort or a foreign body sensation. The patient may describe a sectoral redness to the eye with lens awareness over time. There may be increased epiphoria as well as noticeable lens decentration. Subsequently, the patient may describe dry eye–type symptoms and increasing lens intolerance. Additionally, the patient may exhibit an incomplete or erratic blink reflex when utilizing lenses.

Dellen appear as pale–keratinized white "saucerlike" depressions within, usually the 3- to 9-o'clock area intralimbal juxtaposed to the edge of the lenses. Rarely are these lesions larger than 2 mm. If the overlying epithelium is intake, they will not stain. They may have a slightly vascularized surface with adjacent sectoral conjunctival injection. Fluorescein may appear to "gutter" and surround the base of the dellen. The staining, at or near the 3- and 9-o'clock positions, appears on or adjacent to the limbus of rigid lens wearers. Breaks in the epithelium may allow for peripheral bacterial contamination leading to a keratitis or ulceration or inflammatory infiltration. Because of the localized dehydration, subsequent cell desiccation occurs and necrosis of the epithelial cells. This leads to epithelial hyperplasia similar to corneal scarring. Epithelial hyperplasia is observed as a mound of tissue that becomes eroded and irritated by the lens edge due to chronic dehydration of tissue exposure.

◆ Differential Diagnosis

Several potential differentials need to be considered when observing a dellen or epithelial hyperplasia. If there is significant sectoral conjunctival injection, then one should also consider vascularized limbic keratitis, episcleritis, phlyctenulitis, pinqueculitis, pterygium, or early marginal degenerations such as Terrien's. The most important differential would be marginal ulceration, particularly if epithelium compromise is observed. If the adjacent conjunctiva is quiet, then one may consider ruling out a preexisting scar or postoperative scar from cataract or extraocular muscle surgery, filtering blebs, and scleritis, obviously differentiated by history.

◆ Management

Therapy focuses on the proper reepithelialization and rehydrating the cornea. Copious lubrication every 1 or 2 hours and bland ointment at night are recommended. In particular, nutrient-based therapy is most appropriate utilizing an electrolyte-balanced or antioxidant-based drop. In addition, a demulcent such as Systane (Alcon Laboratories) or Endura (Allergan), which forms a network gel-like consistency on the ocular surface and acts as a temporary bandage enhancing epithelial healing and revitalizing the microvilli and surface glycocalyx. Initial treatment will demonstrate efficacy in 48 to 72 hours, but reinsult occurs easily. Topical cyclosporine can also be considered in short- or long-term care.

Topical antibiotics are unnecessary, except in extreme cases involving significant epithelial compromise to prevent infection and ulceration. In these cases, the inflammatory component is raised, and therefore a combination tobramycin with dexamethasone or loteprednol may be appropriate in a short course of 7 days at four times a day.

Once there is proper resolution, the gas permeable lenses can be refit with a diligent reevaluation of the peripheral corneal anatomy versus the peripheral curve and edge profile of the lens. Additionally, blinking exercises encouraging the patient to force a complete lid closure, once every 2 or 3 seconds, are essential. Also, continue proper lubrication with rewetting drops complementary to the material of choice. Consider higher dK materials with plasma treatment for enhanced wettability.

Epithelial hyperplasia may resolve following discontinuation of lens wear. When poor resolution occurs and is an obstruction to lens refitting and PTK excimer laser procedure may be considered to flatten the area and elevate the devitalized cells.

◆ Contact Lens-Induced Corneal Warpage Syndrome

The syndrome of "corneal warpage" implies that the contact lens has iatrogenically induced anatomical changes to the corneal surface. The warpage is visualized as an irregular retinoscopic reflex, distortion to topography, and keratometric mires, induced irregular corneal astigmatism, and observable distortions to the corneal surface upon lens removal.

Contact lens–induced corneal warpage is more frequently associated with polymethyl methacrylate (PMMA), more so than gas-permeable lenses; however, ~27% of reported cases of corneal warpage have been attributed to hydrogel lens wear. Corneal contour–induced irregularities are considered the result of probable mechanical deformation, chronic metabolic insult, or a combination of both. Additionally, warpage is seen as secondary to lens binding or stagnation due to lens dehydration or a CLIDE syndrome. Also, some solution interactions may tend to induce lens immobility due to the level of solution viscosity leading to lens binding.

More commonly, hard PMMA or rigid gas-permeable lenses are recognized for the induction of corneal warpage or iatrogenically induced reshaping of the cornea when improperly fit or aligned to the corneal surface. The corneal epithelium, having a very "plastic" or "moldable" character, is easily reshaped by the high modulus or stiffness of the lens, which molds the cornea to the shape of the lens curvature(s) unintentionally. This can be intentionally accomplished in a process called *orthokeratology.*

Rigid contact lens–induced corneal warpage is easily documented and monitored via observation of topographic abnormalities. There will be induced central irregular astigmatism, inferior steepening or smile-like pattern (pseudokeratoconus-like images), superior flattening, loss of radial symmetry, highly irregular patterns with loss of surface symmetry, or an impression of a demarcation contour line consistent with the lens edge. Induced warpage with hydrogels are considered more transient; however, gas permeable may be transient to permanent.

Hydrogel-induced deformations are related to a weakened epithelium due to lesser than optimal oxygen transmissibility through various hydrogel lens materials. Subsequently, a misaligned, tight, ultrathin lens or extreme variants in elastic modulus of lenses can induce hydrophilic corneal warpage syndrome. In a positive effect, a high elastic modulus lens worn in reverse can actually induce a subtle flattening–orthokeratological effect to the cornea of 0.50 to 1 diopter (**Fig. 16.9**).

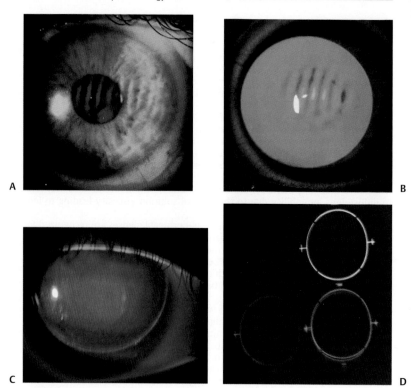

Fig. 16.9 **(A)** Corneal wrinkling (convolutions) induced by ultrathin hydrogel lenses. **(B)** Hydrogel corneal warpage as seen with sodium fluroscein stainage. **(C)** Corneal impression ring induced by orthokeratologically fit lens. **(D)** Irregular keratometric mires by induced corneal warpage from a rigid gas permeable lens.

◆ Presentation

Patients will complain of poor or distorted vision with lenses with subsequent reduction in visual acuity. They will tend to utilize more rewetting drops that tend to assist in clearing the vision momentarily, yet do not resolve the visual decrement. The unintentional molding or warpage of the cornea leads to subjective visual distortion and complaints of postlens removal spectacle blur or inability to wear glasses and objective measures of regression of power if the lens is fit flat and reduction of astigmatism can be made. In many cases, particularly with hydrogel lenses, subtle distortions cannot be observed by biomicroscopy but may be more obvious on topography and aberrometry. In these cases, history of poor vision or nonoptimal vision is the only descriptor by the patient. This will often occur when one is refitting from older conventional designs to frequent-replacement, thinner lens designs that may lack the proper alignment to the corneal topography.

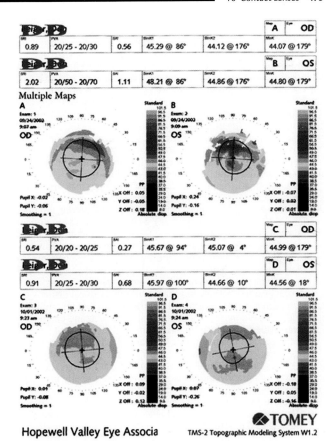

					A · OD
0.89	20/25 - 20/30	0.56	45.29 @ 86°	44.12 @ 176°	44.07 @ 179°

					B · OS
2.02	20/50 - 20/70	1.11	48.21 @ 86°	44.86 @ 176°	44.80 @ 179°

Multiple Maps

					C · OD
0.54	20/20 - 20/25	0.27	45.67 @ 94°	45.07 @ 4°	44.99 @ 179°

					D · OS
0.91	20/25 - 20/30	0.68	45.97 @ 100°	44.66 @ 10°	44.56 @ 18°

Hopewell Valley Eye Associa   TMS-2 Topographic Modeling System W1.2   **E**

Fig. 16.9 (*Continued*) **(E)** Topography of warpage—RGP-induced corneal warpage at present and at 1 week lens discontinuance.

Clinical signs of corneal warpage are first documented by reduced, subjective and objective, visual acuity with contact lenses and subsequently persistent acuity reduction with spectacles. The visual reduction may be subtle (20/20 minus) or pronounced. Once the lenses are removed for an adequate period, the patient's manifest refraction returns to normal with consistent improvement in acuity measures. During the examination, retinoscopy reflexes will appear "warped" or yield a "scissor" reflex often seen in keratoconus. Keratometry and topographic measures demonstrate variant levels of irregularities. Particularly, descriptive statistics with topography will be highly variable as compared with prefit measures, sometimes mimicking a disease state.

◆ Differential Diagnosis

History of lens use and subjective complaints will define the concern. However, a spectacle blur from lens-induced warpage occurs either due to the mechanical distortion or from corneal edema with corneal haze. If there is a weakened endothelium, particularly with the extended-wear patient or an older individual, corneal edema may occur secondary to imbibement of fluid through endothelial cell junctions and may lead to associated central corneal striae, folds, or clouding. Therefore, endothelial polymegathism, polymorphism, and reduced endothelial cell count may be the underlying cause.

Advanced or uncontrolled glaucoma with significant corneal edema can also cause corneal warpage or distortions, particularly with a lower than normal (540 μm) central corneal thickness. Once the IOP is controlled, the distortion of the cornea dissipates and refractive recovery occurs rapidly.

Highly astigmatic, nondiseased, corneal anatomy may also demonstrate topographic irregularities. The irregular corneal astigmatism may have a decentered corneal cap or a high asymmetry of superior versus inferior, temporal versus nasal, sections of the cornea. In these cases, a contact lens is very difficult to center on the unusual landscape of the corneal topography and when done so, it will have a higher propensity to decenter towards the steeper meridian and bind, causing induced molding to the cornea. Reduced vision in these patients is not always induced by the contact lens, but will have an enhanced appreciation for visual aberrations and may also have a meridional amblyopia.

Scarring or other pathologies that induce mechanical distortions to the cornea can also mimic corneal warpage. In particular pterygium, pulling across the corneal surface, has a more global than localized effect, and pannus or aberrant conjunctival tissue may induce similar mechanical distortions.

Ectactic corneal degenerations such as pellucid or keratoconus may not have been determined at the initial lens fitting of the patient many years prior. Forme fruste keratoconus (absence of classic anatomical findings) is often missed in the initial fit if topography and aberrometry are not properly utilized. Due to the increased interest in refractive surgical procedures, many of these patients are being discovered in preoperative care and justly denied the procedure. Literature suggests that PMMA and gas-permeable lenses at one time induced keratoconus. In fact, the lenses did not induce the disorder, but instead caused a "pseudokeratoconic" distortion of the cornea, which, in some cases, is permanent. Pseudokeratoconus induced by contact lenses warping of the cornea produces a pattern that mimics keratoconus evidenced in a localized area of inferior corneal steepening. Upon lens discontinuance the induced steepening will regress to a normal "bow tie" or "hourglass-shaped" topography with symmetry, much unlike a true keratoconic eye.

◆ Management

Diagnosis by history, refraction, retinoscopy, and corneal imaging is critical. Serial measures after lens discontinuance will determine the severity, transience, or permanency and the final end point prior to refit or surgical procedure. If concerns of corneal edema arise, serial pachymetry is a required measure.

If there is significant corneal edema, lens discontinuance is recommended with the incorporation of hyperosmotic agents with repeat pachymetry till the patient demonstrates refractive recovery and stable central corneal thickness (CCT) measures.

If the corneal distortions are induced by hydrogel soft lenses, the simple discontinuance for a few days and refit to a slightly thicker or intermediate elastic modulus, high-water, high-oxygen permeability, and parameter-stable lens is appropriate. These would include a group 2 lens such as Proclear (CooperVision, Fairport, NY), Extreme Water (Hydrogel Vision Corp., Sarasota, FL) or a lower elastic modulus silicone hydrogel. In these cases, the induced distortion is transient and resolves in a few hours. Monitor with topography and aberrometry until stability of refraction and vision occurs prior to completing a refitting of the contact lenses.

In treating corneal deformity or warpage induced by gas-permeable lenses, one could take several approaches. Simply discontinue contact lenses and revert to eyeglass wear for several days to weeks until the stability of the cornea can be determined. In the majority of cases, this is not an attractive option for the patient because vision will dynamically change and the patient likely does not have a pair of glasses to wear during this period. Or first observe the lens on eye, then remove and perform a dry refraction, pachymetry, and topographic or aberrometry measures. These measures will be repeated several times in the "rehabilitation process" until stability of measures occurs. Defer cycloplegia until resolution after several serial measures. During the "recovery" or "corneal rehabilitation" period, refit the patient with hydrogel soft lenses to their best achievable acuity. On aftercare, repeat diagnostic measures and refit with soft lenses according to the results. Continue this process until corneal and refractive stability is achieved. A critical point in patient care is to warn the patient of the dynamic change to vision and the frustration that will probably pursue. Patient reassurance is vital, encouraging them to immediately return for continued care if the vision becomes unacceptable.

Stabilization of the cornea is defined as the point that the manifest refraction is consistent two to three times within a −0.50 diopters sphere and cylinder, with axis within 10 to 15 degrees of original manifest, proper symmetry to the topography and pachymetry within normal ranges of prefit estimates or measures. Noting that, based on the extent and severity of corneal warpage, 20/20 (6/6) may no longer be achievable by the patient. Once stable, the patient can be refit to any lens that is deemed appropriate, be it soft hydrogel or gas permeable or orthokeratology or a refractive surgical procedure.

If considering orthokeratology or refractive surgery, even cataract procedures on patients who have worn gas-permeable lenses for any extent of time, a "corneal rehabilitation" should be incorporated into the prefit or preoperative care. There is no single rule for preoperative care. Some might suggest that corneal stability is achieved between 8 and 20 weeks, or even up to 6 months. In my experience it is suggested that approximately 1 to 2 weeks' discontinuance of gas permeable lenses for every year of wear be observed prior to a refractive surgical procedure, more time if the patient had worn PMMA lenses only.

◆ Contact Lens Deposits

Deposits are the accumulation of debris on the surface. The various types of deposit accumulate based on the material chemistry characteristics such as water content, ionic versus nonionic surface treatments, or physiological interactions of the constituents of the tear film or the ability of the lids to spread the tear film and cleanse the contact lens surface. Deposits are multifactorial with a variety of types (**Fig. 16.10**).

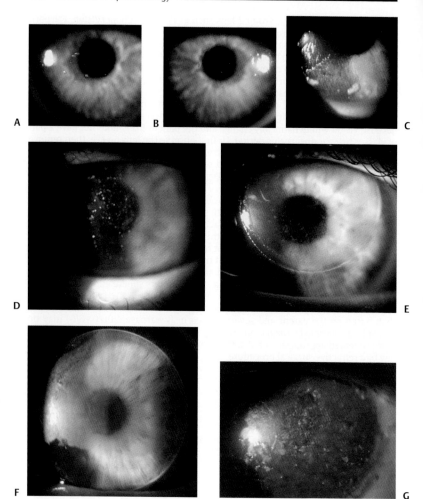

Fig. 16.10 **(A)** Mucin balls and surface film silicone hydrogel lenses. **(B)** Mucin balls and surface film silicone hydrogel lenses. **(C)** Severe lipid–protein –mucous surface film on soft hydrogel lenses. **(D)** Severe lipid protein calcium deposits—lens calculi. **(E)** Severe protein film rigid gas permeable (RGP). **(F)** Severe nonwetting secondary to surface film RGP. **(G)** Filming of a prosthetic eye.

◆ **Presentation**

The underlying problem is the improper clearance of metabolic and/or exogenous debris that accumulates on or penetrates within the lens material. This accumulation of debris and waste is due to poor tear chemistry, inappropriate or incomplete cleaning by the lens care product, or a poor lid interaction to spread the tear film and cleanse the lens surface. This leads to deleterious interactions with the palpebral conjunctiva of the superior eyelid that leads to a mechanical and antigenic response causing CLPC.

Proteins in the tear film are composed of organic amino acids of various electrolytes. Oxidation by heating or ultraviolet exposure encourages the denaturing (chemical transformation) or alteration of the proteins, the most predominant being lysozyme, which has a strong antimicrobial characteristic. When the proteins change their character, they now become foreign to the system, initiating an autoimmune hypersensitivity response. Antibodies are stimulated leading to subsequent inflammation, injection or erythema, and pruisitis. As the deposits accumulate, they become "space occupying" nodules on the back surface that lead to localized impressions on the corneal epithelial surface, seen as discrete punctate staining. Also, the denatured proteins can lead to a cytotoxic response and a generalized superficial punctate keratitis. The surface proteins can also act as nutrition to normal flora, whereas mucus can encapsulate and nurture the colony. As such, the flora replicate into a larger colony, which is beyond the normal balance and defenses of the ocular surface. If there is a break in the epithelium, a sequela of infiltration with resultant microbial keratitis or ulceration may occur.

The patient, in many cases, is asymptomatic other than describing variable dryness, itch, redness, and visual concerns with the lenses. In the majority of cases, when frequent replacement lens modalities are properly used, the deposits do not become significant enough to cause a noticeable problem. Rarely, in few patients, lens deposits form quickly due to their poor tear chemistry. In frequent-replacement lenses, lenses used less than 30 days, deposits tend to create a "film" that cleans off easily with the proper care product, yet reaccumulates more rapidly each day of lens wear until it is discarded.

In patients where deposits become excessive, the lens will interact aggressively against the lid, leading to inflammation such as CLPC. The patient will once again be somewhat asymptomatic other than describing a lens that frequently decenters or even dislodges. There will also be a "conjunctivitis type" discharge and redness without discomfort. In these cases, very often, the PCP is consulted and will prescribe an antibiotic inappropriately (see CLPC and ARE).

In other cases, the patient will present with an acute red eye, with discomfort to pain, copious watery or purulent discharge, with possible effects on visual ability. This would imply a secondary bacterial contamination due to a contact lens–associated nutrient- and protein-rich biofilm. The biofilm allows bacteria, even normal flora, to "feast" and increase colonization beyond levels in which the eye can defend itself. Also, with the lack of tear lysozyme, the bacterium has a great ability to populate and invade. In these cases of usual abuse to the contact lens and lack of proper care, the cornea is also compromised, allowing for a vast opportunity for bacterial infiltration and subsequent ulceration of the cornea. The most common are *Staphylococcus epidermidis* and *aureus*, followed by *Pseudomonas aeruginosa*.

As microorganisms spread, they will either immediately attack the cornea or serpiginously spread over the lens surface. These are gray, black, brown, or white growths in the lens matrix. Fungi or yeast will appear in a filamentary pattern, observed as having a central density and translucent fronds protruding from the core. Most commonly, surface microorganisms are associated with contamination from various nonsterile water sources, such as pools, recreational waters (ponds, rivers, lakes), contaminated tap water, nonpreserved saline, or, as more recently seen, ineffective contact lens care products. Catastrophic infections related to the acanthameoba (a protozoa) and fusarium (a fungal infection) have been cited in an outbreak of cases worldwide in 2005 through 2006.

◆ Differential Diagnosis

Protein Deposits
The most common type of deposit is protein based originating from tear components of albumin, globulin, and lysozyme. The deposit is characterized by its opaque, thick, dense, white film with striations, found on hydrogel lenses, predominantly on the anterior surface versus gas permeables that accumulate these deposits on both surface and particularly in the peripheral curves. Protein uptake occurs within moments upon lens insertion and varies to the time of matrix saturation. Saturation of the matrix is highly dependent on the polymer characteristic. Ionic lenses will tend to absorb and bind a great amount of protein, nonionic as well as plasma or surface-treated lenses tend to retard the absorption.

Lipid Deposits
Lipids are a component of the tear film arising from the meibomian glands to prevent tear evaporation. When lipids accumulate on the lens surface they have a smeared, greasy, whitish appearance. Individuals with dietary or metabolic deficiency in potassium, have dry eye, use diuretics or alcohol, have poor tear osmolarity, or have higher-fat diet tend to be more prone to these forms of deposits.

Lens Calculi or Jelly Bumps
Combination deposits of lipid and proteins accumulate as more discrete, round bumps and localized "droplets" that bore into the lens matrix. As a combined deposit, various minerals such as calcium from the tear film may also be part of the composition. These types of deposits are most common in ionic, high-water-content lenses used in a continuous or extended-wear modality.

Mucin Balls
Most synonymous with silicone hydrogel lenses, these are recognized as small, round, discrete particles or plugs seen between the contact lens and corneal surface. They are composed of a combination of mucin, tear proteins, and lipids. The appearance will vary in size from 10 to 20 μm in diameter and is typically transparent, similar to the appearance of microcysts. They are differentiated from microcysts by their impregnation of the lens surface, versus microcysts, which are intraepithelial. Mucin balls may accumulate and clump; thus they may not move as the lens moves, appearing trapped against the corneal surface. Upon lens removal or subsequent blinking, they will dislodge, leaving an indentation in the corneal surface that also appears similar to discrete punctate staining associated with back surface debris.

Exogenous Deposits
These types of deposits can be from foreign bodies such as rust, cosmetics, paint, lotions and creams, and other forms of airborne debris. These deposits will be discrete and obvious upon observation. Rust or metallic foreign bodies appear round, small, and brown-red that have become embedded in the lens surface. Cosmetics tend to spread across the lens surface in a vortex manner, whereas paint (and some oil-based cosmetics) tend to variably "spot" the surface. In general, exogenous debris is usually airborne or physically impaled onto the lens surface and will quickly bind without patient symptoms.

Medications

Medications can also create deposits or lens discoloration. This is due to the water solubility of hydrophilic soft lenses that allow for the ease of absorption by the by-products that circulate into the tear film. Antibiotics such as phenazopyridine or nitrofurantoin (urinary infection) will discolor lenses to a yellow or pink. Phenyl-ephrine, propine (prodrug), and epinephrine will appear as brown-black deposits on the lens surface (adenochrome staining), which can also be found on the conjunctiva and lid margin. Tetracycline, used for dermatological concerns or upper respiratory infection, may be observed as grayish brown dots. Rifampin used in the treatment of tuberculosis–meningococcal infections causes orange-pink tear excretion that absorbs into the lens. Iodine and sulfa-based drugs such as sulfasalazine (treatment for ulcerative colitis and Crohn disease) as well as stool softeners such as phenolphthalein will yield a yellow discoloration of the lens. These are easily defined by medical history. Any suppression of the lacrimal or exocrine system will allow for increased lens depositing.

◆ Management

The treatment is simple but the hardest thing for many patients to complete. It is called proper lens care and hygiene. The simplification of care systems is a double-edged sword. On the positive side, it is easier, less cumbersome, and more user friendly with good effectiveness in microbial challenge multi-item testing. On the negative, simplicity is followed by complacency and worsened by the commoditization of contacts through third-party vendors. The general public does not look at contacts as a medical device that requires proper care until something goes wrong. The best treatment for deposits is good education and instructions on the proper use of the recommended and prescribed lens care product. In recent studies, peroxide, acting as a solvent cleanser and high efficacious antimicrobial solution, has been shown to be the most efficient for cleansing and microbial reduction. Multipurpose solutions, which at one time recommended no rub, have since gone back to "rub." Rubbing can reduce the bacterial load by 90% and purges the lens surface of the protein–lipid accumulation.

Ophthalmic Instruments and Diagnostic Tests
Samuel Boyd and Amar Agarwal

◆ Cover Testing

Cover/Uncover Tests

◆ Cover Test

The cover test is done to confirm the presence of a manifest squint. The patient is asked to look at the fixation target (a flashlight should never be used as a fixation target because it fails to control accommodation—an accommodative fixation target held at 33 cm is used for near and the Snellen 6/9 visual acuity symbol is used for distance fixation). The apparently fixating eye is then covered and the behavior of the uncovered eye is noted. Each eye is tested in turn for near (33 cm) and distance (6 m). It is performed in all nine positions of gaze. Head posture should be straight. The test is performed with and without eyeglasses. In the presence of squint, the uncovered eye moves to take up fixation. If there is no movement of the uncovered eye, that eye is then covered and the other eye observed. No movement of either eye is seen in pseudosquint.

◆ Uncover Test

Cover the apparently fixing eye and observe the other eye (apparently deviating eye). If movement is seen, then there is heterotopia.

◆ Cover/Uncover Test

This test tells about the presence and type of heterophoria. The patient looks at the fixation target and one eye is covered with an occluder. The occluder is then removed, and the eye under cover is observed. The findings vary depending on the diagnosis:

- ◆ In a person with normal vision, covering either eye will not produce any movement of the other eye. On removing the occluder, there is no movement of the uncovered eye, which continues to look straight ahead.
- ◆ In heterophoria, the eye under cover will deviate in the direction of the heterophoric position. On uncovering, it will move in the opposite direction to reestablish binocular fixation. The opposite eye continues to maintain fixation and makes no movement. Thus only one eye moves in case of a heterophoria.
- ◆ In heterotropia, on covering the fixating eye, the opposite eye, provided it is able to do so, will make a movement from the heterotropic position to take up fixation, and the covered eye will make a corresponding movement in accordance with the Hering law. On uncovering the formerly fixating eye, it will either move again to take up fixation or may continue to remain deviated de-

pending on whether it is a unilateral or an alternate heterotropia. One can also make out the fixation pattern, that is, whether there is strong fixation preference for one eye, free alternation (formerly deviated eye continues to maintain fixation indefinitely), weak alternation (formerly deviated eye maintains fixation for some time, such as until a blink), or eccentric fixation (on covering the fixating eye, the deviated eye makes no movement or an incomplete movement) is present.

Prism Bar Cover Test

This is an objective method of measuring the deviations. Apply the following rule: the apex of the prism should point toward the deviation:

◆ *Esodeviations*: Place the prism base out.
◆ *Exodeviations*: Place the prism base in.
◆ *Right hypertropia*: Place the prism base down in front of the right eye.
◆ *Right hypotropia*: Place the prism base up in front of the right eye.
◆ *Combination of vertical and horizontal deviation*: Place horizontal prisms in front of one eye and vertical prisms in front of the other eye.

Alternate Cover Test

In this test, the patient looks at the fixation target with both eyes open, and the occluder is alternately moved between the two eyes to produce maximal dissociation of the two eyes. This prevents fusion between the two eyes and decompensates any latent squint. The patient should not be allowed to regain fusion while the cover is being transferred. It can be used to diagnose a latent squint of even 2 degrees and small degrees of heterotropia. It also differentiates concomitant squint from paralytic squint.

◆ Rod Tests

Maddox Rod Test

The patient is asked to fix on a point light in the center of the Maddox tangent scale at a distance of 6 m. A red Maddox rod (which consists of many glass rods of red color set together in a metallic disk) is placed in front of one eye with the axis of the rod at a right angle to the axis of deviation. The Maddox rod converts the point light image into a line. Thus the patient will see a point light with one eye and a red line with the other. Due to dissimilar images of the two eyes, fusion is broken and heterophoria becomes manifest. The number on the Maddox tangent scale where the red line falls will be the amount of heterophoria in degrees (**Fig. 17.1**).

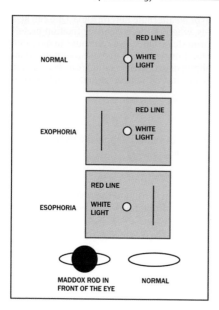

Fig. 17.1   Maddox rod test.

Double Maddox Rod Test

This test helps in detecting and measuring cyclodeviations. Place a red Maddox rod vertically in front of the patient's right eye and a white Maddox rod also vertically in front of the other eye in a trial frame. The axes of the Maddox rod(s) are rotated until the two lines seen by the patient are parallel. The degrees of cyclodeviation and direction are measured from the trial frame with excyclodeviation having outward rotation and incyclodeviations having inward rotations.

Maddox Wing Test

The Maddox wing is an instrument by which the amount of heterophoria for near (at a distance of 33 cm) can be measured. It is based on the principle of dissociation of fusion by dissimilar objects. It has two slit holes in the eyepiece. The fields that are exposed to each eye are separated by a diaphragm in such a way that they glide tangentially into each other. The right eye sees a white arrow pointing vertically upward and a red arrow pointing horizontally to the left. The left eye sees a horizontal row of figures in white and a vertical row in red. These are calibrated in diopters of deviation. The arrow pointing to the horizontal row of figures and the arrow pointing to the vertical row are both at zero in the absence of a squint or in the presence of squint with a harmonious abnormal retinal correspondence.

Clinically important points are as follows:

◆ The Maddox wing should be held pointing 15 degrees inferiorly, as for reading.
◆ It is important to do the test with and without correction for refractive errors.
◆ The ability of the patient to give an answer on the Maddox wing does not mean the patient has normal binocular vision because the patient can have abnormal retinal correspondence (ARC) or rapid alteration.

◆ Stereopsis and Fusional Testing

◆ Stereopsis

Stereopsis is the visual appreciation of three dimensions during binocular vision. It is a function of spatial disparity and arises when horizontally disparate retinal elements are stimulated simultaneously. The fusion of these disparate retinal images will result in a single visual impression perceived in depth, provided the fused image lies within the Panum area of binocular single vision.

◆ Tests for Stereopsis

Titmus Test
The titmus test consists of a three-dimensional Polaroid vectograph—two plates in the form of a booklet, which has to be viewed through Polaroid spectacles. On the right there is a large fly and on the left a series of circles and animals. The working distance is 16 inches (40 cm).

Fly Test
The fly test is for gross stereopsis (degree of disparity is 3000 seconds of arc). The fly should appear solid and the subject should be able to pick up one of the wings of the fly. On inverting the book, the targets will appear to recede. If the fly appears as a flat photograph, the subject is not appreciating stereoscopic vision.

Circles Test
The circles test measures fine stereopsis (degree of disparity is 800 to 40 seconds of arc). There are nine squares, each of which contains four circles. One of the circles in each square will appear forward of the plane of reference in the presence of normal stereopsis. The subject that perceives the circle to be shifted off to the side is not appreciating stereoscopic vision but is using monocular clues instead.

TNO Test (degree of disparity is 480 to 15 seconds of arc)
The TNO test consists of seven plates to be viewed with red-green spectacles. Each plate has various shapes created by random dots in complementary colors. Some shapes are visible without glasses, whereas others can be appreciated in the presence of stereopsis only. It has no monocular clues.

Lang Test (degree of disparity is 1200 to 600 seconds of arc)
The targets are seen alternately by each eye through the built-in cylindrical lens system; hence there is no need for special spectacles.

Frisby Test (degree of disparity is 600 to 15 seconds of arc)
There are three transparent plates of varying thickness. On the surface of each plate there are printed four squares of small random shapes. One of the squares contains a hidden circle in which the random shapes are printed on the reverse of the plate. The subject must identify this hidden circle.

◆ Base-Out Prism

This is a quick and simple method using a 20 diopter base-out prism to detect binocular single vision (BSV).

◆ Synoptophore

All types of heterophorias and heterotropias can be measured accurately with a synoptophore (both objective and subjective angle of squint). In the synoptophore the rays of light from the target hit a mirror and then pass through a convex lens of + 6.5 diopters to reach the eye. Thus the image is seen behind the mirror, for example, at a distance of 6 m, which will be equal to the focal length of the lens. Thus the synoptophore images are seen at a distance and not near. This is because we do not want the patient to use his or her accommodation. The technique for using the synoptophore is as follows (**Fig. 17.2**):

◆ Interpupillary distance (IPD) is checked and adjusted.
◆ Angle kappa is measured.
◆ Simultaneous macular perception is tested for.

We use the simultaneous paramacular perception slides. Both the objective and subjective angles of squint are checked in all nine cardinal positions of gaze (one is the primary position and the other eight are 15 degrees from the primary position).

To test the objective angle, one arm of the synoptophore is fixed at zero degrees. The other arm is moved until there is no movement of the eyes when the tester alternately switches on and off the lights of the two arms. The point where the eyes do not move is the objective angle.

To test the subjective angle, one arm of the synoptophore is fixed at zero degrees. The patient is shown slides of a lion and its cage. The slide of the cage is kept in the arm that is fixed. The patient is asked to move the other arm (containing the slide of the lion) so as to put the lion in the cage. The angle at which this is done is the subjective angle of squint.

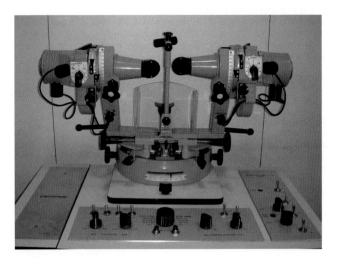

Fig. 17.2   Synaptophore

To detect abnormal retinal correspondence (ARC) with the synoptophore, the objective angle (OA) and the subjective angle (SA) of squint are first determined, which gives the angle of anomaly (AOA).

$$AOA = OA - SA$$

In the case of normal retinal correspondence (NRC), the SA is equal to the OA, and the AOA will be zero. In unharmonious ARC, the subjective angle will be less than the objective angle, and the difference between the two should be at least 5 degrees or more. In the case of harmonious ARC, the subjective angle will be zero. Thus the angle of anomaly in a harmonious ARC will be equal to the objective angle.

◆ *Fusion*: For testing fusion, two slides are used: one is that of a rabbit without a tail and the other is that of a rabbit without ears. The two slides are kept in each arm of the synoptophore and the arms are fixed at the angle of squint. If the patient sees both the ears and the tail, then fusion is present. If the patient sees either the tail or the ears, fusion is absent.
◆ *Stereopsis*: Stereopsis can be tested with slides containing paratroopers with a plane in the background. The patient should be able to tell whether the paratroopers are in front of the plane or not, which indicates good stereopsis.
◆ *After images*: After images can also be done.

◆ Visual-Field Testing

The visual field is the portion of space that is visible to the fixation eye. Visual-field examination is the examination of the function of the visual system in the field and not only the determination of the limits of the field. The difference threshold is the smallest measurable difference in luminance between a stimulus and the background (**Fig. 17.3**).

Automated Static Perimetry

The different tests in autoperimetry are as follows:

◆ *Suprathreshold test*: This test is used as a screening device for severe or moderate defects.
◆ *Threshold related strategy*: The actual threshold is determined at a small number of points and they are used to extrapolate the hill of vision.
◆ *Threshold testing*: Threshold testing is the standard of care for glaucoma management. Many points are tested and there are different strategies used to accurately define the visual field. These tests can be long and the patients can become fatigued.
◆ *SITA*: Because full threshold can be time consuming, shorter algorithms have been developed. The Swedish Interactive Thresholding Algorithm (SITA) uses mathematical modeling and present understanding of the visual field to increase accuracy while speeding up the test.
◆ *Short-wavelength automated perimetry (SWAP)*: This selectively tests the short-wavelength pathway by presenting a blue target on a yellow background. SWAP may be able to show defects 1 to 3 years before standard techniques.

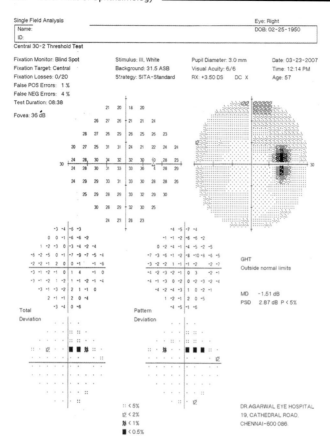

Fig. 17.3 Humphrey autoperimetric 30–2 test.

The various field defects seen in glaucoma are generalized depression, baring of the blind spot, isolated paracentral scotoma, Seidel scotoma, Bjerrum scotoma or arcuate scotoma, double arcuate scotoma, Ronne nasal step (which respects the horizontal midline), temporal wedge defect, peripheral breakthrough, altitudinal defect, central and temporal islands, and split fixation.

◆ **Automated Corneal Topography**

Imaging techniques of the cornea are developing rapidly, mainly because of continuous advances in refractive and cataract surgery. It is crucial to understand the significance of new imaging techniques and the relevant principles of corneal optics. The discussion of the most common clinical method of Placido-based corneal topography emphasizes important concepts of its clinical interpretation (**Fig. 17.4**).

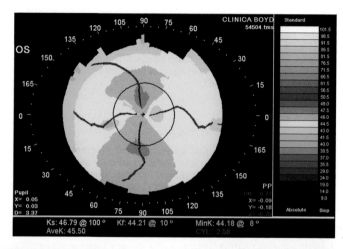

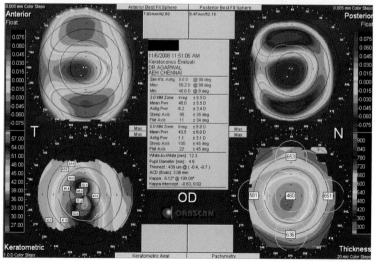

Fig. 17.4 **(A)** Astigmatic corneal topography. **(B)** Orbscan topography of an eye with keratoconus.

Optical Properties of the Cornea

Several concepts are used to characterize optical properties of the cornea, such as curvature, shape, local surface, power, expressed as refraction in diopters, thickness, and three-dimensional structure. The keratometric value is a concept inherited from keratometry and is calculated simply from radii of curvature as follows:

$$K = \text{refractive index of } 337.5/\text{radius of curvature}$$

The intact central corneal thickness of ~560 μm is considered enough to ensure long-term mechanical stability of the cornea. The peripheral thickness (~600 μm) is certainly clinically important in some refractive procedures such as intracorneal rings, astigmatic keratotomy, and cataract surgery. With the advances in corneal imaging and widespread refractive surgeries, corneal behavior will likely be better understood. Corneal topography instruments used in clinical practice most often are based on Placido reflective image analysis. This method of imaging of the anterior corneal surface uses the analysis of reflected images of multiple concentric rings projected on the cornea.

Interpretation of Topographic Maps

Every map has a color scale that assigns particular color to a certain keratometric dioptric range. Never base an interpretation on color alone. The value in keratometric diopter is crucial in the clinical interpretation of the map and has to be looked at with the interpretation of every map. Absolute maps have a preset color scale with the same dioptric steps and dioptric minimum and maximum assigned to the same colors for particular instrument.

Normalized maps have different color scales assigned to each map based on instrument software that identifies the actual minimal and maximal keratometric dioptric value of a particular cornea. The dioptric range assigned to each color is generally smaller compared with the absolute map, and, consequently, maps show more detailed description of the surface. The disadvantage is that the colors of two different maps cannot be compared directly and have to be interpreted based on the keratometric values of their different color scales.

◆ Specular Microscopy

This is an important part of the preoperative evaluation, especially if corneal guttata or other signs of a low endothelial cell count are found. It is clinically and medical-legally important to document a low endothelial cell count before LASIK, rather than worry later whether LASIK caused it. It must be done before any examination that might roughen or dry the corneal surface. Although endothelial cell changes following lamellar surgery (including LASIK) have not been reported clinically, they have been seen experimentally when excimer ablation of greater than 90% depth was achieved. This depth is of course entirely contraindicated in patients, but two cases of corneal perforation during LASIK have recently been reported, and one would assume that other cases with deep ablation must also exist (**Fig. 17.5**).

Focus: 0.50 mm

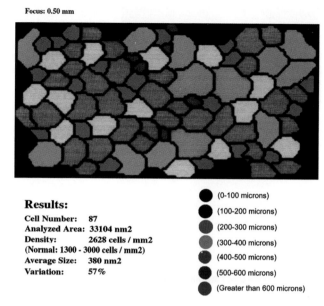

Results:

Cell Number: 87
Analyzed Area: 33104 nm2
Density: 2628 cells / mm2
(Normal: 1300 - 3000 cells / mm2)
Average Size: 380 nm2
Variation: 57%

(0-100 microns)
(100-200 microns)
(200-300 microns)
(300-400 microns)
(400-500 microns)
(500-600 microns)
(Greater than 600 microns)

Fig. 17.5   A normal specular microscopy.

◆ Corneal Pachymetry

Study of the central cornea with ultrasound pachymetry is fundamental. The surface of the ultrasonic pachymeter probe is wiped with alcohol and does not need to be sterilized. This instrument is used to take a very careful and accurate reading of the thickness of the central cornea. The pachymeter probe is placed on the center of the cornea, perpendicularly, to determine corneal thickness. The pachymeter has a console displaying the corneal thickness reading (**Fig. 17.6**).

Clinical Importance

Ideally, we must preserve a minimum of 250 µm in the posterior stromal bed. Other investigators consider that preservation of a minimum of 50% of the preoperative central pachymetry is essential. This is referred to as the *Barraquer law of corneal thickness.* This is particularly important in the treatment of high refractive errors with the excimer laser and in "enhancement" procedures. Unless sufficient corneal stroma remains, as determined by Barraquer's basic principle, there is an increased risk of developing corneal ectasia. It is generally estimated that 10 µm of ablation corrects one diopter of myopia.

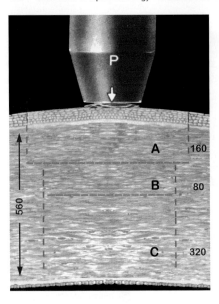

Fig. 17.6 Illustration of a corneal pachymetry in a patient undergoing LASIK. P, ultrasound pachymeter; A, flap depth in case of LASIK; B, amount of stroma ablated for correction of refractive error; C, residual bed thickness. (From Boyd, BF. Preoperative evaluation and considerations. In: Atlas of Refractive Surgery. Highlights of Ophthalmology, 2000, 45. Courtesy Jaypee Highlights Medical Publishers Inc., Panama.)

◆ A-Scan Ultrasonography

Ocular biometry must be performed prior to cataract surgery. Biometry is the discipline in charge of the physical parameters of the eyeball and includes two fundamental explorations, keratometry and the axial length measurement of the eye. Usually, in clinical practice, the term *biometry* refers to the latter and considers keratometry to be a separate procedure.

There is no question that when well selected and properly done the modern methods of partial coherence interferometry (optical coherence biometry), the pentacam (Oculus, Inc., Lynnwood, WA) and the advance contact and immersion ultrasonography afford us the best way of achieving the desired postoperative refraction. Determination of intraocular lens power through meaningful keratometric readings and axial length measurements has become the standard of care. This is a challenging technique to obtain good visual results and patient satisfaction (**Fig. 17.7**).

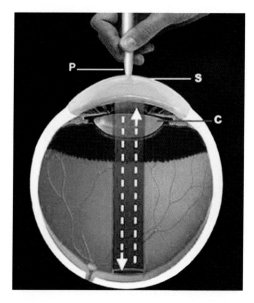

Fig. 17.7   Determination of intraocular lens power in patients with normal axial length (normal eyes)—mechanism of how ultrasonography measures distances and determines axial length. The use of ultrasonography to calculate the intraocular lens power takes into account the variants that may occur in the axial diameter of the eye and the curvature of the cornea. The ultrasound probe (P) has a piezoelectric crystal that electrically emits and receives high-frequency sound waves. The sound waves travel through the eye until they are reflected back by any structure that stands perpendicularly in their way (represented by *arrows*). These *arrows* show how the sound waves travel through the ocular globe and return to contact the probe tip. Knowing the speed of the sound waves and based on the time it takes for the sound waves to travel back to the probe (*arrows*), the distance can be calculated. The speed of the ultrasound waves (*arrows*) is higher through a dense lens (C) than through a clear one. Soft-tipped transducers (P) are recommended to avoid errors when touching the corneal surface (S). The ultrasonography equipment computer can automatically multiply the time by the velocity of sound to obtain the axial length. Calculations of intraocular lens power are based on programs such as SRK-II, SRK-T, Holladay, or Binkhorst, among others, installed in the computer. (From Boyd, BF. IOL power calculation in normal cases. In: The art and science of cataract surgery. *Highlights of Ophthalmology*, 2001, 41. Courtesy Jaypee Highlights Medical Publishers Inc., Panama.)

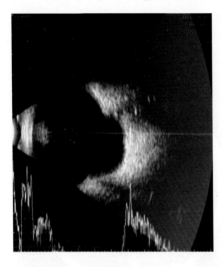

Fig. 17.8 Mode B-scan showing retinochoroidal coloboma.

◆ B-Scan Ultrasound

Linear A scans are summated in the B-scan. This gives a two-dimensional cross-sectional image of the eye and orbit. It is of great value in evaluating the posterior segment in eyes with opaque media (**Fig. 17.8**).

◆ Potential Acuity Meter Testing

The Potential Acuity Meter (PAM; Marco Ophthalmic Inc., Jacksonville, FL) is an instrument that attaches to a slit lamp. It serves as a virtual pinhole by projecting a regular Snellen visual acuity chart through a very tiny aerial pinhole aperture ~0.1 mm in diameter. The light carrying the image of the visual acuity chart narrows to a fine 0.1-mm beam and is directed through clearer areas in cataracts (or corneal disease), allowing the patient to read the visual acuity chart as if the cataract or corneal disease were not there. The PAM is taken from its stand and placed directly onto the slit lamp in the same manner as the detachable type of Goldmann tonometer. The examination takes from 2 to 5 minutes per eye, depending on the density of the cataract (**Fig. 17.9**).

As pointed out by Guyton, for the PAM to work adequately, there must be some small hole in the cataract for the light beam to pass through. You may find such a hole even in cataracts that have media clouding of up to 20/200 and better. When you find it, then you can avoid the light scattering produced by the opacities. It is this light scattering that washes out the retinal image and decreases vision behind cataracts. By projecting the image of the visual acuity chart through one tiny area, we avoid the scattering effect, and the patient can see the chart.

Fig. 17.9 Potential Acuity Meter Guyton Test. C, cornea; R, retina. (From Boyd, BF. Preoperative evaluations. In: The art and science of cataract surgery. *Highlights of Ophthalmology*, 2001, 16. Courtesy Jaypee Highlights Medical Publishers Inc., Panama.)

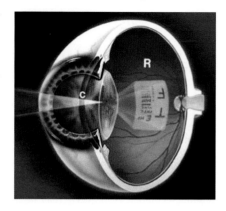

◆ Color Vision Tests (Ishihara Plates, Depth Perception Tests)

People with normal cones and light sensitive pigment (trichromasy) are able to see all the different colors and subtle mixtures of them by using cones sensitive to one of three wavelengths of light—red, green, and blue. A mild color deficiency is present when one or more of the three cones' light sensitive pigments are not quite right and their peak sensitivity is shifted (anomalous trichromasy—includes protanomaly and deuteranomaly). A more severe color deficiency is present when one or more of the cones' light sensitive pigments is really wrong (dichromasy—includes protanopia and deuteranopia).

The Ishihara test, for example, is composed of a series of colored cards on which numbers or lines of equal shade can be read by a person with normal color vision but not by someone with defective color vision. It makes use of the peculiarity that in red-green blindness, blue and yellow appear remarkably bright compared with red and green. The color plates are encased in a specially designed album-type book for ease of handling. The set includes four special plates for tests to determine the kind and degree of defect in color blindness. This color blindness test is accepted by leading authorities (**Fig. 17.10**).

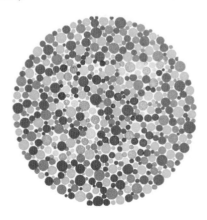

Fig. 17.10 Ishihara plate.

◆ Fluorescein Angiography

Fluorescein angiography can be a very useful procedure for assessing retinal disease by delineating areas of involvement, guiding treatment, and formulating a prognosis for changes in the patient's vision.

To interpret fluorescein angiographic images, knowledge of retinal/choroidal anatomy and circulation is essential. Arterial and venous circulation differences, as well as the retina's barriers against the passage of sodium fluorescein (NaFl) dye, including the retinal pigment epithelium (RPE) (outer blood–retinal barrier) and the retinal vascular endothelium (inner blood–retinal barrier), must be understood. Knowledge of fundus pathophysiology and anatomy has been greatly enhanced by research using fluorescein angiography (**Fig. 17.11**).

For purposes of angiogram interpretation, the sensory retina can be divided into vascular and avascular portions. The vascular portion is composed of the internal limiting membrane (ILM), nerve fiber layer (NFL), ganglion cell layer (GC), inner plexiform layer (IPL), and inner nuclear layer (INL). These portions of the retina receive direct metabolic support from retinal blood vessels.

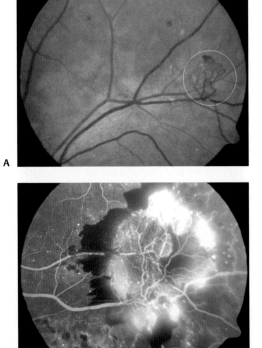

Fig. 17.11 (A) Fundus photo of neovascularization.
(B) Fluorescein angiography of neovascularization.

The sensory retina's avascular portion consists of the outer plexiform layer (OPL), the outer nuclear layer (ONL), and rod and cone photoreceptor cells. These structures receive metabolic support from the choroidal vessels via the pigment epithelial cells.

◆ Optical Coherence Tomography

Optical coherence tomography (OCT) is an imaging modality that performs high-resolution, micrometer-scale cross sections of the eye and other biological structures.

At this time the technology is analogous to B-scan ultrasound. Its utility to the clinician lies in the ability to accurately make noninvasive anatomical measurements in vivo (**Fig. 17.12**). Prior to the development of OCT, the mainstays of clinical examination for many retinal diseases were slit-lamp biomicroscopy, fundus photography, fluorescein angiography, and indocyanine green angiography. Although these diagnostic techniques remain essential to diagnosis and management, OCT has emerged as an invaluable diagnostic tool as well, providing quantitative and qualitative information that was previously unattainable.

In addition to presenting a clearer picture of the pathophysiology of disease, OCT has been extremely useful in determining response to therapy. Multiple studies, for example, have used OCT to examine ocular response following macular treatments determining that there is an initial increase in subretinal and intraretinal fluid, followed by a gradual decline over the next days.

◆ Lasers In Ophthalmology

Laser Peripheral Iridectomy

Because of the coagulating effect of argon laser light, iridectomy performed by argon laser offers advantages over incisional iridectomy or neodymium:yttrium-aluminum-garnet (Nd:YAG) laser iridectomy in patients predisposed to bleeding conditions, such as those taking anticoagulants or with known blood-clotting disorders. The laser iridectomy is performed as an office procedure in a closed eye—a considerable advantage over surgical iridectomy (**Fig. 17.13**).

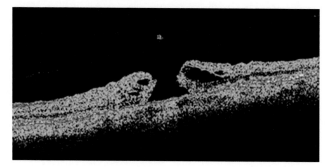

Fig. 17.12   Optical coherence tomography of a macular hole.

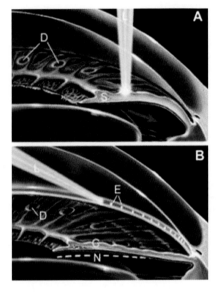

Fig. 17.13 Iridectomy with argon laser—opening a narrow angle in chronic, narrow angle glaucoma. A laser iridectomy is the procedure of choice for narrow angle glaucoma except in cases such as **(A)** where the peripheral iris lies too close to the cornea for treatment. Laser applications (D) are placed in the midstroma area of the iris to open the angle. These nonperforative laser applications cause heat, which in turn causes shrinkage of the iris collagen fibres in the direction of the arrow. The iris sphincter muscle (S) and the laser beam (L) are shown in **(B)**, shrinkage from laser applications (D) has opened the angle to an acceptable position (C). A peripheral laser iridectomy is then executed. The normal iris location is shown on dotted line (N). The angle is now sufficiently open for laser trabeculoplasty if indicated. Laser beam (L) is shown producing burns (E) in the now visible trabeculum. (From Boyd, BF, Luntz, M. Acute and chronic angle closure. In: Innovations in the glaucomas. *Highlights of Ophthalmology*, 2002, 277. Courtesy Jaypee Highlights Medical Publishers Inc., Panama.)

It is an effective way of producing an opening in the iris but should not be used while the eye is congested or inflamed. Clear media are essential. The eye is prepared with topical anesthesia. The surgeon should have comfortable arm supports.

The Abraham technique is highly useful and effective. These burns immediately cause iris contraction and put the iris crypt on stretch. Other surgeons find that the stretch burn is generally unnecessary if the Abraham contact lens is used.

In the majority of cases, an iridectomy is achieved at the first session. As penetration of the iris stroma reaches the pigmented epithelium of the iris, bursts of pigment appear in the anterior chamber ("smoke signals"). Power is then reduced, and further burns are applied until a mushroom cloud of aqueous and pigment balloons through the iridectomy, indicating penetration of the iris.

Argon Laser Trabeculoplasty

The Glaucoma Laser Trial, a major prospective, randomized study, concluded that laser trabeculoplasty as an initial treatment for open-angle glaucoma is as safe and as effective as medical treatment. In some cases, it may be more appropriate as initial therapy. These cases include (1) patients who cannot or will not comply with prescribed medical therapy, (2) areas of the world where adequate medical treatment is unfeasible because of poverty.

In all cases, to be successful, the angle does have to be open, the media must be clear, and one must have access to the trabecular meshwork. James B. Wise, M.D., who developed argon laser trabeculoplasty (argon laser trabeculoplasty), has observed that population groups of phakic patients do better than aphakic. It appears that aphakia does interfere with response to the laser, probably by the influence of vitreous in the anterior chamber and the trabecular meshwork. Interestingly enough, pseudophakic patients respond to the laser very similarly than phakic patients. That is, the presence of the posterior chamber lens implant keeping the vitreous out of the anterior chamber greatly improves the response to the laser. Eyes with anterior chamber lenses and glaucoma usually show a poor laser response due to uveitis and trabecular damage from the lens (**Fig. 17.14**).

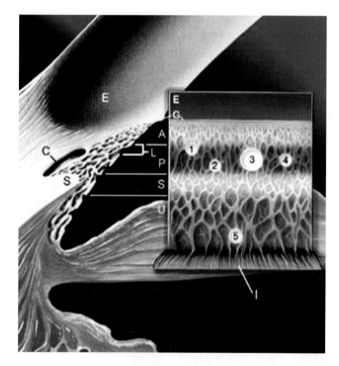

Fig. 17.14   Applying laser burns correctly in argon laser trabeculoplasty. Cross section to the left; cornea (E), Schlemm canal (C), scleral spur (S), Schwalbe line (G), anterior corneoscleral meshwork (A), pigmented band (P), and uveal meshwork (U). Proper placement of the 50 μm laser burn (L) is shown at the posterior margin of the pigmented band (P). To the right is a gonioscopic view with iris (I) below. Properly placed 50 μm laser burn at the posterior pigment band (P) shown at (1). Another burn is shown at (2) along the posterior margin of the pigment band (P). An oversized burn is shown at (3), spanning the entire pigment band. A slightly misplaced burn is shown at (4) in the middle of the pigment band. A seriously misplaced burn into the uveal meshwork (5). (From Boyd, BF, Luntz, M. Argon laser trabeculoplasty. In: Innovations in the glaucomas. *Highlights of Ophthalmology*, 2002, 149. Courtesy Jaypee Highlights Medical Publishers Inc., Panama.)

Retinal Laser Photocoagulation

Many significant applications have been discovered for clinical use of the laser in ophthalmology. The unique features of the eye allowing intraocular transmission and selective absorption of light energy account for a wide range of laser treatments.

Essentially, treatment may be categorized into five general effects: (1) induction of chorioretinal burns or retinal scar that lead to (possible pharmacological) neutralization of ischemia-induced retinal neovascularization; (2) reduction in retinal vascular permeability via direct vascular closure or unknown mechanisms; (3) ablation of undesired tissue such as choroidal neovascularization, tumors, abnormal native vessels, or aqueous-producing tissue; (4) induction of a chorioretinal scar that may serve as a barrier to extension of subretinal fluid; and (5) lysis of traction-inducing or media-opacifying tissues (**Fig. 17.15**).

The techniques of laser photocoagulation include the following broad categories: scatter treatment, focal treatment, ablative treatment, demarcating treatment, and cutting treatment.

Focal Macular Treatment

Macular edema occurs from a variety of disease mechanisms, but the feature common to each is increased retinal vascular permeability. Contributing factors include retinal ischemia, inflammation, and traction. Some entities in the first of

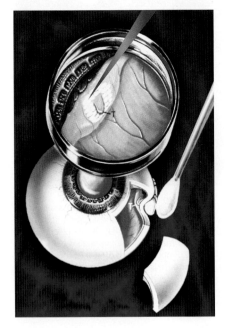

Fig. 17.15 Argon laser treatment of a retinal tear (T). (From Cortez, R. Management of retinal detachment. In: Retinal and vitreoretinal surgery. *Highlights of Ophthalmology*, 2002, 402. Courtesy Jaypee Highlights Medical Publishers Inc., Panama.)

these categories are responsive to focal laser treatment: clinically significant diabetic macular edema and branch vein occlusion-associated macular edema. Macular edema due to central vein occlusion may resolve after treatment, but this is not usually accompanied by a visual benefit.

Nd:YAG Laser Posterior Capsulotomy

Posterior capsule opacification (PCO) is currently the most frequent postoperative complication in cataract surgery.

The use of hypotonic solution and preservative free lidocaine are being investigated in the prevention of PCO. Studies with in vivo specular microscopy suggest that a hydrophilic acrylic intraocular lens would have higher biocompatibility than the hydrophobic acrylic lens, contrary to some previous studies, which affirmed that hydrophobic acrylic lens had higher biocompatibility.

Opacification of the posterior capsule is an inadequate term because it is not the capsule that opacifies but an opaque membrane that grows, originating from the epithelial cells that were retained, which proliferate and migrate on the posterior capsule (**Fig. 17.16**).

The pearls of Elschnig originate from the superimposed epithelial cells of the flexible wing of the anterior capsule and migrate to the posterior capsule.

Opacification of the posterior capsule is treated with Nd:YAG laser, which is a photodisruptor laser. In other words, it uses a high pulse of ionizing electromagnetic energy to break the tissue.

To achieve the opening of the capsule, begin from the periphery at 12 o'clock and go to 6 o'clock with a size larger than the pupil (undilated). Make the incision going from 3 o'clock to 9 o'clock using the Abraham lens. Finally clean the residues to avoid leaving floating fragments.

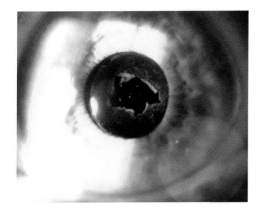

Fig. 17.16 Nd:YAG laser posterior capsulotomy.

◆ Cryoprobes

Cryoprobes are used for peripheral retinopexy in patients with peripherally located retinal breaks and tears, in the treatment of retinal tumors and retinal vascular malformations. They have also been used for performing cyclocryotherapy in
end-stage glaucomas.

   The tip of the probe is placed over the globe at the edge of the break while visu-
alizing with the indirect ophthalmoscope. The freezing is then applied until there
is whitening of the retina (freezing of the vitreous should be avoided). Once the tip
has thawed, it is removed and the next application is made (**Fig. 17.17**).

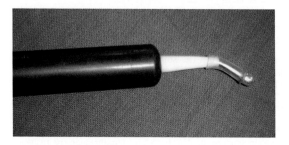

Fig. 17.17   Cryoprobe.

Ophthalmic Office Procedures
Samuel Boyd

◆ Corneal Staining with Fluorescein

Corneal epithelial abrasion is a relatively common occurrence among contact lens wearers. Abrasions are defined somewhat loosely as areas of coalesced epithelial staining or defects, without infiltration, often (but not always) with the symptom of ocular pain. (Any infiltration associated with an epithelial defect should be considered to be a corneal microbial infection until proven otherwise.) The clinician can expect to spend ~1% of contact lens–related office visits treating abrasions, more in practices where keratoconic patients are numerous. Other causes include lens defects (chips, bad edges), retained foreign bodies, overwear, and flat-fitting gas permeables. Many non–contact lens problems cause abrasions as well.

Corneal abrasions can be classified as either microform or macroform. With the latter, severe pain persists from hours to days as a result of a large area of the epithelium being separated from the cornea. In posttraumatic cases, the microform type of erosion always occurs at the site of the original abrasion. Microform recurrent erosions are characterized by intraepithelial microcysts with a minor break in the epithelium. These erosions are usually associated with brief episodes of pain lasting from seconds to minutes (**Fig. 18.1**).

Lesions, such as corneal abrasions or erosions, are stained mainly by fluorescein, whereas devitalized but intact epithelium is stained exclusively by rose bengal. One drop of 1% rose bengal placed on the upper bulbar conjunctiva while the patient looks down is generally sufficient.

A careful slit-lamp examination often reveals corneal affections. Many times, there may be associated generalized or localized patches of corneal edema. In some cases, there may be associated microbial keratitis, which can be diagnosed with bacterial cultures of these corneas.

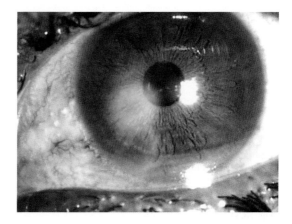

Fig. 18.1 Corneal staining with fluorescein.

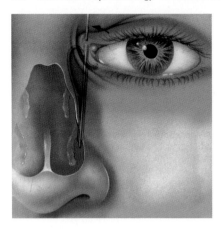

Fig. 18.2 Bowman probe through the lacrimal sac.

◆ Nasolacrimal Duct Patency

Clinical observation of the tearing patient will reveal considerable diagnostic information. Tears and mucus may be accumulating in the medial canthus and on the lower eyelid margin. Palpation in the area over the lacrimal sac may reveal pain or tenderness, a distended sac, or regurgitation of mucoid or mucopurulent material from the puncta.

Probing and irrigation should be performed after the dye disappearance test. First, the clinician anesthetizes the puncta by placing a cotton pledget soaked with topical anesthetic into the medial canthus between the eyelids. A no. 0 or no. 1 Bowman probe is passed through each canaliculus or the medial orbital wall. If a soft stop is felt, the probe is removed, and the distance to the obstruction is measured to determine whether the obstruction is in the canaliculus or the common canaliculus. The canaliculi are then irrigated with a 27-gauge blunt needle on a 5-mL syringe containing irrigating solution.

Regurgitation of fluid indicates that the obstruction is within the canaliculus. Fluid flowing from the opposite canaliculus indicates an obstruction beyond the common canaliculus (**Fig. 18.2**).

◆ Subconjunctival/Sub-Tenon Injections

This is a highly effective way to inject medications or anesthesia, mostly used in combination with topical anesthesia. This combination is also the procedure of choice by surgeons who perform small incision cataract surgery or other minor procedures. Prospective, randomized studies have concluded that single-quadrant, direct sub-Tenon injection of anesthetic is as rapid and effective as retrobulbar injection for cataract surgery. It provides better anesthesia with comparable akinesia (**Fig. 18.3**).

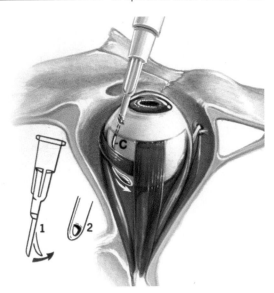

Fig. 18.3   Local sub-Tenon infiltration. (From Boyd, BF. Proceeding with surgery. In: The art and science of cataract surgery. *Highlights of Ophthalmology*, 2001, 73. Courtesy Jaypee Highlights Medical Publishers Inc., Panama.)

The most common complications are chemosis and subconjunctival hemorrhage, but no major complications are encountered. The dispersion of medications or anesthetic fluid under Tenon's capsule is effective enough to diminish lid discomfort substantially. For these reasons, sub-Tenon anesthesia using a flexible cannula has replaced retrobulbar and peribulbar injection except in very unusual cases.

Performing a sub-Tenon local infiltration is made under topical anesthesia. A small incision is made in the fused conjunctiva/Tenon capsule 3 mm from the limbus. If the surgeon is right-handed, it is easier to perform the incision at the inner lower quadrant between the rectus muscles in the right eye and at the lower temporal quadrant in the left eye. If the surgeon is left-handed, it would be the opposite. The surgical plane of the Tenon capsule attachment to the sclera is carefully dissected and the cannula is advanced through this aperture.

◆ Retrobulbar Injection

A blunt-tipped retrobulbar needle on a syringe containing a 50:50 mixture of 4% lidocaine and 75% bupivacaine, with hyaluronidase, is inserted at the junction of the middle and lateral third of the inferior orbital rim. With the patient looking straight ahead and the bevel facing up, the needle is inserted through the orbital septum. Once it reaches the equator of the globe, the needle is redirected toward the apex of the globe. On reaching inside the muscle cone, it is gently moved from

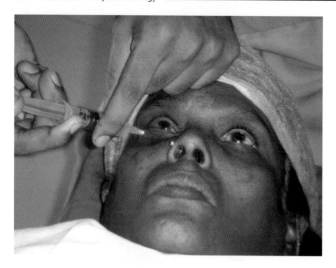

Fig. 18.4   Retrobulbar block being given.

side to side to make sure that there is no globe penetration. After withdrawing slightly to make sure that one is not intravascular, the anesthetic is injected, the needle is removed, and firm pressure is applied for 5 to 10 minutes (**Fig. 18.4**).

◆ Placement of Punctal Plugs

Dry-eye syndrome, the most frequent condition in ophthalmology, has many different causes. The most frequent of these are the natural aging process and hormonal factors, in particular the menopause. The side effects of many medications, such as antihistaminics, antidepressants, certain blood pressure drugs, antiparkinsonians, and birth control pills also play a role in some patients. Dry eye is also a manifestation of some systemic autoimmunologic diseases, the most frequent of which are Sjögren syndrome, which include in type II the triad of dry eyes, dry mouth, and rheumatoid arthritis, or sometimes lupus, rosacea, or others. Many other types of dry eyes are associated with blepharitis, LASIK surgery, lids/eye incongruity, and contact lens wear. In fact dry eyes are the most common complaint among contact lens wearers. Most dry eyes are multifactorial (i.e., they have several etiologic causes).

There are a variety of plugs for punctual occlusion in the market. There are absorbable transitory punctum plugs, which ascertain if during the period of the punctal occlusion the symptoms and signs of the dry eye improve, and there are permanent punctal plugs, which maintain the occlusion as long as desired and can be removed. However, plugs for punctum occlusion are not an etiologic treatment, but they may be very useful in dry eye as an additional measure because they maintain a larger meniscal trough (the central part of the lower tear meniscus), which facilitates the reformation and maintenance of a normal precorneal tear film when the patient is blinking (**Fig. 18.5**).

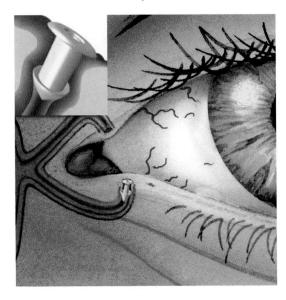

Fig. 18.5   Punctum plugs for dry eyes. (From Murube, J. Management of dry eyes. *Highlights of Ophthalmology Journal*, 2005:33:2–5.)

◆ Corneal Foreign-Body Removal and Use of the Bur

Superficial foreign bodies can be removed in the outpatient department during slit-lamp examination. Deep foreign bodies should be removed in a sterile operating room with sufficient magnification and adequate instrumentation and adequate anesthesia. If there is any sign of aqueous leak during the procedure, therapeutic contact lens or tissue adhesive can be used as a tamponade to seal the leak.

The rust ring surrounding an iron foreign body can be removed using a battery-operated dental bur under topical anesthesia (**Fig. 18.6**).

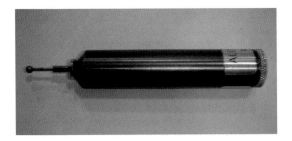

Fig. 18.6   Corneal foreign body bur.

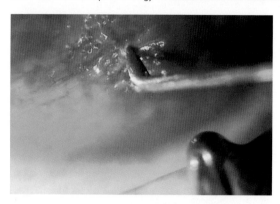

Fig. 18.7 Anterior stromal puncture.

◆ Anterior Stromal Puncture

Anesthetize the eye with topical drops and place a speculum. Have the patient seated on a slit-lamp and instill fluorescein to help to visualize the puncture marks. A bent 27-gauge needle with bevel up is mounted onto a 1-mL syringe, and the tip is penetrated in a perpendicular manner past the Bowman membrane to the level of the superficial stroma. This is repeated over the entire affected area. Because the procedure causes scarring, it is not performed over the visual axis. A pressure patch or a bandage contact lens may be used postoperatively (**Fig. 18.7**).

◆ Pterygium Excision with Conjunctival Graft

Surgery is done under a peribulbar block. The eye is prepped and draped in a sterile manner. Saline is injected into the pterygium to delineate it. The apex of the pterygium is then held with a forceps and stripped from the corneal surface in a rhexis-like manner. Any tags left on the cornea may be removed. The pterygium is then separated from the undersurface of the conjunctiva and cut, along with a part of the conjunctiva. Make sure not to damage the medial rectus muscle. Light cautery is applied to stop bleeding. Saline is again used to balloon the conjunctiva in the donor site and an appropriately sized graft is cut taking care not to incorporate Tenon tissue. It is then sutured into the recipient site or stuck using fibrin glue, taking care to maintain the right alignment and orientation. The donor site can also be closed using fibrin glue (**Fig. 18.8**).

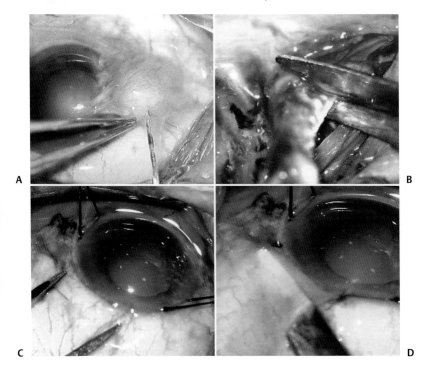

Fig. 18.8 **(A)** Pterygium is grasped with forceps and xylocaine is injected sub-onjuncti-vally. **(B)** The pterygium is excised. **(C)** The donor site conjunctiva is measured for taking the graft. **(D)** Donor conjunctiva is undermined with scissors and then transposed to recipient site and sutured or glued. (Courtesy Amar Agarwall, Dr. Agarwal's Eye Hospital, Chennai, India.).

◆ Pneumatic Retinopexy

Pneumatic retinopexy (PR), first introduced by Dominguez in Spain and then by Hilton in the United States, is an operation for reattaching the retina by injecting an expanding intravitreal gas bubble, postoperative positioning, and transconjunctival cryopexy or laser photocoagulation. PR is performed in an office setting and may be the most cost-effective means of retinal reattachment (**Fig. 18.9**).

◆ Indications

Pneumatic retinopexy is a good alternative for treatment of retinal detachments with a single retinal break, or a group of retinal breaks confined to the superior two thirds of the fundus. Pseudophakic patients can be handled with PR if the view of the peripheral retina is adequate. Some contraindications to this procedure have

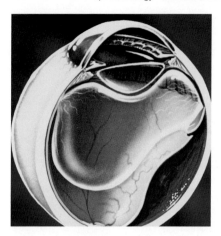

Fig. 18.9 Intraocular gas (pneumatic retinopexy) in a retinal detachment. (From McPherson, A, Schwartz, S, Kuhl, D. Principles of retinal re-attachment surgery. In: Retinal and vitreoretinal surgery. *Highlights of Ophthalmology*, 2002, 364.)

been identified: (1) breaks larger than 1 clock-hour, or multiple breaks extending more than 3 clock hours; (2) breaks located in the inferior 4 clock-hours of the eye; (3) significant traction on the retinal tears; (4) patients who are unable to maintain adequate position; (5) patients with advanced glaucoma who are at risk of further deterioration due to the brief elevation of intraocular pressure; and (6) cloudy media, which prevent identification and treatment of the breaks.

The injection is usually performed temporally, 4 mm behind the limbus, unless the pars plana is detached or large retinal breaks are present in that area, in which case another site is selected. In a patient with retinal detachment in whom there is intraocular fluid the gas is placed under the anterior hyaloid. The needle is directed toward the center of the vitreous and inserted to a depth of 7 to 8 mm and then is partially withdrawn, so that ~3 mm of the needle is left inside the eye. To create a single gas bubble, the gas is injected moderately briskly. As the needle is withdrawn from the eye, a sterile cotton-tipped applicator is rolled over the needle tract, and the head of the patient is rotated to the opposite side to prevent leakage of gas. Then indirect ophthalmoscopy is performed to corroborate the patency of the central retinal artery.

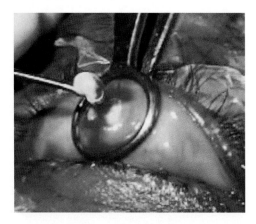

Fig. 18.10   Chalazion incision and curettage.

◆ Chalazion Excision

The acute inflammatory phase is managed by warm compresses, appropriate lid hygiene, scrubbing, and topical antibiotic, or antiinflammatory.

Chronic chalazion requires surgical management to facilitate clearing of the inflammatory mass. Posterior marsupialization of the lesion is done with cross incision through the tarsus and conjunctiva. Sharp dissection and excision of all necrotic material are done. The lesion is allowed to heal by granulation. Postoperatively, the patient is managed with topical antibiotic and steroid drops (**Fig. 18.10**).

◆ Punctal Ectropion Repair

Punctal malposition leading to epiphora is an indication for punctal ectropion repair. Use of simple thermal cautery of the conjunctiva is used in very mild cases, leading to inward rotation of the lid margin.

Horizontal fusiform excision of the conjunctiva and tarsus 4 mm inferior to punctum with closure utilizing inverting sutures, corrects the punctal malposition. This procedure can be combined with lateral canthal tightening in severe cases.

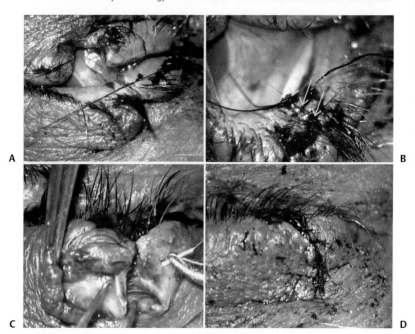

Fig. 18.11 Lid margin repair. **(A)** The lid tear. **(B)** The lid margin sutures with three sets of silk sutures cut long, which are later tied under the skin sutures to avoid cut ends rubbing on the cornea. **(C)** Repair of the tarsus with partial-thickness bites. **(D)** Final appearance. (Courtesy Soosan Jacob, Dr. Agarwal's Eye Hospital, Chennai, India.)

◆ Eyelid Margin Laceration Repair

Local anesthetic is injected into the lids and three marginal sutures are first passed to ensure lid margin apposition: gray line to gray line, meibomian gland orifice to meibomian gland orifice, and lash line to lash line. These three sutures are cut long and tied eventually under the skin sutures to prevent cut ends of the sutures from rubbing on the cornea. The tarsus is then repaired with interrupted 6–0 Vicryl (polyglactin 910) sutures. The skin is then closed (**Fig. 18.11**).

◆ Temporal Artery Biopsy

This is a diagnostic procedure for arteritic anterior ischemic optic neuropathy. Position biopsy is an indication for long-term use of systemic steroids. Negative biopsy does not rule out arteritis. In cases of negative biopsy (false-negative is 3 to 9%) and in cases with strong suspicion, biopsy of the other side is considered.

The biopsy specimen must be 3 to 6 cm long to rule out the biopsy specimen being a skip lesion. The procedure is done under local anesthesia with direct localization of the site. Blunt dissection is done to release the artery from underlying soft tissue. Before cutting the artery, 4–0 silk sutures are applied. The incision is closed with 6–0 suture.

19 Refractive Surgery

David R. Hardten, Natalia Kramarevsky, Louis E. Probst, and Richard L. Lindstrom

◆ Photorefractive Keratectomy

Photorefractive keratectomy (PRK) is one of the refractive procedures using excimer laser to ablate the cornea. It corrects myopia, hypermetropia, presbyopia, and astigmatism. In myopia, the central corneal stroma is ablated to flatten it; in hypermetropia and presbyopia the cornea is made steeper by ablating the desired zone.

◆ Technique

Under topical anesthesia the epithelium is debrided. The patient fixates at the target in the microscope. The desired amount of corneal tissue is ablated using the nomogram made with the patient's data. The eye is taped following the procedure or a contact lens is placed. Postoperative medications include antiinflammatory and lubricating drops.

◆ Selected Complications of Photorefractive Keratectomy

Decentered Ablation

Decentration of the ablation zone by 1 mm or more occurs due to improper patient fixation, centration, or eye movement during the procedure.

◆ Presentation

Patients present with decreased visual acuity, diplopia, glare, halos, induced astigmatism.

◆ Management

Some decentrations will lessen with time and remolding. Those that do not improve require corneal topographic studies. Visual symptom improvement may be attempted with weak miotics, contact lens, or re-treatment.

Central Islands

A portion of the central corneal tissue is raised, leading to area of higher central corneal refractive power surrounded by an adjacent area of paracentral stroma. It has an elevation of at least 1 diopter with a diameter of more than 1 mm as compared with the paracentral flat area. It is seen less often now with the increasing use of flying spot laser systems.

◆ Presentation

Patients present with visual distortion, double vision, decreased vision.

◆ **Management**

Management consists of waiting and watching and corneal topographic study. Re-treatment with the excimer laser may be helpful in selected cases.

Disabling Glare or Halos

◆ **Presentation**

Some patients complain of glare and halos around light, especially in scotopic conditions. These symptoms are more pronounced with smaller ablation zones. They may also be seen with decentered ablations, epithelial ingrowths, and corneal haze.

◆ **Management**

Management consists of constricting the pupil using miotics, topical brimonidine, and secondary ablation with increasing diameter.

Delayed Epithelial Healing

◆ **Presentation**

Nonhealing epithelium even after 3 to 4 days postoperatively is commonly due to a large area of debridement, severe dry eye and prophylactic antibiotic and anti-inflammatory eye drops, diabetes mellitus, and other autoimmune disorders. Patients present with watering, discomfort, redness, pain, and photophobia.

◆ **Management**

Management consists of contact lens wear until reepithelialization, liberal use of lubricating drops, and treatment of the underlying cause. Excess nonsteroidal antiinflammatory drugs and corticosteroids should not be used. The patient may be followed up daily until healing.

Infectious Keratitis

Infectious keratitis is unusual, with bacterial causes most common. The inflammation typically causes redness of the eye with a focal infiltrate. Management includes culturing and antibiotic use directed towards the suspected organism until culture results are known.

Haze and Regression

◆ **Presentation**

The healing process of activated keratocytes laying down new collagen fibers leads to corneal haze. The higher the correction the greater the risk of haze developing. Maximum haze is noticed between 1 and 3 months postoperatively and decreases with time. Corneal steepening leads to regression due to the changes in refractive power of the cornea.

◆ **Management**

Topical steroids reduce the incidence of haze and regression. Patients having decreased visual acuity may benefit from re-treatment.

◆ Laser In Situ Keratomileusis

Laser in situ keratomileusis (LASIK) is keratorefractive surgery for the treatment of high myopia, hyperopia, and astigmatism.

◆ Technique

A corneal flap is created by corneal lamellar incision using a microkeratome or the femtosecond laser. The flap is then reflected and the corneal stroma is reshaped using the excimer laser. The flap is repositioned and realigned correctly after the procedure and allowed to adhere back on its own. It is used in the healing process. Visual recovery is quicker, with less scarring and regression compared with PRK because the epithelial surface is not debrided and the Bowman layer is not ablated.

◆ Selected Complications of Laser In Situ Keratomileusis

Debris after LASIK

◆ Presentation

Interface debris is common and often results from meibomian gland secretions or makeup or mascara. These are typically not visually significant unless they occupy a large area and create an interface scar.

To prevent debris, it is important to operate in a lint-free environment, use non-fragmenting sponges, and have patients clean their lids well before surgery to remove all makeup and mascara (**Fig. 19.1**).

◆ Management

No intervention is needed unless enough debris is present that it is at risk of forming an interface scar or the debris degrades the vision.

Flap Striae

◆ Presentation

The patient with flap striae may have monocular diplopia due to irregular astigmatism in the presence of microstriae. It may be a result of mild or significant LASIK flap displacement (**Fig. 19.2**).

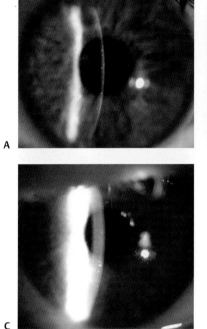

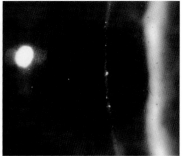

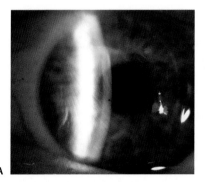

Fig. 19.1 **(A)** Mascara in the interface after LASIK. **(B)** Moderate mascara in the interface. This is typically not visually significant. **(C)** Metal flecks in the interface, which is typically not reactive or visually significant.

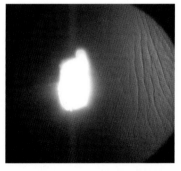

Fig. 19.2 **(A)** Striae across the visual axis from a displaced flap. **(B)** Peripheral striae that are not always visually significant, yet can occasionally cause induced asymmetric astigmatism. (*Continued on page 524*)

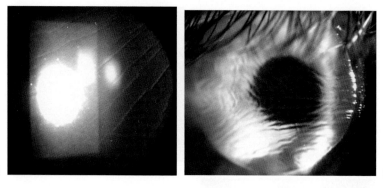

C
D

Fig. 19.2 (*Continued*) **(C)** Significant striae in the visual axis. **(D)** Severe striae from bunching of the flap.

◆ Prevention

Alignment of the created trough by even placement of the corneal cap over the stroma evenly in all directions can help reduce the incidence of striae. Some surgeons advocate making a mark on the epithelium prior to creation of the flap to help with postoperative alignment, yet care must be taken that the epithelium does not shift in relationship to the stroma when using these marks to realign the flap.

◆ Management

Microstriae may be observed if not visually significant. If they are visually significant, the surgeon may need to lift the flap, clean the interface from any cells or debris, and stretch the cap by stroking it with Merocel wipes (Medtronic, Minneapolis, MN www.medtronicophthalmics.com/Ophthalmics Catalog 2007_2008_ LR.pdf) until the gutter is well aligned.

Diffuse Lamellar Keratitis

Diffuse lamellar keratitis (DLK) is a sterile inflammation of the flap interface occurring in the first week after LASIK. The condition has also been known as "shifting sands" phenomenon or "sands of the Sahara."

◆ Presentation

Severe DLK may occur in ~1 out of 5000 cases, and mild DLK in ~1 in 50 cases in most centers.

◆ *Stage 1*: Defined by the presence of white granular cells in the periphery of the lamellar flap, outside the visual axis (**Fig. 19.3**).
◆ *Stage 2*: Defined by migration of cells in the center of the flap, involving the visual axis, in the flap periphery, or in both. It is more frequently seen on day 2 or 3. The result of central migration of cells in stage 1 gives the so-called shifting sands appearance. This occurs in ~1 in 200 cases (**Fig. 19.4**).
◆ *Stage 3*: The aggregation of more dense, white, and clumped cells in the central visual axis, with relative clearing in the periphery. This is often, but not always, associated with a subtle decline in visual acuity by 1 or 2 lines and a subjective description of haze by the patient. The frequency of stage 3 may be as high as 1 in 500 cases (**Fig. 19.5**).

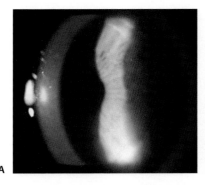
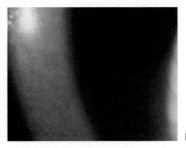

A   **B**

Fig. 19.3 (A) Stage 1 diffuse lamellar keratitis (DLK) with mild cell in the peripheral flap. **(B)** Stage 1 DLK with mild cell in the peripheral flap—high magnification.

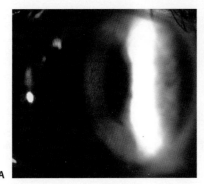
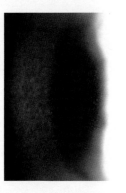

A   **B**

Fig. 19.4 (A) Stage 2 diffuse lamellar keratitis (DLK) with cells in the periphery and central portion of the flap. No significant clumping of the cells is seen in stage 2. **(B)** Stage 2 DLK—high magnification.

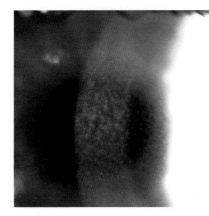

Fig. 19.5 Stage 3 diffuse lamellar keratitis with cells that are now aggregating, typically slightly below the center of the visual axis.

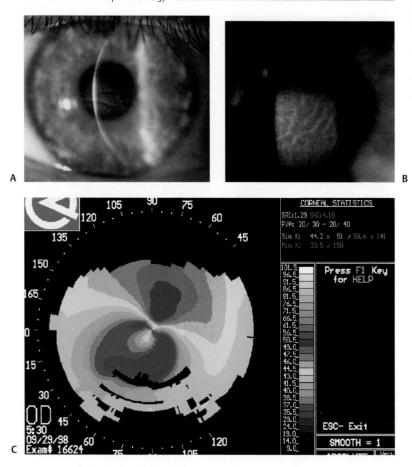

Fig. 19.6 **(A)** Stage 4 diffuse lamellar keratitis (DLK) with stromal melting. **(B)** Stage 4 DLK. **(C)** Stage 4 DLK with irregular astigmatism with flattening due to tissue loss where the cells had aggregated, typically slightly below the visual axis.

◆ *Stage 4*: The presence of stromal melting, often associated with permanent scarring and visual morbidity. There is fluid collection in the central lamellae with bullae formation and stromal volume loss. A hyperopic shift occurs due to central tissue loss, along with the appearance of corrugated "mud cracks," which are a serious finding. The incidence is ~1 in 5000 cases (**Fig. 19.6**).

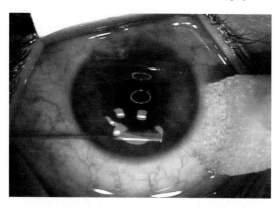

Fig. 19.7   Lifting and gentle irrigation of the flap is ideal management for stage 3 diffuse lamellar keratitis (DLK), typically at day 3 or day 4 after the surgery.

◆ **Management**

◆ *Stages 1 and 2*: Topical prednisolone acetate 1% every hour and steroid ointment (fluoromethalone) at bedtime. Follow up in 24 to 48 hours.
◆ *Stage 3*: Lifting the flap, debulking the inflammatory reaction by careful irrigation of the bed and undersurface of the cap. It is usually done on day 3 or 4 after the procedure (**Fig. 19.7**).
◆ *Stage 4*: No definitive successful treatment identified. If white cells are still present, then gentle irrigation may be helpful in reducing tissue necrosis. Otherwise, waiting for epithelial hyperplasia may allow improvement in irregular astigmatism. Rigid gas-permeable contact lenses are often helpful for visual rehabilitation. Wavefront-directed surface treatment with mitomycin C can be considered after full epithelial hyperplasia has occurred, usually at ~1 year postoperatively.

Epithelial Ingrowth

Growth of epithelium into the interface between the flap and the stroma results in irregular astigmatism and loss of best corrected visual acuity. The presence of the epithelial cells in the interface can be safely followed without intervention in the majority of cases. The epithelial cells in the interface can block the supply of nutrients to the underlying stroma and result in necrosis of the flap, extrusion of the epithelium, and a depressed scar.

The epithelial ingrowth can potentially happen in the presence of an epithelial defect created during the procedure. Edema of the LASIK flap overlying the epithelial defect leads to poor adhesion of the cap to the stromal bed and a subsequent route for epithelial cell migration. Epithelial defects are more common in the presence of anterior basement membrane dystrophy (**Fig. 19.8**).

◆ Management

Immediate removal of epithelial cells is not always necessary, yet if the epithelial ingrowth is progressing, then it should be removed before reaching a 6-mm optical zone. The flap is lifted and epithelial cells, which may be strongly adherent to the tissue, are scraped with a blunt spatula or Merocel sponge (Medtronic) from both the back of the flap and the stromal bed. Epithelial cells are also removed from the edge of the flap, along the surface of the flap for ~1.5 mm from the gutter, and in the periphery of the cornea for ~1.5 mm. An absolute alcohol solution can be applied to the stromal bed and the underside of the cap to devitalize the epithelial cells after the scraping. Care must be taken to protect limbal stem cells from alcohol. The flap is replaced in good position and stretched into place to remove any striae. The key to reducing recurrence is to keep epithelial cells from the flap edge until fibrosis has occurred between the flap and the stromal bed. The flap can be sutured to augment this fibrosis, especially in cases with a very high fistula. Typically interrupted sutures of either 10–0 nylon or 10–0 polyglactin are used. Following replacement of the flap, a fibrin/thrombin bioadhesive tissue glue such as Tisseel or Artiss (Baxter, Deerfield, IL) may be applied on the surface side of the stroma and along the gutter between the flap and peripheral stroma.

Epithelial Defect after LASIK

The advantage of LASIK over surface treatment with PRK is that an epithelial defect is typically not a part of the LASIK procedure. If a corneal abrasion does occur, discomfort is usually less painful than after PRK because of relative corneal anesthesia from the flap.

◆ Management

If the defect is central, irregular astigmatism can be induced until the defect heals and epithelium regularizes. Presence of an epithelial defect can also lead to corneal edema and subsequent epithelial ingrowth. Healing of the epithelial defect can occasionally occur with redundancy of the basement membrane. If this happens, irregular astigmatism may persist, and a phototherapeutic keratectomy could be used to reduce this redundancy, paying special attention to methods to reduce haze formation afterward. Mitomycin C 0.02% (0.2 mg/mL) may be used to reduce the incidence of corneal haze (**Fig. 19.9**).

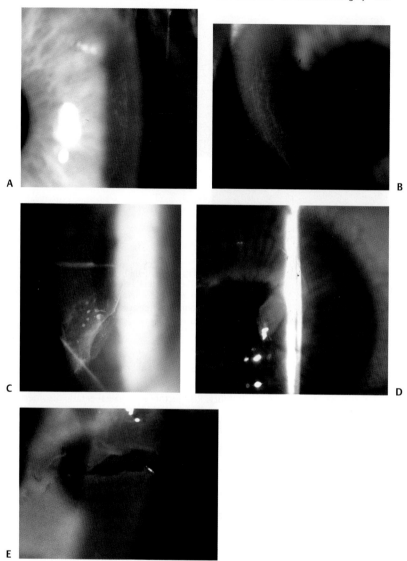

Fig. 19.8 **(A)** Epithelial cells under the flap after LASIK usually start along the peripheral flap edge. **(B)** Epithelial ingrowth can progress along the flap edge, in which case it may not become visually significant. **(C)** Epithelial ingrowth is more common where there are more edges along the LASIK flap, such as following radial or astigmatic keratotomy, or limbal relaxing incisions. **(D)** Epithelial cyst formation is less common after LASIK, yet may result from implantation of epithelium under the flap, and more commonly leads to melting of the overlying flap. **(E)** Epithelial defects along the flap edge are a common cause of flap swelling which can lead to epithelial ingrowth from poor adherence of the flap.

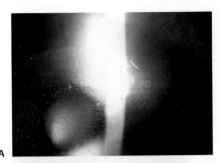

A

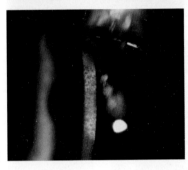

Fig. 19.9 **(A)** Inflammation under an epithelial defect 3 days after LASIK. **(B)** Haze when phototherapeutic keratectomy was done over prior LASIK flap without mitomycin C.

B

Ectasia after LASIK

Post-LASIK ectasia is a progressive central or inferior thinning and steepening of the cornea due to structural instability. Risk factors for corneal ectatic disorders are not well delineated but are likely mainly an underlying predisposition toward keratoconus. Extreme thinning of the cornea or very thin residual stromal bed thickness have also been implicated. Post-LASIK ectasia can present months or even years after the procedure (**Fig. 19.10**).

◆ Management

Management consists of ocular hypotensives, rigid gas-permeable (RGP) lenses, deep anterior lamellar keratoplasty, penetrating keratoplasty, and, recently, also Intacs corneal implants (Addition Technology, Inc., Sunnyvale, CA) and collagen crosslinking treatment with riboflavin and ultraviolet light.

Post-LASIK Infectious Keratitis

Corneal infection after LASIK is a rare complication. Microorganisms isolated from infected corneas following LASIK have been *Staphylococcus aureus*, *Staphylococcus epidermidis*, *Nocardia asteroides*, *Streptococcus pneumoniae*, *Streptococcus viridans*, *Aspergillus fumigatus*, and herpes simplex. Nontuberculous mycobacteria or atypical mycobacterial infections have also been reported. They include *M. chelonae*, *M. abscessus*, *M. fortuitum*, *M. szulgai*, *M. mucogenicum*, *M. fortuitum*, *M. terrae*. One of the peculiarities of *Mycobacterium* spp. is the development of resistance

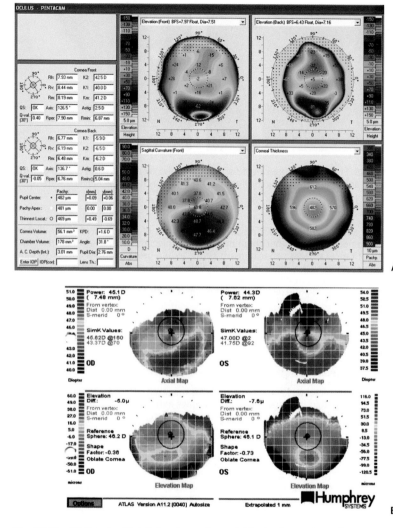

Fig. 19.10 **(A)** Ectasia with inferior steepening and thinning in a patient after LASIK. **(B)** Bilateral ectasia with left eye worse than right eye in a patient with prior LASIK.

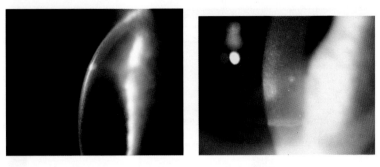

A **B**

Fig. 19.11 **(A)** Infectious keratitis after LASIK. This infectious keratitis cleared with fortified antibiotics. **(B)** Scar in the interface after mycobacterial infection in the interface.

to organomercurials, chlorine, 2% concentrations of formaldehyde and alkaline glutaraldehyde, and other commonly used disinfectants, resulting in difficult disinfections of certain surgical instruments. Iodine-povidone does appear to have some bactericidal activity against these microorganisms. These infections appear to be less common with the prophylactic use of fourth-generation fluoroquinolones such as moxifloxacin and gatifloxacin (**Fig. 19.11**).

◆ Differential Diagnosis

Diffuse lamellar keratitis, epithelial ingrowth, fungal keratitis, and intrastromal crystalline keratitis

◆ Management

Presumed microbial keratitis after LASIK is managed with culture and appropriate frequent antibiotic treatment. Broad-coverage antibiotics (fortified vancomycin 33 mg/mL or amikacin 50 mg/mL and tobramycin 15 mg/mL or gentamicin 15 mg/mL) should be used frequently initially before the culture and susceptibility tests are available to allow more specific treatment. If the infectious process is not controlled and is resistant to treatment, flap lift, debridement, and irrigation of the interface with an antibiotic solution may hasten resolution. Fourth-generation fluoroquinolones (gatifloxacin and moxifloxacin) have been introduced as an alternative or an adjunct to fortified antibiotics. Corticosteroids are typically avoided during the active infectious process yet may reduce the tendency toward scarring.

Application of a periocular skin prep of povidone-iodide 5% and prophylactic antibiotic use may be useful in reducing the incidence of infectious keratitis at the time of refractive surgery.

Buttonhole with Haze

Potential to create a buttonhole during creation of the flap is more likely with a poor suction of the microkeratome or a damaged blade. Increased haze is then typically seen in any area where the Bowman membrane has been violated (**Fig. 19.12**).

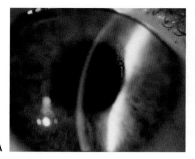 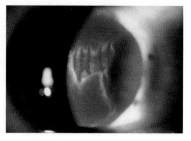

A   B

Fig. 19.12 **(A)** Irregular flap with a hole in the periphery due to poor blade quality. **(B)** Buttonhole in the central portion of the flap.

◆ Management

If buttonholing or a break in the Bowman membrane occurs within the optical zone, the flap should be repositioned and the ablation is postponed.

Haze after Excimer Laser Vision Correction

Central haze or scar can result in loss of BCVA, but haze is extremely uncommon after LASIK. Haze formation is more common when an excimer laser surface procedure is performed after previous lamellar surgery has been performed, especially when used without the addition of mitomycin C to the stroma after the ablation. Haze may be more common in primary PRK or LASIK procedures in deeper ablations (**Fig. 19.13**).

◆ Management

If the patient needs phototherapeutic keratectomy (PTK) or PRK after LASIK or any lamellar surgery careful monitoring for haze should be performed. Some surgeons advocate the use of a solution of mitomycin C 0.02% (0.2 mg/mL) following the ablation. Vitamin C 1 g daily before the procedure is thought to be beneficial. Topical steroids are used for several weeks afterward. Sunglasses with ultraviolet pro-

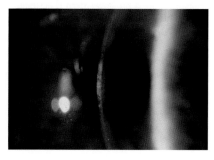

Fig. 19.13 **(A)** Haze seen when photorefractive keratectomy (PRK) was performed over the bed of a previous LASIK without the use of mitomycin C. (*Continued* *on page 532*)

A

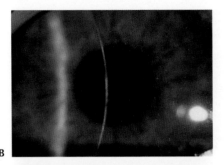

Fig. 19.13 (*Continued*) **(B)** Haze after PRK. **(C)** Haze after LASIK.

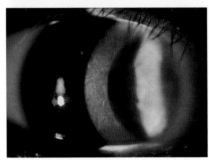

tection are recommended after surface laser procedures. Some surgeons advocate these same haze reduction modalities in primary surface laser procedures also.

Lamellar Interface fluid

Fluid may accumulate in the interface in eyes that have endothelial dysfunction or high intraocular pressure (IOP). Clinically, there is a pocket of fluid in the lamellar interface, decreased vision, and potentially a myopic shift. Microcystic epithelial edema may occur peripheral to the lamellar flap due to the increased IOP. The central corneal pachymetry may be either increased if it reads the entire corneal thickness or reduced if it measures only the thickness of the flap. The IOP may measure quite a bit lower than it actually is when measured over the fluid cyst, due to the tonometer measuring the pressure of the cyst, and not of the eye (**Fig. 19.14**).

◆ Management

The interface fluid usually resolves after lowering the IOP or restoring endothelial health.

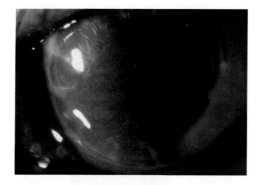

Fig. 19.14 Edema of the interface from poor endothelial function. A similar appearance may occur in a patient with high intraocular pressure.

Irregular Astigmatism after LASIK

Irregular astigmatism after excimer laser refractive surgery can occur for a variety of reasons. Decentration of the excimer laser ablation of the cornea is less common with modern-day surgery because of the availability of pupil trackers and wavefront treatments that shift the ablation zone based on the pupil centroid comparison between the preoperative wavefront acquisition and the intraoperative pupil position. Significant decentration can cause irregular astigmatism with glare, monocular diplopia, and loss of best-corrected visual acuity (**Fig. 19.15**).

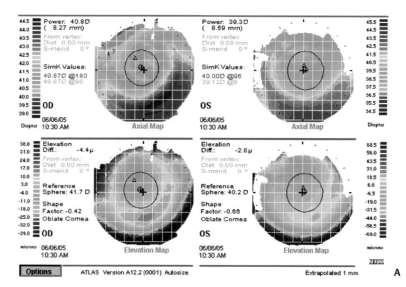

Fig. 19.15 **(A)** This topographic map shows irregular astigmatism due to asymmetry of the ablation zone. (*Continued on page 536*)

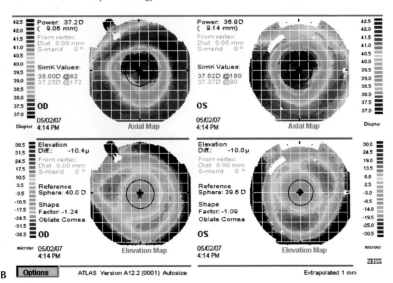

Fig. 19.15 (*Continued*) **(B)** This topography shows a well-centered myopic treatment.

◆ Management

The best method to reduce the incidence of irregular astigmatism is to utilize wavefront technology for the initial treatment. Wavefront technology may also be used to reduce the coma that is associated with a decentered ablation. Asymmetrical ablation using a standard treatment with the excimer laser is more difficult and less predictable.

During the correcting ablation, more tissue is removed from the undertreated area while less tissue is removed from the previously ablated area.

Penetration after LASIK

One of the most feared intraoperative complications is entry into the anterior chamber of the eye during the flap creation. This can happen if the plate was not properly assembled by improper plate positioning or if it was not tightened into place. The use of microkeratomes with fixed plates and femtosecond laser technology such as the IntraLase (Advanced Medical Optics, Santa Ana, CA) should greatly reduce or even eliminate this potential complication (**Fig. 19.16**).

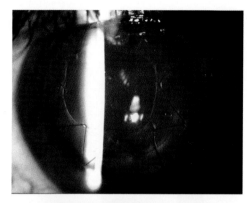

A

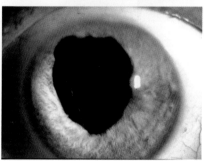

B

Fig. 19.16 **(A)** Perforation with an early keratome with need for suturing of the flap. **(B)** Loss of iris in a patient with a perforation with an early keratome.

◆ **Management**

The damage to other intraocular tissues should be assessed. In addition to corneal tissue, the iris and lens could possibly be involved. The cornea should be repaired with 10–0 nylon sutures. If other damage is found, it should further be repaired in the operating room.

◆ **Wavefront-Guided LASIK**

Wavefront systems such as the AMO/VISX WaveScan WaveFront System (Abbott Medical Optics, Santa Ana, CA) are ophthalmic diagnostic instruments that typically utilize a Hartmann-Shack wavefront sensor to measure the refractive error and wavefront aberrations of the human eye. The system can measure and display aberrations with more complex shapes than just a sphere and cylinder (higher-order aberrations, often described using Zernike polynomials as a mathematical calculation model) (**Fig. 19.17**).

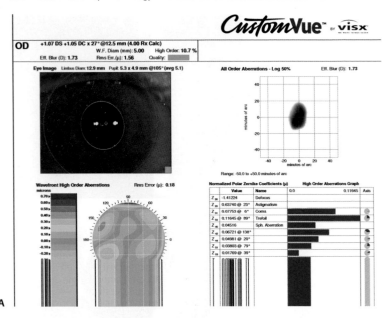

A

Fig. 19.17 **(A)** Information on the wavefront map includes the spherical correction, astigmatic correction, and higher-order aberrations as well as the iris detail used by the iris registration and cyclorotation software.

◆ **Terminology**

◆ Root mean square (RMS) error is the difference between the measured wave-scan and an ideal plane wavefront. RMS is measured in micrometers.
◆ The higher-order aberrations represents the amount or percentage of higher-order aberrations as a value, or as a fraction of the total RMS of aberrations measured.
◆ The point spread function (PSF) attempts to describe the effect of visual aberrations on a point source of light.

◆ **Wavefront as a Screening Tool**

Wavefront diagnostics can be useful in screening for corneal abnormalities that alter the total aberrations of the eye, such as keratoconus, and for assessing treatment options. There is a gradient of visual abnormalities in patients that may cause asymmetric corneas. Some eyes will have corneal or lenticular abnormalities causing distortion of their optical pathway that is apparent on topography or wavefront analysis. In other eyes the irregularities may be more peripheral, and the wavefront may be relatively normal within the central 6 mm.

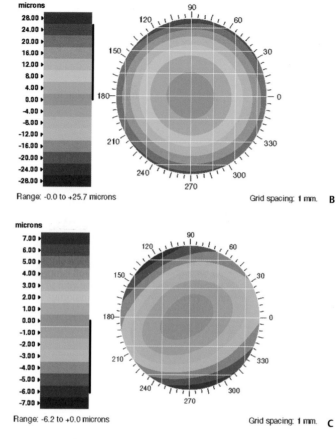

Fig. 19.17 (*Continued*) **(B)** A myopic wavefront is represented by cooler colors such as green in the center surrounded by warmer colors such as yellow or red. **(C)** A hyperopic wavefront map is represented by the warmer colors centrally surrounded by cooler colors in the periphery.

◆ **Lenticular Aberrations**

Wavefront diagnostics can also be used for preoperative screening and can assist in the diagnosis of a lenticular opacity. If the corneal topography is normal but the wavefront shows an increased amount of trefoil, coma and negative spherical aberrations, it suggests that the lens is the source of these aberrations.

Index

Note: Page numbers followed by *f* and *t* indicate figures and tables, respectively.